Cooking the RealAge® Way

Cooking the

RealAge® Way

Turn Back Your Biological Clock *with*
More Than 80 Delicious *and* **Easy Recipes**

MICHAEL F. ROIZEN, M.D.
and **JOHN LA PUMA,** M.D.

HarperCollins*Publishers*

HarperCollins books may be purchased for educational, business, or sales promotional use. For information please write: Special Markets Department, HarperCollins Publishers Inc., 10 East 53rd Street, New York, NY 10022.

RealAge is a federally registered trademark of RealAge, Inc.

FIRST EDITION

DESIGNED BY DEBORAH KERNER/DANCING BEARS DESIGN

Library of Congress Cataloging-in-Publication Data has been applied for.

ISBN: 0-06-000935-7

05   06   07   WBC/QW   10   9   8   7   6   5   4   3   2

FROM MIKE:

To my family, for their enthusiasm for RealAge, and for their patience with the project, and my endless kitchen and food experiments. They not only help me stay young but also are the reason I want to be young. And to those who've logged onto www.RealAge.com, may you change your health and share with others so you can help change the health of the world.

FROM JOHN:

To my patients, for their creativity and spirit, and for allowing me to believe in them and their success. May the pleasures of the healthy table and the energy of feeling younger be theirs.

Contents

All case studies presented in this book are based on real people. Some details insignificant to the examples in this book have been changed to protect the identities of the individuals. In some cases, two or more similar stories have been combined into one story. Only references to my daughter and myself remain clearly identifiable. Any other likenesses are purely coincidental.

In certain instances, I have listed products by their brand names—for example, specific cooking oil sprays, since that is how they are commonly known. I have occasionally also included names of companies and products if I thought that mentioning those names provided relevant information for the reader. To my knowledge, I have no connections to any of the companies or brand-name products listed in this book, with the exception of RealAge, Inc., the company that I helped found for the express purpose of developing the RealAge scientific evidence and computer program, and other RealAge programs. RealAge, Inc., currently directs the RealAge Web site www.RealAge.com.

Note About the Format of the Book

We've written this book in the first person ("I") to make it easier to read. But everywhere you see an "I," you can assume a "we."

Acknowledgments

FROM MFR:

My patients and the thousands of people who read the prior *RealAge* books and logged onto the RealAge.com Web site, and sent questions, notes, cards, and e-mails, inspired this book; I would like to thank them first and foremost. They compelled me to be passionate because they taught me that RealAge and this process of thinking about health have meaning to them. I hope this book will motivate them and the rest of its readers to live younger longer. That would be the best reward any physician could want.

I am especially indebted to the members of the staff and faculty of the Department of Anesthesia and Critical Care at the University of Chicago, and of the Office of the Dean and Vice President at Upstate, who afforded me the time to do this project and who had the vision to understand that the best medicine happens before a patient ever gets sick. I am grateful to the many, many other people who contributed to this book. Some deserve a very specific thank you: Shelly Bowen and Maurina Sherman of the RealAge team, who rewrote and helped develop the early editions of several chapters; Sukie Miller, whose passion proved to be the consistent encouragement I needed; Anita Shreve, for saying the RealAge book was possible, and that the chapters were just what she wanted to read; Candice Fuhrman, for making it happen; Elsa Hurley,

Acknowledgments

for making it clearer, much, much clearer; Pauline Snider for keeping the English crisp and the grammar and style appropriate and consistent; Jennifer DeFrancisco for her excellent editing and contributions; the many gerontologists and internists who read sections of the book for accuracy; Jack Rowe, Linda Fried, the many investigators of the Iowa, Nurse's Health, and the Physician's Health Studies, for invaluable research and advice helped make the science better; others on the RealAge team who helped edit; the many chefs who contributed recipes, including Rich Tramonto and Gail Gand of Tru in Chicago; Marisa Curatolo of the Cooking Studio in Winnipeg and now Vancouver; Linda DeFrancisco of Syracuse, and those whose recipes we modified to make them make you younger, including the chefs of the Canyon Ranch; our amateur chefs who tested the recipes, especially Donna Szymanski (she must have incredible patience—she taught me how to cook); our tasters, especially Nancy (my wife), Jennifer, and Jeffrey, the Wattels of Lettuce Entertain You, the Shermers, the Pelligrinis, and many others who tasted only occasionally; the research associates who worked tirelessly to analyze the nutrients and calculate the RealAge effect of each recipe, Shivani Chadha and Kate Poneta; Norm Faiola, for his suggestions about food safety; Michelle Lewis, for her endless patience and good humor in producing the manuscript; Briisa Kilvoy, who worked late into the night, tirelessly and enthusiastically, to produce corrections to many of the more than forty editions of each chapter, and the final copies of the manuscript; Anne-Marie Ruthrauff Prince, for doing so much so well and doing it so calmly in the midst of a constant storm; Shara Storandt and William Germino, who each made this a better book than it would have been; Arline McDonald, Tate Erlinger, Linda Van Horne, Jeremiah Stamler, and especially Keith Roach, Axel Goetz, and Harriet Imrey, as the scientific partners in the process of evaluating the data and scientific content of RealAge; Sidney Unobskey and Martin Rom, who inspired the process and named it; Charlie Silver, who funded the research and assembled the innovative RealAge team that continually evaluates and updates RealAge and its Web site; Diane Reverend, whose faith in the work inspired it to be better; Kathryn Huck who tirelessly edited the book and made it better and improved it, not just a little, and not just once; and especially Megan Newman, who believed in this book and made it happen. She conveyed her excitement to me and to the book. And of course to my partner, John La Puma, who really taught me that nutrition could and should be delicious.

Finally, I would like to thank my wife, Nancy Roizen, for her constant love and support, and my children, Jeffrey and Jennifer, for their encouragement and patience. The book is dedicated to them.

FROM JOHN:

The people to whom I am most grateful are my patients and clients, especially those of CHEF Clinic. They gave me the courage to champion the pleasures of healthy eating, too often buried beneath the fear and uncertainty about what to eat.

When I returned to Santa Barbara to create a new medical practice in nutrition, my work in writing this book and nearly all of these recipes was made easier and tastier by Bill Coleman of Coleman Family Farms and Barbara Spencer of Paso Robles (and her brilliance with heirloom tomatoes)—two farmers who know and love their delicious plants, their flavors and medical uses, and their customers. Drs. Chris Donner and Andy Binder opened their arms and Rolodexes to welcome me to the medical community, and Drs. Allison Mayer-Oakes, Helmuth Billy, and Tony DeFrance invited me to integrate *RealAge Diet* recipes into medical practice. Michael, Kim, and Emilio De Paolo kept a glass of red wine (soon, their own Zinfandel) waiting for me as I edited and wrote, and Emma Cantu and her husband Rex offered from their hearts and gorgeous organic garden luscious exotic chilies of which I can only dream. Al Kuntz saw that I needed small goals in a beautiful setting, and helped me set them. Bill Ashby modeled the RealAge way, and offered UCSB's extraordinary College of Creative Studies as a home base. Willa Seldon started the Healthy Weight Program Executive Coaching business in my mind. Kathy Zant developed its Web site, www.drjohnlapuma.com, brilliantly and passionately, and Marsha Marcoe helped me believe that it could run, and in her kindness and generosity, worked hard to make her friends as young as they could be.

I had many other wonderful teachers and incurred several large debts of gratitude in writing this book. Gary Hopmayer of the AIWF National Board promotes understanding of others' needs as a way of success in life and is first on that list. His wife and my friend Meme is second. Gary is an inspirational mentor who gives generously and from his heart, and has creativity, insight, tact, and perseverance to which I can only aspire. His belief in my abilities allowed me to give myself to this work.

I thank Karen Levin of Highland Park, Illinois, for her terrific recipe development and testing skills. Karen's carefulness and care, and our mutual passion for great ingredients and new flavors, made every kitchen session a delight. Executive Chef Kimberly Schor of Nordstrom's, so filled with enthusiasm and possessed of a terrific palate, also assisted with the development and testing of recipes. Both women bear no responsibility for any recipe I offer that doesn't taste great.

Christian DeVos of Kendall College provided a first-class culinary setting for an executive CHEF Clinic program—many of the techniques in this book were honed in that special, one-day seminar. Don Newcomb and Jim Price worked to create the unity of food and health, and Scott Warner of the Chicago Medical Society helped me make two transitions, one to my own weight loss of 30 pounds in 1992, and the second to ChicaGourmet's special Kendall program "There's a Doctor in the Kitchen." Theresa Roti captured it all and inspired some of the best home cooking I've ever done. Beth Shephard and Lisa Ekus helped to create ways of integrating my work in RealAge within the fabulously fun business of food, and Kathleen Gallagher, Howard Gilbert, and Roger Fox made sense of it on paper.

Lisa M. Drayer, now of www.dietwatch.com in New York City, did much of the original research to create a running start on this work. And Laura Walsh, R.D., a thoughtful, first-rate clinical dietitian in private practice in Elmhurst, Illinois, did a brilliant job of researching and assembling resources for nearly all of the kitchen equipment.

John Reyes, remarkably wise and humanistic and so solidly grounded, helped me put one foot in front of the other. Bill Rayner did the same—with his ambitious and friendly way of helping me create food that everyone will want to eat, whether at a stadium or in a store.

I am also grateful to dietitians Jennifer Becker and Judy Kolish and physician-assistant-extraordinaire Jeanne McMahon for permission to allow me to devote stolen time to completing the book. They are excellent clinicians to whose care I would trust any member of my family. Natalie Giacomino, Kathi Kardos, Kelley Clancy, Dean Grant, and Nancy Hellyer of Alexian Brothers Medical Center in Elk Grove Village deserve many thanks for providing the space and time to allow me to continue this work and conduct hands-on private classes and tutorials for my patients. Chef Chris Stoye melded great professionalism and great knife skills with great hands-on teaching.

Milo Falcon, Stefanie Lewis, and Brenda Mooney of American Health Consultants deserve special credit for allowing me the freedom to create medical meeting meals for two hundred physicians. So do Dennis Wentz, Charles Willis, Jacquelyn Craig, and Regina Littleton of the AMA, and Jill Keenan and executive chef Kevin Randles of the Baltimore Marriott. Working with Galveston's Moody Hotel Executive Chef Klaus and Garvin O'Neill on a conference menu plan was a huge pleasure—great chefs like Klaus love making food that is good for you taste good. Visionary Vic Sierpina put it all together. Paula Cousins and Leslie Coplin have my deep daily gratitude for their faultless work on Alternative Medicine Alert.

I also owe special thanks to Chefs Rick Bayless, Tracey Vowell, Kevin Karales, and Geno Bahena, and the staff of Chicago's Frontera Grill and Topolobampo, for opening their hearts and sharing so generously what they knew. This food honors their commitment to local farmers, to flavor first, and to seasonal foods. Deborah Madison, so long a culinary inspiration, lives her values and inspires the promise of the local flavors sprinkled here. Patricia Greenberg's passion for social change and eye toward achievement do the same. Manny Valdes of Frontera Foods offered regular, welcome sparks of entrepreneurial encouragement. David and Kim Schiedermayer continued to offer their kindness and editorial support (and in season, David's eye for steelhead, morels, and wild asparagus); it was my privilege to try out some of these recipes at their nephew Jack's birthday party.

Tuscan cooking school teacher Pamela Sheldon Johns encouraged me from the beginning to try my hand at a complementary partnership. Juliana Middleton inspired me with her love of plants grown with care, and then prepared with her magic hands. Dun Gifford and Sara Baer-Sinnott of Oldways are champions who know the synergy of traditional diets and great health. Walter Willett, Susan Bowerman, David Heber, and John Foreyt's pioneering research in weight loss; Dan Nadeau's enthusiasm for food as medicine; and Bill and Erin Arnold's insight into the science behind an arthritis pain alleviating diet all promise to take nutrient-rich, calorie-lean food and meals to the next level.

And finally, I would like to thank Mike Roizen for the exceptional opportunity to work with, learn from, and most of all, become part of the RealAge team. His absolute focus and visionary leadership move and excite me. Mike's passion for science is now joined by the pleasures of the table—and of a healthy, younger RealAge.

Cooking the RealAge® Way

1

Cooking the RealAge Way

*Control Your Genes Simply by
the Way You Set Up Your Kitchen*

You do not have to feel or be your calendar age. Seventy percent of premature aging is caused by the choices we make. By making some good choices, such as eating well, you can slow down or even reverse the signs of aging. And the best way to eat well is by revising key elements of the most important room in your home—the kitchen.

Just as what you eat makes a big difference in how old you feel and how old you actually are, it also amazingly makes a difference in what proteins your genes produce. As we learn more about genes, we learn how much we can modify their actions. The specific proteins they produce and the ratio of proteins any two genes make is at least partially under your control. This chapter is about how we can stock our kitchens and change what we eat to control our genes, ultimately keeping us and our families energetic and younger.

The response to our first book, *RealAge,* which provided consistent scientific data that you can control your rate of aging, has been overwhelming. Thousands of e-mails have told me that knowing the effect of a healthy choice—for example, knowing that eating an ounce of nuts a day makes the average 55-year-old man more than 3.3 years younger—was empowering. Such knowledge motivated individuals to make healthier choices. For the first year after that book was published, I received an average of 1,500 e-mails a day from readers. People told me they loved having a way of measuring their rate of aging and, even better, had found some simple steps for slowing that process.

As explained in *The RealAge Diet,* consistent scientific data show that eating the RealAge way—great-tasting, healthy food that is colorful—can make you younger. The scientific advisory group of RealAge has a strict standard to follow: no food choice (and no other health factor, for that matter) is said to have a RealAge effect (e.g., "Enjoying a half-ounce of dark—cocoa based—chocolate before each meal can make you 1.9 years younger") unless that effect has been shown to occur in at least four studies on humans. In addition, each RealAge food choice should be (and is, as confirmed by taste tests) every bit as satisfying and delicious as the energy-sapping, aging foods so widespread in the American diet. My patients and readers love knowing that simple, easy changes in food choices make a measurable difference in their health.

This is where cooking the RealAge way comes in. Perhaps a patient story helps: Steve I. was a 52-year-old hard-driving executive. His wife, Nancy, cared deeply about him, so when he was home for dinner (he ate out or was away two or three nights every week), Nancy cooked his favorite roasts or steaks. She punctuated every meal with great vegetables and a good salad, but Nancy always had his favorite coffee ice cream (to make him feel like home was a comfortable spot); and on planes or on the road he ate whatever was being served (he traveled in first class often, owing to his frequent flyer status); Mrs. Field's cookies and ice cream for dessert were rewards. And he ate whatever everybody else was eating at meetings. He and his wife exercised two or three times a week when he was at home. But he was getting more tired, enjoying the work less, and his arthritis started to act up. So his wife forced him to see me.

We found his RealAge was thirteen years older than his calendar age; he was really 65, not 52, and he felt it. So he made small changes that made a big difference. Just changing to nuts and chocolate-covered fruit as a snack, ordering fish or vegetarian meals in advance on planes, asking for olive oil, throwing the creamy dressings out, and stocking the kitchen with a balsamic vinegar he adored, his wife making RealAge dishes he loved, and prioritizing 20 minutes of exercise a day, he transformed himself easily into someone who felt 45 not 65. Actually, he became 45 (his RealAge decreased to 45 over three years). He became vigorous and regained his zest for life, and he looked it. So did his wife, who became transformed as well.

And it was easy, they say. It started by understanding why we feel and get older, and how easy it is to deliciously transform our eating. It just started and was (and is) done with easy changes in the kitchen. Nancy looked and felt younger, too—Steve and she each lost weight (18 and 9 pounds, respectively)—but that was not their goal. They wanted to feel the zest for life and energy that had gradually slipped away. They wanted the energy to help their children build families and to enjoy their grandchildren. They just didn't know how easy it was; neither did I until I started to learn about how we can control our genes—how solid that science was—that started for me more than twenty years after I was a doctor, and more than ten years ago.

Now many of us wish we could be 9 or 18 pounds lighter, or feel and be twenty years younger. And we can. That it is easy and predictable is the great news. Steve and Nancy's story is not unique and their transformation is not unusual or different. Many others (myself and my wife included) have done it. And it is not even hard; it is even fun. I want you to learn what I've learned—it's too easy and too important not to learn it. *RealAge: Are You As Young As You Can Be?* and *The RealAge Diet: Make Yourself Younger with What You Eat* reveal the scientific principles and strategies to help you make yourself younger. The goal of the first two *RealAge* books was to help you understand the science behind control of your genes. This book does only a little of that. Much more of the book applies these concepts to preparation of food—how to cook food so it tastes great and makes your RealAge younger. Reading this book and cooking the RealAge way is an easy way to look, feel, and be at least five to eight years and probably fourteen years younger than your calendar age.

I'm a medical doctor and a research scientist. My co-author, John La Puma, is also a medical doctor, as well as a professionally trained chef. We take enormous pride in knowing that the RealAge concepts have helped so many people add extra, vigorous, quality-filled years to their lives. It's not just about living longer. It's about enjoying a higher quality of life at all ages.

Unfortunately, too many of us have come to think of cooking and eating in the wrong way. We eat food out of habit and convenience, instead of making our meals a joyful focal point in our lives. Instead of celebrating food, we feel ambivalent about it. Time spent sharing a meal with loved ones should be a celebration. Food nourishes us, sustains us, makes us grow, and gives us energy. It is a positive force in our lives, making us feel good, alive, and younger every day. Grow old gracefully? Not you. You'll live life to your youngest!

In this book, we show how to take our healthy concepts and bring them into your home, literally. The best way to begin eating well is by revising key elements of the most important room in your home—the kitchen. Simply put, transforming your kitchen is an easy way to transform your health. A little science will slip in, especially in this chapter, but the book aims primarily to make healthy cooking easy and the results delicious.

With some effort and a little practice, you can create RealAge-smart and energy-giving meals that are as delicious as those created by a top chef but without all the cream and butter. But before you learn how, you might want to know something about the RealAge concept and a little of the science behind it. Then you'll understand how much you can control how well and how long you will live.

The RealAge Concept

Those who have read *RealAge* and *The RealAge Diet* are already familiar with the RealAge concept, which states that the fundamental source of your overall good health is the good maintenance of two of the most important systems in the body: the cardiovascular system (the heart and blood vessels) and the immune system. While we do not know the molecular basis of aging, we do know what ages. The aging of your arteries is responsible for such potentially disabling conditions as strokes, heart attacks, memory loss, impotence, decay in the quality of orgasm, and wrinkling of your skin. And aging of the other major system, the immune system, can lead to autoimmune diseases, such as arthritis; to serious infections, such as pneumonia; and to cancer. RealAge identifies what factors are important in your aging processes for these systems, how you can change those factors to keep yourself younger, and the relative value of such choices. For example, eating an ounce of nuts a day keeps the average 55-year-old man 3.3 years younger. Similarly, consuming less than 20 grams of saturated and trans fats a day (see below) makes the average 55-year-old woman 2.7 years younger. RealAge is really like money: it places a value on your choices. There are many choices you can make to keep your arteries and immune system younger.

The good news is that to a large extent we do not have to be at the mercy of fate or heredity. Seventy percent of premature aging is caused by the choices we make. By making some easy choices, you can slow—or even reverse—aging, regardless of your inherited genetics. The choices that can easily make you younger include food choices.

Getting Back to the Basics

A walk down the aisle of any grocery store will reveal the predominance of foods high in the kinds of fat that age you (not all fat ages you), and in simple sugars and salt. Although this quickly reveals the extent to which the quality of the average American diet has declined, it also shows to what extent most of us have forgotten, or have never experienced, the most fundamental pleasures of cooking and enjoying our kitchens.

The existence of prepared mixes for bread machines is a perfect example. To make bread in a bread machine, you measure flour, water, yeast, milk, and salt and then press a button. Nothing could be simpler. However, the fact that Nancy (of Steve and Nancy above) served her family bread made in this machine with a commercially packaged mix that is full of added chemicals, stabilizers, and sodium—just to save the time necessary for collecting and measuring ingredients—shows the extent to which many of us feel too busy to spend time measuring, pouring, and mixing in our own kitchens. Nancy just didn't know. She did care. Probably this predominance of packaged food is partly due to the prevalence of busier-than-ever two-career families. Many busy working people regard grocery shopping and cooking as just two more chores at the end of a stress-filled day. This need not be the case. Armed with a "smart" kitchen—one that has the right ingredients and equipment—and an understanding of simple cooking techniques, you can quickly and easily create a great-tasting, healthy, and energy-giving meal. How you stock your kitchen can result in a high IQ: a kitchen with a high IQ is smart enough to help control your genes and make your RealAge younger.

Like everything else that is important in life, learning to change habits, such as switching from aging to age-reducing food choices, takes a little dedication and persistence. In a short time, your new RealAge-smart habits will become such a natural part of your life that you'll wonder how you ever lived any other way. Learning how to cook and how to enjoy a great-tasting, RealAge-smart meal will take some practice, it's true. But you wouldn't expect to break 90 on your first day on the golf course. Similarly, it will take time to retrain your taste buds (a key to enjoying great tasting food). Soon, however, your RealAge dishes will taste better than the artery-aging bucket of greasy fried chicken or the energy-sapping take-out food you would have chosen. I know because I, too, had to work to change bad eating habits. It was also challenging for a doctor whose food specialty was toast to learn how to cook. But now I'm full of energy, I keep my weight at a steady low level, and best of all, I've made myself *younger*—and I enjoy the extra vitality.

The Science Behind the Numbers

If you chart the health, longevity, and, ultimately, *youth* of a "population age cohort"— a group of people all born in the same year—you will find that, with few exceptions, people age at a similar rate until they reach their late twenties or mid-thirties. With the exception of those who have inherited rare genetic disorders or have been in serious accidents, everyone is basically healthy and able. Men reach the peak of their performance curve in their late twenties, women in their mid-thirties. At that time, our bodies have fully matured, and we are at our strongest and most mentally acute. Then, somewhere between 28 and 36 years of age, most people reach a turning point, a transition from "growing" into "aging."

If you examine the population as a whole and track any one biological function— be it kidney function or cognitive ability—performance declines as we age. In general, after the age of 35, each biological function decreases about 5 percent every ten years. That decrease is a measure of the *average* for the population as a whole. Although these kinds of measurements have been the standards used by scientists to calculate the rate of aging, the averages don't take into account variation between individuals. The variation is so great among people over 40 that it is often meaningless to calculate an average at all. Averages are statistically meaningful only if the values for the people or things being measured actually congregate closely around the midpoint (that is, if everyone is pretty much the same).

When we age, there is so much variation between individuals over age 40 that the "average" obscures more than it shows. Rather than gathering around a mean (the midpoint), there are people in every age group who manifest every level of functioning. Some show dramatic decline, others show virtually no decline. What you eat contributes mightily to this difference between people. Twins who choose different lifestyles or foods age at different rates. People with genetic diseases such as type II diabetes can age at different rates if they make different choices.

Our genes matter. Genes simply make proteins—that is how genes cause their effects. But how much of each protein a gene makes changes as we grow older and the ratio of some proteins to other proteins changes as we grow older. But changing what we eat, for example from red meat to fish, might change the ratio of proteins from that typical of an older person to one typical of a younger person. Feeding your genes more B_6, B_{12}, and folate may make them less vulnerable to chromosome breaks or substitutions. This type of change in what your genes produce or how they function with a change in your habits exemplifies the control you can exert over your genes and the diseases that are characteristic of aging. And you do not have to memorize long lists—it is easy to put it into everyday choices.

First, a Little Science

Aging of the Arteries

Keeping your arteries young and healthy is the single most important thing you can do for your health. Simply put, you're as young as your arteries. When your arteries are not taken care of properly—for example, when your diet is high in saturated or trans fats—they get clogged with fatty buildup, diminishing the amount of oxygen and nutrients that can get to the cells.

There are four major types of dietary fat: saturated, polyunsaturated, monounsaturated, and trans fat. The first three occur naturally. The fourth, trans fat, is usually an artificially created product that mimics saturated fat. Trans fat—also called trans fatty acid—is created when unsaturated fats are hydrogenated (combined with hydrogen). The purpose of this chemical process is to create fats that are solid at room temperature rather than liquid, their normal state at room temperature. For example, most solid margarine is produced by transforming (through partial hydrogenation) good vegetable oils into bad vegetable oils. Even though a food label doesn't use the exact words "trans fat," if you see "partially hydrogenated vegetable oils"or "hydrogenated oils" as an ingredient, you can be sure the product contains trans fat. Any fat that is liquid when heated but hardens when cooled to room temperature is probably made of either saturated or trans fat. If the fat is solid when cool, it will age you. For example, most stick margarine is trans fat, as is much of the glaze on doughnuts.

Since food producers are not required to list trans fats on their nutrition labels, trans fat is called "the hidden fat." The FDA has proposed that the trans fat content of food be listed on labels by mid-2003. Some food manufacturers are fighting this requirement. Many packaged foods—cookies, crackers, and chips—contain these oils because they give food a longer shelf life (and you a shorter life filled with more disability). Many cookies and crackers claim to be "baked, not fried," or to have "no saturated fat" or "no cholesterol." This implies they're low in fat, when in fact they're often full of trans fat. It doesn't matter if the product is cholesterol-free; if it contains trans fat, it will age your arteries and immune system.

When your arteries get clogged with fatty buildup, not only your cardiovascular system but also your entire body ages more quickly. Cardiovascular disease, which is brought on by aging of the arteries, is the major cause of heart attacks, strokes, many types of kidney disease, and memory loss. Even mild forms of vascular disease that won't actually kill you can sap your energy and make you feel old and tired.

Aging of the arteries also causes impotence, diminished quality of orgasm, and even wrinkling of the skin.

Luckily, small, easy-to-make changes in food choices and in lifestyle can profoundly improve your arterial health and can reverse a great deal of the aging that has already taken place. Simply eating certain foods, such as a little garlicky olive oil in a pasta dish or a great-tasting tomato sauce, can reduce the fatty arterial-wall buildup that can lead to vascular disease. More than six studies in the highest-quality peer-reviewed medical literature have reported that both garlic and olive oil decrease aging of the arteries, and that the two, eaten together regularly, can make you over three years younger if you're a 50-year-old man or two years younger if you're a 50-year-old woman. What's more, garlic and olive oil taste great.

These foods can also decrease the likelihood that a cell will have a break in its DNA that could lead to cancer. That's right; just switching from one fat (butter or margarine) to another (olive or nut oil) can make your arteries and immune system many years younger.

Aging of the Immune System

In addition to taking care of your arteries, don't let your immune system make you old. As you age, your immune system begins to get sloppy, ignoring important warning signals and becoming negligent. You can end up with cancer or another disorder caused by a malfunction of the immune system. For example, when you are young—except in relatively rare cases—genetic controls in your cells protect your cells from becoming cancerous. If one of these cellular controls slips up, all is not lost. Your larger immune system can identify precancerous cells in the body and eliminate them. Thus, your body has a double block against cancer, one on the cellular level and one on the organism-wide level.

As you age, both the cell-based genetic controls and your immune system become more likely to malfunction, and you are more likely to develop a cancerous tumor. Also, many types of arthritis are examples of a breakdown of the immune system, which is why arthritis is another disease associated with aging. Luckily, some food choices, such as having a bowl of fresh mixed berries as an afternoon snack, can help your body shed free radicals (substances that can cause cell damage), which lessens your chance of getting arthritis, macular degeneration (a disease that destroys vision), and even cancer. (Nature got it right: the best foods are almost always the most naturally delicious and the most colorful.) The RealAge kitchen program also helps reduce the stress in your life; stress can upset the balance of the immune system.

Getting Younger with Lycopene

The tomato-sauce story is even more important to aging, and even more scientifically solid than the garlic–olive oil story. There are more than thirty studies in humans showing that consumption of 10 tablespoons of tomato sauce a week decrease the likelihood of cancer. Breast and prostate cancer are the two cancers for which the most evidence exists for prevention of cancer by consumption of tomato sauce or, more precisely, lycopene, the carotenoid in tomato sauce that is believed to be the active ingredient for health. Although lycopene is also found in guava, watermelon, and pink grapefruit, it is most easily absorbed from cooked tomatoes combined with a little oil.

Although we do not use test-tube data when calculating a RealAge effect—we use only data from studies on human beings—it should be noted that the addition of lycopene (from tomatoes) to human cells in test tubes and cell cultures has decreased the number of breaks that occur in DNA. Such breaks are thought to be the precursors of cancer. So, in addition to a substantial amount of data in human beings that tomato sauce decreases the risk of cancer, biologic evidence from test tubes gives us a mechanism for the effect. These data may not thrill your taste buds, but tomatoes can. Having 10 tablespoons of tomato sauce a week makes the typical 55-year-old man 1.9 years younger and the typical 55-year-old woman 0.7 years younger.

There may be a bonus to keeping your RealAge younger with lycopene, whatever the source. As of this writing, three studies in humans have shown that lycopene is associated with an impressive reversal, or slowing, of aging of the arteries. Because we must have four supporting studies in humans before we claim that a factor produces an effect on RealAge, we cannot say that consumption of lycopene decreases aging of the arteries. If, however, the data from these three studies are corroborated in a fourth study, that will increase tomato's RealAge effect, making 10 tablespoons a week of tomato sauce give you a three-year benefit. Eating tomato sauce is a pretty easy and delicious way to make your RealAge younger, don't you think? And maybe realizing just that—that it was easy and fun to make yourself more than half a year younger—is why it's so enjoyable to make a few RealAge-smart choices.

What's Your RealAge *Now*?

If you'd like to know your RealAge, and you have access to the Internet, you can take the RealAge quiz online at www.RealAge.com. There is no charge for this service. Your account stores RealAge information about you that can be accessed and updated by you as many times as you like. All information is completely confidential and accessible only by you through a password you choose as you use the Web site to chart and update your progress.

The computer test takes about thirty-five minutes to complete. You'll need to know your blood pressure, heart rate, weight, height, cholesterol values (both total cholesterol and high density lipoprotein cholesterol), triglyceride value, c-reactive protein, and the amounts of any vitamins or supplements you take. (If you do not know these values, the average for your gender and age will be used until you provide your values.) After you've answered all the questions, the computer calculates your RealAge. This rarely takes more than two minutes. Similarly, you can determine your kitchen's IQ, and see the effect of your kitchen's IQ on your RealAge. After completing either test, you are also given a list of suggestions tailored to your health and behavior profile, how to make your RealAge younger, and how to stock your kitchen.

Planning to Get Younger

These suggestions are a list of possible choices you can adopt to make your RealAge younger. Select the suggestions you would consider incorporating into your life—for example, eating 5 ounces of nuts a week, substituting an olive oil and balsamic vinegar salad dressing for one containing saturated fat, or adding three 4-ounce portions of fish to your diet every week. The computer then recalculates your RealAge in light of these new behaviors. In this way, you can see how much of a difference each choice would make. For example, adopting the suggestions on nuts, fish, and salad dressing might make you 5.4 years younger three years after you adopted those behaviors. The computer thus helps you set goals, showing what your RealAge would be in three months, one year, and three years if you follow your plan. One of the easy ways that most of us can slow our aging is to make small changes in the way we set up our kitchen.

How to Implement the RealAge Concept in Your Kitchen

The Goals of RealAge

Learning to live the RealAge way is like learning to do anything—riding a bike, using a computer, reading. Practice and a little coaching go a long way. Changing your kitchen habits and your eating habits (and other food-related habits, such as cooking regularly at home or being a smarter grocery shopper) requires just a little time and just a little consistency. If you aren't used to cooking healthy meals for your family, it isn't second nature. But to make healthy eating an enjoyable, natural part of your life, you just have to take the first step. It's easier and more fun than you ever imagined!

The goal of increasing your kitchen IQ and RealAge cooking is age reduction—giving you a higher quality of life and more vigor every day. Weight reduction is a side effect of this diet that many find an unexpected bonus. However, feeling better every day, and feeling the power of more energy every day, are the benefits patients tell me I can guarantee if you cook the RealAge way for ninety days.

Making Every Calorie Delicious and Nutrient-Rich

If you are aware of the amount of saturated and trans fat you consume and make everything you eat nutrient-rich, calorie-poor, and delicious, it will be hard for you to gain weight unless you are malnourished. It will be easy to maintain or lose weight.

You won't go far astray if you remember the RealAge mantra: whenever you eat, *make every calorie delicious and nutrient-rich.* Learn the pleasure of spending time in a well-stocked, RealAge-smart kitchen, or what we call a "high-IQ kitchen." Include your friends and loved ones, so that you have the pleasure of their company and, at the same time, the satisfaction of seeing them become more vibrant and energized as a result of the healthy foods you're serving them.

The food choices of the average American are responsible for approximately one-third of his or her rate of aging. Other choices, which are discussed in the RealAge books or on the Web site, determine the other two-thirds of the rate of aging: stress, group participation, family history, job choices, physical activities, and good and bad habits, such as flossing, wearing a helmet when you bike, or smoking. Regularly eating nutrient-poor, calorie-rich choices such as "Cinnabons," "Bloomin' Onions," or "Cheesecake Factory Carrot Cake" can make your RealAge as much as thirteen years older than your calendar age. In contrast, eating delicious foods that are nutrient-rich (our Warm Spinach Salad with Chicken, Apples, and Toasted Almonds—the recipe is in *The RealAge Diet,* page 351, or any of the recipes in this book) can make you fourteen years younger than your calendar age. Every item you choose to eat should be world class in taste and nutrients. If you choose great-tasting foods that are full of vitamins, minerals, nutrients, and fiber rather than empty calories, you're eating the RealAge way.

My friends have asked me to summarize the principles of RealAge cooking on a card or foldover set of sheets they could carry in their breast pocket or purse for the first ninety days. The following 27 points are those principles, followed by a brief explanation of each.

Eating the RealAge Way

If you follow these practices, your food choices can make your RealAge fourteen years younger:

1. Make every calorie you eat delicious and nutrient-rich. Don't eat foods that taste just "okay." If they're not special, don't let them touch your lips. You deserve to treat yourself well.

2. Eat foods that aren't processed. If you rarely eat packaged goods or prepared foods, you'll usually know what's in your food.

3. Eat breakfast—preferably, a whole grain and a little healthy fat. You'll start the day off with energy, avoid hunger pangs that lead to unwise food choices, and have more stable blood sugar levels. Try real peanut butter on toasted rye or on a chewy whole wheat bagel, or a Kashi cereal.

4. Eat some healthy fat first at every meal. The ideal amount represents approximately 60–75 calories: ½ tablespoon of olive oil or canola oil, 6 walnuts, 12 almonds, 20 peanuts, or ½ ounce of cocoa-based chocolate or avocado.

5. Read the labels for serving size. Determine exactly how many servings you will be eating, and how many grams of saturated and trans fat that amount contains. Avoid products that put you over your daily limit of 20 grams, or that have more than 6 grams in a serving you'll eat.

6. Read the labels for whole-grain content. Look at the first six items in the label. The first that involves grains should say "whole wheat," "oats," "oats, unprocessed," "brown rice," "corn," etc. Choose products that have more whole-grain content than processed-grain content.

7. Tally your saturated and trans fat consumption every day. Try to keep it to less than 20 grams a day. No matter what the special interest lobbyists say, eating more than 20 grams a day of saturated and trans fat (we call these two together the "Aging Fats"; see earlier in this chapter) correlates with the development of arterial aging (heart disease, stroke, memory loss, impotence, decay in orgasm quality, wrinkling of the skin) and cancer (the evidence is strongest for increases in saturated and trans fats being associated with the development of breast and prostate cancers). And aging fats sap your energy acutely when they prevent your arteries from dilating as your muscles need more oxygen. The risk of arterial disease and cancer seems to increase substantially as your intake of saturated and trans fats combined exceeds 20 grams a day.

8. Limit red meat consumption to 4 ounces a week. This includes "the other white meat." Use red meat as a side dish or condiment, not a main course.

9. Read the label when you buy baked goods. Choose those with whole grains, and no aging trans or saturated fats, and great texture. Baked goods tend to make you older because they contain tons of trans fats and processed flour. One Cinnabon, I'm told, contains 75 grams of aging fat—not a four-pack, but just one Cinnabon; a slice of whole-grain cinnamon-flavored bread made by our local Montana Bread Company or by P and C contains no aging or other fat and no processed flour, tastes great, and if you want to make it even healthier, add some peanut butter or pure avocado spread.

10. Substitute healthier foods. Assess your foods and meals in terms of how they could be made healthier by additions, subtractions, or substitutions. A few substitutions can make a big difference in your rate of aging. They also make food taste great! Try substituting olive oil for butter or margarine on bread, or prune purée or drained applesauce for 1 to 3 tablespoons of butter in smaller recipes; fruit for cookies; real (dark) chocolate for milk chocolate; nuts for chips; and cooked garlic salsa or marinara sauce for a cream sauce.

11. Make eating, and the place you eat, special. Only eat sitting down at one of your special places. (Usually, designate no more than three places as "special"—one at home and perhaps two at work). Only eat food on plates and on 9-inch plates, not giant ones. My most successful patients (and their families) have *a special place in their home that is the only place for eating.* Not eating anyplace else was and is their rule—not the TV room, not standing up, not in the car, not out of the refrigerator.

12. Take a 30-minute walk every day with a friend. I call this a RealAge double dip. Not only do you get the anti-aging benefit that physical activity and exercise give you, but also you build the strong social support networks that can help you prevent needless aging through times of stress.

13. Plan menus and learn to cook. Cooking can be a true pleasure; in addition, you will know what's in your food, and you will also have the fun of learning how to use herbs and spices to make food taste fabulous.

14. Be a smart shopper. If you don't *buy* food that's bad for you, you won't *eat* food that's bad for you.

15. Eat nonfried fish three times a week. Any fish, not just fatty fish, makes you younger.

16. Eat 10 tablespoons of tomato sauce a week. Try marinara sauce, salsa, and other varieties. The carotenoid found in tomatoes, watermelon, guava, and pink grapefruit—lycopene—when eaten with a little oil, provides an immune-strengthening antioxidant that seems to inhibit growth of prostate, breast cancers, and maybe other cancers, and may make your arteries younger.

17. Add variety to your diet and the way you cook vegetables. Why is variety in your diet so important? Many people don't eat a balanced diet. Forty percent of Americans don't eat fruit daily, and 30 percent don't consume any dairy or soy products regularly. On average, Americans get less than half of the 25 to 30 grams of fiber they need a day. Eating a diverse diet that is low in calories and high in nutrients decreases aging from arterial and immune dysfunction and makes your RealAge as much as four years younger. If you eat from all five food groups daily, you can be as much as five years younger than if you ate from only two. (The five groups are whole-grain breads and cereals; fruits; vegetables; dairy and dairy-substitute products; and meats, nuts, legumes, and other proteins). Adding variety to the way you cook is what you'll learn when you read Chapter 5. And variety will make all vegetables taste better, great even. It makes more fun to try new ways of cooking—and that makes you younger.

18. Be the CEO every time you eat out—why should you pay for something that ages you? Learn to ask questions of the wait-staff when you eat out. Then learn to ask for healthy, great tasting choices—"Would you ask the chef to substitute the marinara sauce for the Alfredo sauce?"

19. Keep your portions energy-giving, not energy-sapping. The usual restaurant entrée is not an acceptable meal size. Use your fist or a pack of cards as a measure of a serving.

20. Stop eating as soon as you *start* to feel full. Because your stomach is roughly the size of your fist, eating meals larger than your fist can stretch your stomach beyond what's comfortable or healthy. Eat a little healthy fat first. Then pause before the rest of the meal. And remember: stop eating as soon as you first sense you might be getting full—before the full feeling hits.

21. Don't eat absentmindedly. All too often, eating is an unconscious act. We lift the fork, swallow absentmindedly, and lift the fork again. Sometimes we overeat because we just aren't paying attention. We're bored, nervous, or busy. Often, we're not even hungry. Instead, eat mindfully. Be actively conscious of what you're eating and why. Use all of your senses to enjoy the color, texture, smell, and flavor of your food. Not only will you enjoy your food more, but you'll also slow down your rate of consumption.

22. Do resistance exercises for 10 minutes every other day. You replace a pound of your muscle with a pound of fat about every five years after age 35 if you do not do resistance exercises. And a pound of muscle uses about 150 calories a day, compared to 3 calories a day for a pound of fat. Whether you use free weights, resistance bands, or machines, it takes just 10 minutes three times a week to maintain muscle mass. (You can go to www.realage.com/realagecafé/myfitnessplan to see these resistance exercises and design a plan for yourself, but I recommend consultation with a trainer for at least the first three times you do resistance exercises and then at least once every three months thereafter.)

23. Be a savvy snacker. Think nutrient rich and calorie lean. Try a few nuts and a piece of whole fruit. Try not to snack at night.

24. Avoid simple carbohydrates and simple sugars. Remember that carbohydrates were meant to be complex. Simple sugars in food are absorbed quickly in the intestine and increase the amount of sugar in the blood for at least one to two hours. A high concentration of sugar in the blood eradicates the natural protective control your body has over the usual, everyday variations in blood pressure. High blood-sugar levels also increase triglyceride levels in the blood.

What about honey and natural sugars? Unfortunately, these are not healthy substitutes for white sugar. So avoid foods that are laden with carbohydrates from brown sugar, corn sweetener, dextrose, fructose (high fructose corn sweetener), glucose, corn syrup, honey, invert sugar, lactose, maltose, malt syrup, molasses, raw sugar, sucrose, syrup, and table sugar.

25. Drink alcohol in moderation. Women benefit from one drink a day; men, from one or two. Avoid making this choice if you or your family are at risk of alcohol or drug abuse.

26. Drink lots of water. Drink a glass of water between every glass of wine or other alcoholic drink you have. Also, at food events, carry a glass of water in one hand.

27. Take the right vitamins and minerals twice a day and avoid the wrong ones. See Chapter 12 of this book (page 334) to find what vitamins you should consider taking and in what amounts.

RealAge Kitchen Recipes

ncluded in this book are delicious RealAge recipes I know you'll enjoy. Each recipe carries with it a RealAge effect. I tell you how much younger (or older) enjoying each recipe twelve times a year will make you. For example, enjoying Barbecued Red Snapper with Spicy Red Beans and Rice (page 297) twelve times a year will make you 11.4 days younger. Although these calculations are approximations, they clearly provide a direction and magnitude of health effect for each recipe. In addition, each recipe was selected for great taste and ease of preparation, and all were tested repeatedly by several amateur and professional chefs for ease of cooking and for taste ratings from multiple audiences (see Chapter 9, page 145, for rating scale). Think of these recipes, and of your new, healthy lifestyle, as a giant menu of possibilities: a menu of choices for growing younger and staying young. Think of it as a menu for a lifetime— a long and healthy lifetime—of great-tasting foods.

In *Cooking the RealAge Way* I also address simple cooking and healthy eating as a joyful lifestyle, full of the pleasures of creative cooking; the blessing of sharing sensuous, delicious foods and a glass of fine wine with loved ones; and the relief and relaxation of stress-free time spent in a well-stocked, well-equipped kitchen.

2

Kitchen of Youth

What Is Your *Kitchen's IQ?*

How smart is your kitchen now? How smart could you make it? Learn how to calculate your kitchen's IQ: By answering 25 questions about your habits and behaviors, and the way your kitchen is stocked and equipped, you can determine if your kitchen is smart enough to help you age more slowly. By choosing from the recommendations in this book or on the Web site, you can develop a step-by-step Age Reduction™ plan based on food choices customized to your needs and lifestyle.

The Nuts and Bolts of the RealAge Kitchen of Youth

What's Your Kitchen's IQ?

In this questionnaire, we ask you detailed questions about a variety of your behaviors and the contents of your kitchen and pantry. These are behaviors and food choices known to affect aging. For example, at home, do you eat only in places and with dishes you consider special? Do you have seasonal fruit attractively displayed in your kitchen or at the places you're most likely to eat? Do you have applesauce, prunes, and bananas in your kitchen, and do you try to use these foods as substitutes for butter and shortening when baking? Do you purchase only baked goods that are low in saturated and trans fats? (These are aging four-legged and partially hydrogenated vegetable fats.)

When you entertain, do you try to keep your dishes simple? Do you frequently serve nuts, fish, tomato products, and whole grains? Do you eat a little healthy fat before each meal? And we ask questions about these habits such as: When eating out, do you ask about the way dishes are prepared? Do you usually walk 30 minutes a day? We ask you questions about 125 food-related factors that affect your health and youth.

For each question, choose the answer that best describes your situation and *circle the corresponding points.* Then write that number in the "Tally" box. For some of the questions, you will need to add several numbers together. In each case, we tell you exactly how to figure out what number to write in the box.

After you finish all the questions, see page 59 to see how to calculate the tallies. This is your current kitchen's IQ. The higher the number, the more likely your kitchen is making you younger. After you finish all the questions, we discuss how to calculate the effect your kitchen's IQ has on your rate of aging and your RealAge.

How can you raise your kitchen's IQ? You will notice that each question has two parts. The second part shows what you can do to increase your kitchen's IQ for that particular factor. Are you willing to change that behavior, and to what degree? You again choose the correct answer and *circle the number of points.* Next, determine how many additional Kitchen IQ points you'll be gaining and write that number in the "Increased Tally" square. If you already make a lot of RealAge choices, you won't have much of an increased tally—but if you have room for improvement, and are willing to make changes, you should have a higher number than the original tally. Again, in each instance, we'll tell you exactly how to determine what number to write in the square.

For Cooking at Home

1A. Do you have the following in your kitchen?

	Kitchen IQ Points
• Mixer or blender	1
• Toaster oven	1
• Microwave oven	1
• Stove-top grill or grill pan	1
• Steamer	1
• Poacher	1

Possible points: 0 to 6   **Tally** [   ]

Explanation: These items make it easy for you to decrease the amount of saturated fat and trans fat in your food. Decreasing those kinds of fat makes your RealAge younger.

My Plan to Increase My Kitchen's IQ (and Make My RealAge Younger)

1B. I don't have them now, but I will purchase the following items for my kitchen:

	Kitchen IQ Points
• Mixer or blender	1
• Toaster oven	1
• Microwave oven	1
• Stove-top grill or grill pan	1
• Steamer	1
• Poacher	1

Possible additional points: 0 to 6   **Increased Tally** [ ]

2A. Do you have ample applesauce, prunes or prune purée, and bananas on hand, and do you try to use them as a substitute for some of the butter or shortening when baking; or do you purchase only baked goods that are low in saturated and trans fats?

	Kitchen IQ Points
• Yes, always	6
• One-third to two-thirds of the time	3
• Less than one-third of the time	1
• No, never	0

Possible points: 0 to 6   **Tally** [ ]

Explanation: Keeping your saturated fats and trans fats to less than 20 grams a day will make your RealAge as much as 6.4 years younger. At the present time, food manufacturers are not required to list trans fat ("the hidden fat") on food labels. However, if you see "partially hydrogenated" vegetable oil on the label— or more fat than you can account for by adding up all the saturated, polyunsaturated, and monounsaturated fats—you can assume the rest is artery-aging trans fat. When baking, substitute applesauce, prunes, prune purée, or bananas for some of the butter and shortening to produce a rich and moist texture and make you substantially younger.

My Plan to Increase My Kitchen's IQ (and Make My RealAge Younger)

2B. I will have ample applesauce, prunes or prune purée, and bananas on hand and will try to use them as substitutes for some of the butter and shortening when baking; or I will purchase only baked goods that are low in saturated and trans fats.

	Kitchen IQ Points
• I will always do this.	6
• I will do this one-third to two-thirds of the time.	3
• I will do this less than one-third of the time.	1
• I will never, or hardly ever, do this.	0

Possible additional points: 0 to 6   **Increased Tally** ☐

In the Increased Tally box above, write the result of subtracting the tally number in Question 2A from the circled number above.

3A. Have you retrained your palate to enjoy healthy fats?

	Kitchen IQ Points
• Yes, in many ways. Skim milk, baked potato chips, nuts, olive oil, canola oil, avocados, fish, soy, cocoa-based chocolate, and flax seed are my major fats and fat substitutes.	10
• Yes, in some ways. Whole milk never touches my lips, but sometimes I eat saturated fat (animal fat) and trans fat (Crisco-like and stick margarine-like fat).	3
• Huh? What do you mean "healthy" fat?	0

Possible points: 0 to 10   **Tally** ☐

Explanation: Retraining the palate to prefer olive oil, cold-pressed canola oil, or fish is just that, retraining. If you drink whole milk and switch to skim, it will probably take eight weeks before you prefer the skim milk. For baked goods, try this switch for four weeks: If a recipe calls for 3 tablespoons of butter, try 2 table-spoons of butter and 1 tablespoon of an oil substitute (drained applesauce or prune purée). Then, for the next four weeks, try 1 tablespoon of butter and 2 tablespoons of an oil substitute. In eight weeks, you and your family will love the taste, and your RealAge will be 6 to 12 years younger. That's why this particular habit gets so many IQ points.

My Plan to Increase My Kitchen's IQ (and Make My RealAge Younger)

3B. I will retrain my palate to enjoy healthy fats.

	Kitchen IQ Points
• I will retrain my palate to enjoy many healthy fats. Skim milk, baked potato chips, nuts, olive oil, canola oil, avocados, fish, soy, cocoa-based chocolate, and flax seed will become my major fats and fat substitutes.	10
• I will retrain my palate to enjoy some of the healthy fats. I won't drink whole milk but will probably still eat some saturated fats and trans fats.	3
• I'm not going to be able to retrain my palate.	0

Possible additional points: 0 to 10   **Increased Tally***

In the Increased Tally box, write the result of subtracting the tally number in Question 3A from the circled number above.

4A. Do you routinely read labels and try to choose foods without simple sugars or aging fats?

	Kitchen IQ Points
• Always	10
• Usually	7
• Sometimes	2
• Never	0

Possible points: 0 to 10   **Tally** [ ]

Explanation: Being aware of and avoiding hidden fats, simple sugars, and needless calories will make your RealAge substantially younger. For all prepared foods, learn to read the serving size first. Then read the list of ingredients: It tells you which ingredients are first, second, third, fourth, and fifth in quantity for that item. Although saturated fats, trans fats, and sugars are often "hidden ingredients" in processed foods, the package label will give you the clues you need about the fats, carbohydrates, etc.

My Plan to Increase My Kitchen's IQ (and Make My RealAge Younger)

4B. I will routinely read labels and try to choose foods without simple sugars or aging fats:

	Kitchen IQ Points
• I will always do this.	10
• I will usually do this.	7
• I will sometimes do this.	2
• I will never, or hardly ever, do this.	0

Possible additional points: 0 to 10   **Increased Tally*** [ ]

*In the Increased Tally box, write the result of subtracting the tally number in Question 4A from the circled number above.

5A. Do you prepare for more than one meal and plan to freeze extras for an additional one to three meals?

	Kitchen IQ Points
• Always	6
• One-third to two-thirds of the time	3
• Less than one-third of the time	1
• No, never, or hardly ever	0

Possible points: 0 to 6   **Tally** [　　　　]

Explanation: Preparing in advance is an easy way to reduce stress, which is the leading cause of aging. If you freeze only the fresh food, give yourself an additional 3 Kitchen IQ points; and if you always use frozen food in a timely manner, give yourself another bonus of 3 Kitchen IQ points. Both strategies are key to ensuring that your frozen dishes also excite your taste buds.

My Plan to Increase My Kitchen's IQ (and Make My RealAge Younger)

5B. I will prepare for more than one meal and plan to freeze extras for an additional one to three meals.

	Kitchen IQ Points
• I will always do this.	6
• I will do this one-third to two-thirds of the time.	3
• I will do this, but less than one-third of the time.	1
• I will never, or hardly ever, do this.	0

Possible additional points: 0 to 6   **Increased Tally*** [　]

In the Increased Tally box, write the result of subtracting the tally number in Question 5A from the circled number above.

6A. Do you separate food into individual serving sizes before freezing?

	Kitchen IQ Points
• Always	6
• One-third to two-thirds of the time	3
• Less than one-third of the time	1
• No, never, or hardly ever	0

Possible points: 0 to 6   **Tally** [ ]

Explanation: If you separate food into individual serving sizes before freezing, you are much less likely to eat too much at any one time.

My Plan to Increase My Kitchen's IQ (and Make My RealAge Younger)

6B. I will separate food into individual serving sizes before freezing.

	Kitchen IQ Points
• I will always do this.	6
• I will do this one-third to two-thirds of the time.	3
• I will do this, but less than one-third of the time.	1
• I will never, or hardly ever, do this.	0

Possible additional points: 0 to 6   **Increased Tally*** [ ]

*In the Increased Tally box, write the result of subtracting the tally number in Question 6A from the circled number above.

7A. Do you squeeze excess air out of the package before you freeze food items?

	Kitchen IQ Points
• Always	3
• One-third to two-thirds of the time	2
• Less than one-third of the time	1
• Never, or hardly ever	0

Possible points: 0 to 3   **Tally** [   ]

Explanation: Frozen food will stay fresher longer and will taste better if excess air is eliminated before freezing. If you always "freeze fast and thaw slowly," give yourself 3 extra Kitchen IQ points.

My Plan to Increase My Kitchen's IQ (and Make My RealAge Younger)

7B. I will squeeze excess air out of the package before I freeze food items.

	Kitchen IQ Points
• I will always do this.	3
• I will do this one-third to two-thirds of the time.	2
• I will do this, but less than one-third of the time.	1
• I will never, or hardly ever, do this.	0

Possible additional points: 0 to 3   **Increased Tally*** [ ]

*In the Increased Tally box, write the result of subtracting the tally number in Question 7A from the circled number above. If you adopt the "freeze first and thaw slow" rule, give yourself an additional 3 points.

8A. When appropriate, do you "reduce" sauces in order to accentuate their flavor?

	Kitchen IQ Points
• Yes, often	3
• Occasionally	1
• Never, or hardly ever	0

Possible points: 0 to 3   **Tally** [   ]

Explanation: "Reducing" sauces (and soups) is a great way to increase flavor without having to change anything else.

My Plan to Increase My Kitchen's IQ (and Make My RealAge Younger)

8B. I will learn how to "reduce" sauces in order to accentuate their flavor.

	Kitchen IQ Points
• I will reduce sauces often.	3
• I will reduce sauces occasionally.	1
• I will probably never, or hardly ever, do this.	0

Possible additional points: 0 to 3   **Increased Tally*** [ ]

In the Increased Tally box, write the result of subtracting the tally number in Question 8A from the circled number above.

9A. Do you routinely buy fresh herbs and keep only herbs and spices in your kitchen that are less than six months old?

	Kitchen IQ Points
• I keep only fresh herbs or dried herbs and spices under six months old.	6
• I keep mostly fresh herbs or dried herbs and spices under six months old.	3
• I rarely discard herbs or spices, even if very old.	1
• I never buy fresh herbs or toss old ones.	0

Possible points: 0 to 6   **Tally**

Explanation: Fresh herbs and recently dried herbs and spices taste bright and clean. Dried herbs and spices lose a lot of their aroma and flavor by the time they are six months old.

My Plan to Increase My Kitchen's IQ (and Make My RealAge Younger)

9B. I will routinely buy fresh herbs and will keep only herbs and spices in my kitchen that are less than six months old.

	Kitchen IQ Points
• I will keep only fresh herbs or dried herbs and spices under six months old.	6
• I will keep mostly fresh herbs or dried herbs and spices under six months old.	3
• I will rarely discard dried herbs and spices, even if very old.	1
• I will almost never buy fresh herbs or spices or toss old ones.	0

Possible points: 0 to 6   **Increased Tally***

In the Increased Tally box, write the result of subtracting the tally number in Question 9A from the circled number above.

10A. Do you have seasonal fruit attractively displayed in your kitchen or other common areas in your home, or at the spot where you are most likely to be eating?

	Kitchen IQ Points
• Always, and mostly seasonal fruit	6
• One-third to two-thirds of the time, and usually seasonal fruit	3
• Less than one-third of the time	1
• Never	0

Possible points: 0 to 6   **Tally** [   ]

Explanation: Having nutritious food handy makes it more likely you will eat healthfully. The lengthening of the average life span in America has paralleled the availability of fresh fruit. Fresh fruit is rich in vitamins, fibers, carotenoids, flavonoids, and other phytonutrients. Remember to wash fruit well but to keep the peel on when you can. If you peel an apple or pear, you're tossing most of the fiber. You will make yourself over 3.7 years younger from just the fiber and flavonoids in fruit if you have four helpings a day.

My Plan to Increase My Kitchen's IQ (and Make My RealAge Younger)

10B. I will have seasonal fruit attractively displayed in my kitchen or other common areas in my home, or at the place I'm most like to be eating.

	Kitchen IQ Points
• I will almost always have seasonal fruit available.	6
• I will have seasonal fruit available one-third to two-thirds of the time.	3
• I will have seasonal fruit available less than one-third of the time.	1
• I will never, or hardly ever, have fruit available.	0

Possible additional points: 0 to 6   **Increased Tally*** [ ]

In the Increased Tally box, write the result of subtracting the tally number in Question 10A from the circled number above.

11A. Are your dining areas and the dishes you use "special"?

	Kitchen IQ Points
• Always	10
• One-third to two-thirds of the time	6
• Less than one-third of the time	3
• No, never, or hardly ever	0

Possible points: 0 to 10   **Tally** [ ]

Explanation: My most successful patients (and their families)—that is, those who have the youngest RealAges and who are happy with their weights—have a special place in their home that is the only place for eating. Not eating anyplace else—not the TV room, not standing up in front of the refrigerator—was, and is, their rule.

To make that place special, decorate it beautifully. Make it a great spot. Give it energy. For example, choose bright, colorful plates and accessories that cheer you up and bring a smile to your face. Even whimsical decorations can make the meal more enjoyable.

Also, avoid reading or watching television while you're eating. Mealtime is a great time to enjoy our friends and family, and an opportunity to give thanks for the happy parts of our lives. Savor the smell and sensation of the food, the visual delights of the food, the special dinnerware, the decor of the place where you eat, and the stimulating company of your eating companions. Make eating special. Those who make eating a time of joy for friends and family have a RealAge two to sixteen years younger.

My Plan to Increase My Kitchen's IQ (and Make My RealAge Younger)

11B. I will make my dining areas and the dishes I use "special."

	Kitchen IQ Points
• I will always do this.	10
• I will do this one-third to two-thirds of the time.	6
• I will do this less than one-third of the time.	3
• I will probably never, or hardly ever, do this.	0

Possible additional points: 0 to 10   **Increased Tally*** ☐

*In the Increased Tally box, write the result of subtracting the tally number in Question 11A from the circled number above.

12A. Do you routinely:

	Kitchen IQ Points
• Use juicy low-fat foods for moisturization?	If yes, + 1
• Eat unpeeled vegetables?	If yes, + 1
• Head home right after shopping at farmers' markets or with produce?	If yes, + 4
• Use herbs or vegetables you've grown yourself?	If yes, + 3
• Use fresh herbs and dried herbs and spices?	If yes, + 1

Possible additional points: 0 to 10   **Tally** ☐

Explanation: Using juicy low-fat foods to add or retain moisture in foods that can taste dry, gaining the fiber from washed but unpeeled vegetables, taking produce and other foods home before they can spoil in the trunk of a car, and using fresh herbs and dried spices help protect you from food borne illness, add great flavor, and make your RealAge younger. One Kitchen IQ point is awarded if you remember that "herbs are best fresh, spices are best dried"; give yourself another (extra) Kitchen IQ point if you use the rules "Fresh–Quick–Fresh" and "Dried–Slow–Dried," which mean that if your food is fresh and cooked only briefly, use fresh herbs. If your food started out as dried (from beans, for example) or is to cook for more than a few minutes, use dried herbs and spices.

My Plan to Increase My Kitchen's IQ (and Make My RealAge Younger)

12B. I will routinely:

	Kitchen IQ Points
• Use juicy low-fat foods for moisturization.	1
• Use unpeeled vegetables.	1
• Head home right after shopping at farmers' markets or with produce.	4
• Use herbs or vegetables I've grown myself.	3
• Use fresh herbs, and dried herbs and spices.	1

Possible additional points: 0 to 10   **Increased Tally***

In the Increased Tally box, write the result of subtracting the tally number in Question 12A from the circled number above.

13A. Do you frequently serve nuts, fish, tomato products, and whole grains?

	Kitchen IQ Points
• Yes, always	12
• At least one-third to two-thirds of the time	8
• Less than one-third of the time	2
• What? No red meat for the guests?	0

Possible points: 0 to 10   **Tally**

Explanation: Eating nuts five days a week for three years makes the RealAge of a typical woman 3.4 years younger and of a typical man 4.4 years younger. Eating fish three times a week makes a person 1.6 to 3.4 years younger, depending on age and gender. Eating ten servings of tomato products a week helps prevent prostate, breast, and up to ten other cancers. When eaten with a little oil, lycopene—the carotenoid found in tomatoes—provides an immune-strengthening antioxidant that seems to inhibit many cancers. The age benefit from tomatoes can be as much as 1.9 years younger for men and 1.1 years younger for women. In addition, lycopene, which is also found in watermelon, guava, and pink grapefruit, may make your arteries younger. Whole grains contain not only many vital nutrients that seem to inhibit both arterial and immune aging but also contain fiber. If you have 25 grams of fiber a day, your RealAge can be at least 2.4 years younger.

My Plan to Increase My Kitchen's IQ (and Make My RealAge Younger)

13B. I will frequently serve nuts, fish, tomato products, and whole grains.

	Kitchen IQ Points
• I will always serve these foods.	12
• At least one-third to two-thirds of the time	8
• Less than one-third of the time	2
• I will probably hardly ever serve these foods.	0

Possible points: 0 to 10   **Increased Tally*** ☐

*In the Increased Tally box, write the result of subtracting the tally number in Question 13A from the circled number above.

14A. Do you have a few favorite delicious dishes that are RealAge-smart that you commonly serve guests?

	Kitchen IQ Points
• I almost always do so.	10
• I do so one-third to two-thirds of the time.	7
• Yes, but less than one-third of the time.	2
• No, never. I save those recipes to cook for myself!	0

Possible points: 0 to 10   **Tally** ☐

Explanation: Having favorite RealAge-smart dishes to serve others means you will always have great-tasting, easy-to-prepare dishes that are stress-free for you and will make your RealAge younger.

My Plan to Increase My Kitchen's IQ (and Make My RealAge Younger)

14B. I will have a few favorite delicious dishes that are RealAge-smart to serve guests.

	Kitchen IQ Points
• I will always do this.	10
• I will do this one-third to two-thirds of the time.	7
• I will do this, but less than one-third of the time.	2
• I will probably never, or hardly ever, do this.	0

Possible additional points: 0 to 10   **Increased Tally*** ☐

*In the Increased Tally box, write the result of subtracting the tally number in Question 14A from the circled number above.

15A. When entertaining, do you prepare simple dishes rather than elaborate ones?

	Kitchen IQ Points
• Always	10
• One-third to two-thirds of the time	7
• Less than one-third of the time	2
• Never, or hardly ever. I'd be embarrassed.	0

Possible points: 0 to 10   **Tally** [   ]

Explanation: Making dishes that are simple, yet tasty and rich in nutrients, helps relieve the stress of entertaining.

My Plan to Increase My Kitchen's IQ (and Make My RealAge Younger)

15B. When entertaining, I will strive for simplicity rather than elaborateness.

	Kitchen IQ Points
• I will always do this.	10
• I will do this one-third to two-thirds of the time.	7
• I will do this, but less than one-third of the time.	2
• I will continue to prepare only elaborate dishes for guests.	0

Possible additional points: 0 to 10   **Increased Tally*** [   ]

In the Increased Tally box, write the result of subtracting the tally number in Question 15A from the circled number above.

16A. Do you enjoy one half hour of rest prior to your guests' arrival?

	Kitchen IQ Points
• Always	10
• I try to, at least one-third to two-thirds of the time.	7
• At best, one-third of the time	2
• You're kidding?	0

Possible points: 0 to 10   **Tally*** [   ]

*In the box, write the circled number.

Explanation: Anything that decreases stress and provides time to meditate and rest is highly beneficial to you, making your RealAge younger.

My Plan to Increase My Kitchen's IQ (and Make My RealAge Younger)

16B. I will enjoy one half hour of rest prior to my guests' arrival.

	Kitchen IQ Points
• I will always do this.	10
• I will do this one-third to two-thirds of the time.	7
• I will do this, at best, one-third of the time.	2
• I will never, or hardly ever, do this.	0

Possible points: 0 to 10   **Increased Tally*** [ ]

*In the Increased Tally box, write the result of subtracting the circled number above from the tally number in Question 16A.

17A. Do you feel *no* guilt when you serve RealAge-smart (healthy) food versus the expected aging dishes that contain saturated or trans fat?

	Kitchen IQ Points
• No, I don't feel any guilt.	10
• I feel a little guilty.	7
• My mom took "Jewish Guilt" training lessons. I always feel guilty.	2
• I always give my guests what they want, even if it will kill them.	0

Possible points: 0 to 10   **Tally** [   ]

Explanation: Your friends should want to eat healthy food, but you may feel guilty if you don't have something that is elaborate, expected, and fat ladden. Getting over that guilt and actually showing love for others by trying to extend their vibrant life will make your own RealAge (and theirs) substantially younger. Your guests will be around longer to share joy with you, too.

My Plan to Increase My Kitchen's IQ (and Make My RealAge Younger)

17B. I will feel *no* guilt when I serve RealAge-smart (healthy) food versus the expected dishes that contain saturated or trans fat.

	Kitchen IQ Points
• I will never feel guilty.	10
• I will feel a little guilty.	7
• I will always feel guilty.	2
• I will continue to give my guests what they want.	0

Possible points: 0 to 10   **Increased Tally*** [ ]

*In the Increased Tally box, write the result of subtracting the tally number in Question 17A from the circled number above.

18A. Do you eat a little "healthy" fat first at each meal?

	Kitchen IQ Points
• Always	10
• At least one-third to two-thirds of the time	7
• At best, one-third of the time, or not healthy fat	2
• What is "healthy" fat?	0

Possible points: 0 to 10   **Tally** [ ]

Explanation: Getting a little monounsaturated or polyunsaturated fat before or first in each meal will make you 1.8 years younger in three years. It might be easy to start dinner off with a few nuts, but what about breakfast? Be inventive. Try nut butter, freshly ground flax seed on your cereal, a granola cereal made with olive oil, or an omelet made with egg whites and a little olive oil.

My Plan to Increase My Kitchen's IQ (and Make My RealAge Younger)

18B. I will eat a little "healthy" fat first at each meal:

	Kitchen IQ Points
• I will always do this.	10
• I will do this one-third to two-thirds of the time.	7
• At best, I will do this one-third of the time.	2
• I'm probably not going to do this.	0

Possible additional points: 0 to 10   **Increased Tally*** [ ]

In the Increased Tally box, write the result of subtracting the tally number in Question 18A from the circled number above.

19A. Do you drink a glass of water between every serving (glass) of alcohol or wine?

	Kitchen IQ Points
• Always	4
• One-third to two-thirds of the time	2
• Not usually—at best, one-third of the time	1
• Never	0

Possible points: 0 to 4　　　　　　**Tally** [　　　　　]

Explanation: By alternating wine with water, you will tend to drink less wine. The right amount is one to two glasses a day for men and one glass for women. By drinking water, you will avoid excessive calories from alcohol and will get the benefits of drinking ample amounts of water. In addition, at cocktail parties try to keep one hand free: avoid having both hands full of food or drink because you are bound to eat more.

My Plan to Increase My Kitchen's IQ (and Make My RealAge Younger)

19B. I will drink a glass of water between every serving (glass) of alcohol or wine.

	Kitchen IQ Points
• I will always do this!	4
• I will do this one-third to two-thirds of the time.	2
• At best, I will do this one-third of the time.	1
• I will never, or hardly ever, do this.	0

Possible additional points: 0 to 4　　**Increased Tally*** [　]

*In the Increased Tally box, write the result of subtracting the tally number in Question 19A from the circled number above.

20A. Do you stop eating when you first start to feel full?

	Kitchen IQ Points
• Always	10
• One-third to two-thirds of the time	7
• What with all those starving kids in Ethiopia? At best, one-third of the time.	2
• I eat everything served.	0

Possible points: 0 to 10   **Tally** [   ]

Explanation: By continuing to eat after you first feel full, you stretch your stomach. That will eventually enlarge your stomach and allow you to consume progressively and gradually a little more at each meal. This enlargement would obviously be bad for the waistline, and will generally sap your energy later on. More important, however, eating more than you need undermines the desirable goal of keeping a constant low weight, which makes your RealAge over three years younger.

My Plan to Increase My Kitchen's IQ (and Make My RealAge Younger)

20B. I will stop eating when I first start to feel full.

	Kitchen IQ Points
• I will always try to do this.	10
• I will do this one-third to two-thirds of the time.	7
• I will do this, at best, one-third of the time.	2
• I will probably not do this.	0

Possible additional points: 0 to 10   **Increased Tally*** [   ]

*In the Increased Tally box, write the result of subtracting the tally number in Question 20A from the circled number above.

When Eating Out

21A. When dining out, do you ask your server about the way dishes are prepared? ("Does the soup contain cream?")

(If you eat out *fewer* than 5 times a week)	Kitchen IQ Points
• I always ask.	12
• I ask about one-third to two-thirds of the time.	9
• I ask, at best, one-third of the time.	3
• Yeah, right. The waiter would embarrass me if I did that!	0

Possible additional points: 0 to 12   **Tally** [   ]

(If you eat out *more* than 4 times a week)	Kitchen IQ Points
• I always ask.	24
• I ask about one-third to two-thirds of the time.	18
• I ask, at best, one-third of the time.	6
• Yeah, right. The waiter would embarrass me if I did that!	0

Possible points: 0 to 24   **Tally** [   ]

Explanation: If you eat out only once a year, these issues will not be a problem. However, most people are eating out more and more often. Therefore, the restaurant experience should be very much a part of your RealAge plan. You can enjoy your food, be satisfied, and still do your body some good. Why pay for food that will age you and sap your energy? The key is being the chief executive officer (CEO) every time you pay for food.

If you ask your server, "Can you ask the chef if it's possible to have my dish with marinara sauce instead of cream sauce?" the answer is usually yes. That's the key to eating out successfully: First ask questions about your food, and then ask if it can be prepared *your* (RealAge) way.

My Plan to Increase My Kitchen's IQ (and Make My RealAge Younger)

21B. When dining out, I will ask the server about the way dishes are prepared.

(If you eat out *fewer* than 5 times a week)	Kitchen IQ Points
• I will always do this.	12
• I will do this one-third to two-thirds of the time.	9
• At best, I will do this one-third of the time.	3
• I'll probably never, or hardly ever, ask.	0

Possible additional points: 0 to 12   **Increased Tally*** ☐

In the Increased Tally box, write the result of subtracting the tally number in Question 21A from the circled number above.

(If you eat out *more* than 4 times a week)	Kitchen IQ Points
• I will always do this.	24
• I will do this one-third to two-thirds of the time.	18
• At best, I will do this one-third of the time.	6
• I will probably never, or hardly ever, ask.	0

Possible additional points: 0 to 24   **Increased Tally*** ☐

In the Increased Tally box, write the result of subtracting tally number in Question 21A from the circled number above.

22A. When eating out, do you ask for olive oil or avocado as a substitute spread for butter or margarine?

	Kitchen IQ Points
• Always	6
• One-third to two-thirds of the time	4
• At best, one-third of the time	1
• Never!	0

Possible additional points: 0 to 6   **Tally** [   ]

Explanation: Even though it seems like a very small thing to ask for olive oil instead of butter or margarine for your bread, it is a significant step toward keeping your RealAge younger. Remember, healthy fats include those in olive oil, canola oil, nut butters, avocados, soy, flax seed, true chocolate, and fish. Although avocado is a great substitute spread for bread, crackers, or tortillas, consume all fats modestly, as all fats contain quite a few calories. You could also ask for sliced vegetables instead of bread. If you do so, give yourself 10 Kitchen IQ points (instead of 6) for this question.

My Plan to Increase My Kitchen's IQ (and Make My RealAge Younger)

22B. When eating out, I will ask for olive oil or avocado as a substitute spread for butter or margarine on bread.

	Kitchen IQ Points
• I will always do this.	6
• I will do this one-third to two-thirds of the time.	4
• At best, I will do this one-third of the time.	1
• I'll never do this.	0

Possible points: 0 to 6   **Increased Tally*** [   ]

*In the Increased Tally box, write the result of subtracting the tally number in Question 22A from the circled number above. If you ask for sliced vegetables instead of bread, give yourself 10 points minus the tally number from question 22A.

23A. When eating out, do you ask that your salad or other dressings be served on the side?

	Kitchen IQ Points
• Always	6
• One-third to two-thirds of the time	4
• At best, one-third of the time	1
• Never—the dressing is the best part!	0

Possible points: 0 to 6   **Tally** [   ]

Explanation: When researchers analyzed the diets of women 20 to 30 years of age, they found that more than half the calories of these women came from salad dressing consumed. Salad dressing is sneakily high in calories. A tablespoon often contains over 100 calories, and it isn't uncommon for restaurants to ladle 4 tablespoons or more (over 400 calories) onto a salad. Avoid this problem by asking for your salad dressing on the side, and then dip your fork into the dressing and then into the salad before each bite. So dip, spear, and enjoy.

My Plan to Increase My Kitchen's IQ (and Make My RealAge Younger)

23B. I will ask that my salad and other dressings be served on the side.

	Kitchen IQ Points
• I will always ask.	6
• I will ask one-third to two-thirds of the time.	4
• I will ask, at best, one-third of the time.	1
• I will probably never, or hardly ever, ask.	0

Possible additional points: 0 to 6   **Increased Tally*** [ ]

In the Increased Tally box, write the result of subtracting the tally number in Question 23A from the circled number above.

Your Kitchen Supplies

24A. Do you have the following items in your kitchen? (These will be discussed in Chapter 3.)

	Kitchen IQ Points
• A saucepan with a heavy bottom	2
• A pan with an unmarred nonstick surface	2
• Two heavy-bottomed cookie sheets or baking pans (1 point for each)	2
• A nonstick muffin pan that makes small muffins	1
• A heavyweight round pan for roasting and baking	1
• A heavyweight square or rectangular pan for roasting or baking	1
• A blender with a substantial motor	3
• An extra blender container	1
• A can opener	1
• Three colanders (small, medium, and large) (1 point for each size)	3
Tally	

Explanation: Although many kitchens have a bewildering array of implements and pots and pans accumulated over the years, only a few really make a huge difference in how well and how long you live. The key to a RealAge kitchen is to simplify by having only the equipment that allows you to cook in a way that makes food nutrient-rich, calorie-poor, and fabulously tasty. It's much easier to do this than you think. See Chapter 3 on how this equipment can make your RealAge younger.

My Plan to Increase My Kitchen's IQ (and Make My RealAge Younger)

24B. I will purchase the following items that I do not now have:

	Kitchen IQ Points
• A saucepan with a heavy bottom	2
• A pan with an unmarred nonstick surface	2
• Two heavy-bottomed cookie sheets or baking pans (1 point for each)	2
• A nonstick muffin pan that makes small muffins	1
• A heavyweight round pan for roasting and baking	1
• A heavyweight square or rectangular pan for roasting or baking	1
• A blender with a substantial motor	3
• An extra blender container	1
• A can opener	1
• Three colanders (small, medium, and large) (1 point for each size)	3

Increased Tally* ☐

*Possible Increased Tally: 0 to 17 points. Write the total of the circled numbers in the increased tally square.

24C. Do you have the following items?

	Kitchen IQ Points
• A Dutch oven	1
• A sauté pan	1
• A saucepan or pot	1
• An oven-safe skillet	1
• A stir-fry pan	1
• A corkscrew	1
• One cutting board for produce	1
• One cutting board for fish and meats (make the two cutting boards of different shape or color for an extra IQ point)	1
• A food chopper	2
• A food mill	1
• A food processor	2
• A garlic press	1
• A grater	1
• Kitchen shears	1
• A steel for sharpening knives	2

Tally [   ]

My Plan to Increase My Kitchen's IQ (and Make My RealAge Younger)

24D. I will purchase the following items that I do not now have:

	Kitchen IQ Points
• A Dutch oven	1
• A sauté pan	1
• A saucepan or pot	1
• An oven-safe skillet	1
• A stir-fry pan	1
• A corkscrew	1
• One cutting board for produce	
• One cutting board for fish and meats	1
(make the two cutting boards of different	
shapes or colors for an extra IQ point)	1
• A food chopper	2
• A food mill	1
• A food processor	2
• A garlic press	1
• A grater	1
• Kitchen shears	1
• A steel for sharpening knives	2
Increased Tally*	☐

Possible Increased Tally: 0 to 18 points. Write the total of the circled numbers in the Increased Tally square.

24E. Do you have the following items?

	Kitchen IQ Points
• A chef's knife	1
• A paring knife	1
• A serrated knife	1
• A butcher's block or wall rack for knife storage	1
• A small (4-ounce) stainless steel ladle	1
• A set of glass measuring cups	1
• A set of plastic measuring cups	1
• A set of measuring spoons	1
• A meat thermometer	1
• A mixer	1
• A 2-quart stainless steel or glass mixing bowl	1
• A 4-quart stainless steel or glass mixing bowl	1
• A 6-quart stainless steel or glass mixing bowl	1
• Six wooden mixing spoons ($\frac{1}{2}$ point each)	3
• A roll of parchment paper	1
• A pepper mill	1
• Clean-up tools, including 6 or more white kitchen cloths (no sponges please) and a pump bottle of hand soap	2
Tally	

My Plan to Increase My Kitchen's IQ (and Make My RealAge Younger)

24F. I will purchase the following items that I do not now have:

	Kitchen IQ Points
• A chef's knife	1
• A paring knife	1
• A serrated knife	1
• A butcher's block or wall rack for knife storage	1
• A small (4-ounce) stainless steel ladle	1
• A set of glass measuring cups	1
• A set of plastic measuring cups	1
• A set of measuring spoons	1
• A meat thermometer	1
• A mixer	1
• A 2-quart stainless steel or glass mixing bowl	1
• A 4-quart stainless steel or glass mixing bowl	1
• A 6-quart stainless steel or glass mixing bowl	1
• Six wooden mixing spoons (½ point each)	3
• A roll of parchment paper	1
• A pepper mill	1
• Clean-up tools, including 6 or more white kitchen cloths (no sponges please) and a pump bottle of hand soap	2

Increased Tally* ☐

*Possible Increased Tally: 0 to 20 points. In the Increased Tally square write the sum of the circled numbers.

24G. Do you have the following items?

	Kitchen IQ Points
• A potato masher	1
• A rice cooker and steamer	1
• Three salad spinners (1 point for each)	3
• A small spatula	1
• A large spatula	1
• A pancake turner	1
• Two pairs of tongs	4
• A vegetable peeler and corer	1
• A wire whisk	1
• A zester	1
• A gas stovetop	4
• An electric oven	3
• A nonstick stovetop grill	2
• Four hot mitts	2
• Two heavy trivets	2
• A freezer, clear containers, and marking pen	5

Tally [ ]

My Plan to Increase My Kitchen's IQ (and Make My RealAge Younger)

24H. I will purchase the following items that I do not now have:

	Kitchen IQ Points
• A potato masher	1
• A rice cooker and steamer	1
• Three salad spinners (1 point for each)	3
• A small spatula	1
• A large spatula	1
• A pancake turner	1
• Two pairs of tongs	4
• A vegetable peeler and corer	1
• A wire whisk	1
• A zester	1
• A gas stovetop	4
• An electric oven	3
• A nonstick stovetop grill	2
• Four hot mitts	2
• Two heavy trivets	2
• A freezer, clear containers, and marking pen	5

Increased Tally* ☐

*Possible Increased Tally: 0 to 33 points. In the Increased Tally square write the sum of the circled numbers.

25A. Do you have any of these specific food items in your pantry? Give yourself ⅓ point for each of the following:

- Applesauce
- Arrowroot
- Artichoke hearts
- Baking powder
- Baking soda
- Broth or stock
- Brown rice
- Canned fish (give yourself credit for up to three varieties)
- Capers
- Chiles
- Chili (vegetarian)
- Cooking oil spray
- Cornmeal
- Couscous (whole wheat) or bulgur
- Dijon mustard
- Dried cereal (whole grain)
- Dried fruit (give yourself credit for up to three varieties)
- Dried or canned beans and legumes (give yourself credit for up to two varieties)
- Evaporated nonfat skim milk
- Flour (whole grain)
- Garlic
- Ginger
- Healthy oils
- Herbs and herb blends (give yourself up to 3 points [total-adding up the ⅓ points for each as for all other items in this question] for the first nine of these in your pantry)
- Honey

- Hot pepper sauce
- Instant coffee
- Ketchup
- Nut and seed butters
- Nuts
- Olives
- Onions
- Pasta (whole-grain)
- Pepper
- Potatoes
- Salsa
- Salt
- Soy sauce
- Spices and spice blends (give yourself credit for up to six varieties)
- Sun-dried tomatoes
- Sweet potatoes
- Tea (give yourself credit for up to three varieties)
- Tofu
- Tomato paste
- Tomatoes (canned)
- Tortillas (corn)
- Vanilla extract, pure
- Vinegar (give yourself credit for up to six varieties)
- Whole-grain crackers
- Whole grains (give yourself credit for up to three varieties)
- Wine (give yourself credit for up to six varieties)
- Worcestershire sauce
- Give yourself $\frac{1}{3}$ point (with exceptions specified) for each of the above items you have in your pantry.

Possible points: 0 to 28   **Tally** [   ]

Explanation: The RealAge pantry principle is that *easy availability begets eating*. If you don't keep bad food choices on hand, you won't be tempted to eat them. How you stock your pantry makes all the difference to your RealAge. The best way to make your kitchen RealAge-smarter is to stock your pantry with foods that will make your arteries and immune system younger and more vibrant. Here's a key corollary to the RealAge pantry principle: *The first appealing thing you see is the first thing you'll eat.* So, make the first appealing thing you see in your pantry a great-tasting healthy food. With a well-stocked RealAge pantry, you will always have a giant menu of delicious and healthy possibilities right at hand. Just keeping your pantry stocked with healthy items can make your RealAge as much as 2.8 years younger.

My Plan to Increase My Kitchen's IQ (and Make My RealAge Younger)

25B. I will purchase the following items that I do not now have in my pantry. (Give yourself ⅓ point for each of the following):

- Applesauce
- Arrowroot
- Artichoke hearts
- Baking powder
- Baking soda
- Broth or stock
- Brown rice
- Canned fish (give yourself credit for up to three varieties)
- Capers
- Chiles
- Chili (vegetarian)
- Cooking oil spray
- Cornmeal
- Couscous (whole wheat) or bulgur
- Dijon mustard
- Dried cereal (whole grain)
- Dried fruit (give yourself credit for up to three varieties)

- Dried or canned beans and legumes (give yourself credit for up to two varieties)
- Evaporated nonfat skim milk
- Flour (whole grain)
- Garlic
- Ginger
- Healthy oils
- Herbs and herb blends (give yourself up to 3 points [total-adding up the $1/3$ points for each as for all other items in this question] for the first nine of these in your pantry)
- Honey
- Hot pepper sauce
- Instant coffee
- Ketchup
- Nut and seed butters
- Nuts
- Olives
- Onions
- Pasta (whole-grain)
- Pepper
- Potatoes
- Salsa
- Salt
- Soy sauce
- Spices and spice blends (give yourself credit for up to six varieties)
- Sun-dried tomatoes
- Sweet potatoes
- Tea (give yourself credit for up to three varieties)
- Tofu
- Tomato paste
- Tomatoes (canned)
- Tortillas (corn)
- Vanilla extract, pure

- Vinegar (give yourself credit for up to six varieties)
- Whole-grain crackers
- Whole grains (give yourself credit for up to three varieties)
- Wine (give yourself credit for up to six varieties)
- Worcestershire sauce

Give yourself ⅓ point (with exceptions specified)

for each of the above items you will purchase.

Possible points: 0 to 28 **Increased Tally***

26A. Do you eat breakfast?

Kitchen IQ Points

Give yourself 3 points for each time you eat

breakfast a week. 0–21

Tally

Explanation: No one is sure how it does it, but consistent studies show that eating breakfast makes your RealAge younger. For the typical man or woman, the RealAge benefit is 1.4 years younger.

My Plan to Increase My Kitchen's IQ (and Make My RealAge Younger)

26B. I will eat breakfast.

Kitchen IQ Points

Give yourself 3 points for each additional time

(additional to what you do now) you plan to

eat breakfast a week. 0–21

Increased Tally*

In the Increased Tally box, write the result of subtracting the tally number in Question 26A from the circled number above.

Develop Your Kitchen of Youth

1. Find Your Current Kitchen's IQ

Add up all your IQ points—that is, your current kitchen's IQ. The higher the number, the more likely those kitchen smarts have helped you control your genes and make your RealAge younger. Add all the numbers in the Tally boxes. (These are the rectangular boxes.)

This number is your current kitchen's IQ:

The higher your current kitchen's IQ and the higher your future kitchen's IQ, the more likely your kitchen and the changes you are going to make have been and will help you make your RealAge younger. As a rough estimate, divide your current kitchen's IQ by 10 and then subtract 10 to find out how much younger your kitchen as it is now is likely to make you. For example, if your kitchen's IQ is 200, then divide 200 by 10, which produces 20, and subtract 10, which produces 10. Your kitchen is likely to make you 10 years younger!

Once you have calculated your current kitchen's IQ, how should you interpret the results? It's as easy to understand as weighing bananas on the grocery store scale. If your current kitchen's IQ is higher than 150, you are taking steps to protect your youth, and you are aging more slowly than most of your peers. See what you can do to make your RealAge even younger.

If your current kitchen's IQ is below 100, the news is not so good. You are aging faster than most of your peers. But do not be disheartened. Instead, be proactive. Now that you know what your kitchen's IQ is, what will you do to get younger? Consider what choices you can make to reduce your risk. You have the opportunity to slow your rate of aging, bring yourself back in line with your peers, and even become younger.

2. Find the Amount You Will Increase Your Kitchen's IQ

Add all the numbers in the Increased Tally boxes. (These are the square boxes.)

*This number is the amount you will increase
your kitchen's IQ, your Increased Tally number:*

3. Find Your Future Kitchen's IQ

*Add both the total Tally number and the total
Increased Tally number together.*

Your future kitchen's IQ:

How to Use the Kitchen IQ Concept

I use the Kitchen IQ concept in my medical practice. In questioning my patients, I am trying to determine their genetic and behavior-related risks. These are the same kinds of questions used to determine RealAge in the first book and on the RealAge Web site. The answers to these questions help reveal whether my patients (and you!) are more likely to develop conditions such as heart problems or prostate or breast cancer. Then, the patient and I design a plan to prevent those specific problems. The degree of aggressiveness of the plan, and of my efforts to bring about the desired results, depends on how great the patient's current risk factors are—that is, what that patient's present RealAge is.

For example, if the patient's RealAge is old because of a strong family history of arterial aging (stroke and heart disease), symptoms related to arterial aging (occasional impotence), a borderline aging blood pressure (130/85 mmHg. as opposed to the optimal of 115/75 mmHg.), an elevated level of bad (LDL) cholesterol (160 mg/dl versus the ideal for aging, less than 100 mg/dl), a low level of healthy (HDL) cholesterol (32 mg/dl versus the ideal of 55 mg/dl or higher), lack of regular physical activity, and aging dietary habits, I am likely to recommend immediate changes in diet and physical activity, with follow-up (reminders) daily and assessments in two months. At that time, if blood pressure is not optimal and significant changes in weight and cholesterol levels have not occurred, I add one or two medications directed at lowering blood pressure and lipid levels. This regimen is more aggressive than the gradual program that would be used for someone with no genetic predispositions and normal levels of healthy cholesterol—a program of dietary changes and physical activity that we (the patient and I) might agree on as a six-month trial period before I prescribe medications.

So, the more habits and genetic predispositions a patient has that make his or her RealAge older, the harder I push for early changes in diet and activity. Note that although management of bad cholesterol is important, it may have, at maximum, a three- or four-year effect on RealAge. In contrast, at maximum, there's a nine-year effect for regular physical activity, a twenty-five-year effect for low blood pressure, a twenty-seven-year effect for healthy dietary habits, and a thirty-two-year effect for stress reduction. So, if you think you can just take drugs like Pravachol (pravastatin), Zocor (simvastatin), or Lipitor (atorvastatin) alone to lower your risk and make your RealAge younger, you are only partially correct. These "statin" drugs represent some of the greatest advances in the treatment of arterial aging in the last decade, but they are not cure-alls. For most of us, changes in diet, stress management, and physical activity are the primary ways of keeping your arteries young and preventing heart disease, strokes, memory loss, impotence, and wrinkling of the skin.

You can use your Kitchen IQ similarly. If you have a large family history of arterial aging diseases (heart attack, heart failure, strokes, memory loss, etc.) or cancer in your family, and have a low Kitchen IQ, you should be even more motivated to try a few things that will increase your kitchen's IQ. And after you've begun to discover how easy and delicious such changes are, add more! That way you'll increase your Kitchen IQ, make your RealAge younger, and begin to enjoy more vitality. How long will it take to feel better, much better? Fewer than ninety days say Steve, Nancy, and a large number of other patients. Try it; you may like the vigor, and you'll certainly like the food. Stocking your pantry is a great place to start.

3

The Well-Stocked RealAge Kitchen

A gleaming, shiny store full of kitchen equipment can be an intimidating maze that causes stress and aging. Sometimes the equipment prices make you swoon. There are hundreds of gadgets, from garlic roasters to nutmeg graters. How do you choose? You choose the ones that make your kitchen's IQ higher and you younger.

This chapter describes the equipment you'll need to cook in the simplest and most effective way. Your kitchenware should make cooking easier and more fun. If you have great equipment and the right tools to make your RealAge younger, and the better stocked your kitchen is, the more apt you'll be to cook well.

Pots, Pans, and Basic Tools

The first step is to evaluate what you have. Pull out all the pots and pans you now have and spread them in front of you. Give each the quality test. Does the saucepan have a heavy bottom? *(2 Kitchen IQ points).* Are all of your nonstick surfaces free of scratches and gouges *(2 Kitchen IQ points)*? These questions imply what I have found true: there is a connection between the quality of equipment and your ability to prepare healthy food easily and without stress. The better your kitchen is stocked, the higher its IQ and the younger your RealAge is likely to be.

Our advice is to invest in high-quality, easy-to-use basic tools. They'll make your time in the kitchen easier, more productive, and more fun. Pick each item carefully. If you're interested in a set of pots or knives, try one out before buying the whole set. A little hands-on experience with a product can show you right away what's right and what's wrong with it. Keep the heaviest and largest pans; you'll probably use these the most. No pot over 6 quarts? Not a problem. You won't need one that's larger than that, although you can put larger ones to use.

Get rid of the very smallest pots and pans; you're probably not going to need them. Donate them to a charity, hold a garage sale, or give them away, but whatever you do, clear them out! Giving things away makes it seem like you have to spend money to replace them, but this is not so. The goal is to simplify so you will be less stressed by crowded space and less likely to have equipment that encourages aging food choices. Living within your means does make your RealAge younger. So put the items you are missing on a wish list for when you can afford to buy them. But do not keep a deep-fryer around, no matter what, as it is aging!

Do the same thing for your kitchen utensils and small appliances. Chances are, you'll find items you'd forgotten all about and don't really need. You can never go wrong investing in good tools that you'll use frequently and that will save you tremendous amounts of time, such as a great chef's knife and a good blender. Here's the basic equipment you'll need to stock a RealAge kitchen.

The Basic Equipment for a RealAge Kitchen

(The Kitchen IQ points listed here are included in the test and calculations of your kitchen's IQ in Chapter 2.)

Equipment	Description and Use
Baking pans (5 points)	➤ Every kitchen needs at least two heavy-bottomed sheet pans (sometimes called jelly-roll pans) (2 points). Opt for the nonstick ones, or buy a roll of parchment paper. The nonstick pans allow less fat to be used, meaning all the fat that is used (healthy fat!) can contribute to taste. A muffin pan is also a necessity. Get a heavy one that makes small muffins and has a nonstick surface (1 point). Then add heavyweight round, square, and rectangular pans for roasting and baking (2 points). Don't bother with cookie sheets (too thin), angel food cake pans (too specialized), or thin aluminum molds (too fragile).
Blender (4 points)	➤ Most kitchens are not complete without a blender. They're great for making breakfast smoothies, creating salsas, and smoothing out sauces. Fruit smoothies, tomato-based dips, and healthy sauces help make food fun, tasty, and RealAge-smart. Buy a blender that has a substantial motor, a large container (44 ounces or more, preferably glass), just a few buttons, and a warranty of at least one year, as they tend to burn out with heavy use (3 points). If you can find one with a graduated dial instead of buttons, buy it—you'll have more control. Get an extra blender container, if you can, just to have on hand (1 point). Not having the hassle of replacing one after it breaks helps keep your RealAge younger.
Can opener (1 point)	➤ Even the most sophisticated chef needs a can opener. Although can openers come in many varieties, a manual one is suitable for most needs. Buy one that has an easy grip.

Equipment	Description and Use
Colanders and strainers (3 points)	➤ A colander is a necessity for every kitchen. Use it to wash foods and to drain pasta and vegetables. Colanders and strainers are so useful, we suggest you have three sizes: small, medium, and large (1 point for each size). Having extra colanders handy to facilitate washing of food is a great way to foster food safety and a younger RealAge. A large basket-sized colander that has a fine mesh and a handle is great when you need to wash vegetables or if you want to press large quantities of sauce through a strainer.
Cookware (7 points)	➤ Cookware comes in a bewildering array of materials, sizes, weights, durabilities, and heat conductivities. There are endless combinations of sets, frequent sales, and various warranties. Buy one piece before purchasing an entire set; it's important to get an item you will use. Larger is better. If you can afford only one piece at a time, start with a high-quality, 6-quart Dutch oven that is heavy-bottomed, 18/10 stainless steel, and dishwasher-safe. Stainless steel is easy to clean and doesn't flake off. It's usually combined with other metals to improve heat conduction. Heavy cast aluminum (not thin, plain, rolled aluminum) is also a good choice: It's easy to clean and reasonably priced. In addition to a Dutch oven (1 point), you'll need these basic pans: a sauté pan (1 point), a saucepan (2 points), a sauce pot (1 point), a stockpot (1 point), and an oven-safe skillet (1 point). A stir-fry pan also comes in handy (1 point). In general, larger is better. (Although nonstick cookware lets you cook with less fat and sticking, cookware that doesn't have a nonstick surface seems to get hotter and, for many foods, produces a better crust.)
Corkscrew (1 point)	➤ Because wine is good to drink and cook with, you need a corkscrew. There are many varieties of corkscrews. Although we like a simple one that looks like a *T,* it requires a bit of strength to remove the cork. Another type of corkscrew slips between the cork and the bottle and is favored by many connoisseurs because it seldom leaves bits of cork in the wine. Another type, the winged corkscrew,

The Well-Stocked RealAge Kitchen

65

Equipment	Description and Use

has two arms that rise as you screw down the device; this requires less strength and experience to extract the cork—its wings just fold down.

**Cutting boards
(2 points)**

➤ No kitchen is complete without cutting boards. You'll need at least two. Food safety is a primary concern with cutting boards, so two—one for produce, and one for meat, poultry, and fish—are necessary to gain any Kitchen IQ points and make your RealAge younger. A high-quality, polyethylene (plastic) cutting board is best. (Glass and marble boards are more decorative than practical for most people.) Look for the NSF (National Safety Foundation) label. Polyethylene boards usually have a slightly rough surface that prevents foods from slipping when cut. Plastic is more sanitary than wood because it's dishwasher-safe. (Do wash your plastic boards in the dishwasher frequently.) Plastic also resists warping. Wood boards are porous and tend to crack and harbor bacteria. They cannot be put in the dishwasher, so they have to be cleaned with bleach and water, a solution that is potentially toxic. If you choose a glass board, select one that can withstand microwaving.

Popular sizes include 8 × 12-inch and 12 × 18-inch. To avoid cross-contamination, remember to use only one board for produce and another only for fish and meats. Grooved edges help keep juices from running onto the counter, but they are not really necessary and decrease the amount of usable surface area; we don't recommend them. Here's a RealAge kitchen tip: Place a damp dishtowel on the counter under your board. The dishtowel will keep the board from slipping as you cut, slice, and dice.

**Food chopper
(2 points)**

➤ This quick and easy tool saves time when you don't want to use a knife or clean your food processor. It's especially good for chopping small amounts of dense foods, such as nuts, seeds, and root vegetables. The food chopper is a plastic (or sometimes glass) cylinder that contains a plunger equipped with a small rotating blade. The finer the chopping, often the more intense the flavor. Buy the most durable unit you can find; it's going to take a lot of abuse.

Equipment	Description and Use
Food mill (1 point)	➤ A food mill is used to purée and strain fruits and vegetables; it separates the meat of the food from the skin and seeds. Large food mills (those having 2- or 3-quart baskets) are great for making jams, jellies, and preserves. Buying one that's easy to clean and dishwasher safe will make your RealAge even younger.
Food processor (2 points)	➤ The food processor goes beyond just chopping. It purées, shreds, grates, dices, kneads, slices, and juliennes. Food processors are great for chopping herbs, grating blocks of cheese, and chopping vegetables. The smaller models are used mostly for chopping and mincing. Choose a size appropriate for your needs. Also, remember: processing can quickly produce a purée, so watch as you do this!
Garlic press (1 point)	➤ Garlic makes your RealAge younger by reducing arterial and immune aging. If you want a garlic press, we recommend one that has large holes and doesn't require that you peel the cloves. Make sure the press is easy to clean. Some presses can be used to crush peeled ginger: all of them leave a little of the flavor and oil behind.
Grater (1 point)	➤ The classic four-sided stainless-steel box helps you make vegetables and fruits, not to mention chocolate, more enjoyable, allowing you to gain intense flavor from just a little cheese (a key to keeping your saturated fat intake to less than 20 grams a day). Specialty graters are also fun—for example, those small, handheld gadgets you operate by turning a handle or a rasp (from a hardware or specialty cooking store) for zesting. These work well on hard cheeses, nuts, and whole nutmegs. Another specialty grater, the mandolin, has adjustable blades and teeth for creating slices and shreds of all kinds. It's ideal for slicing, shredding, and julienning large quantities of vegetables. We recommend steel graters, not plastic ones. Whatever grater you purchase, it should have teeth of different sizes. Small, closely set teeth are good for grating fruits, vegetables, chocolate, and cheeses. Tiny teeth are necessary for zesting citrus fruit and grating whole nutmegs. Some graters have interchangeable blades that store in the unit.

Equipment	Description and Use
Kitchen shears **(1 point)**	➤ Anything that decreases the frustration of opening difficult packages raises your Kitchen IQ. Kitchen shears can be used for general cutting chores and for cutting through food. Kitchen shears have other uses as well: the notched inside edge is used for cutting poultry bones, and the curved, notched inner handle can be used to open jars. You can find shears in stainless steel or chrome-plated carbon. Make sure they're on the large side. We like 8-inch stainless-steel shears (with 4-inch blades) that have coated handles that make them easier to hold.
Knife sharpeners **and steels** **(2 points)**	➤ There's nothing more dangerous than a dull knife. Dull knives can slip and injure you, the cook. If you need to exert a lot of pressure on the knife to cut or slice, your blade should be sharpened. Unfortunately, few knife sharpeners are truly useful. Most act as sharpening stones, but we recommend instead that you have your hardware store sharpen your knife. In contrast, a steel (usually a fluted round rod that has a handle) is quite useful. It's not intended for extremely dull knives. Steels are used to true (straighten) the edges of all kinds of knives except serrated knives, which should never be sharpened or straightened. Buy a steel that is harder and a little longer than your knife. It's very handy to buy a knife and a steel together, from the same maker.
Knives and **their protectors** **(4 points)**	➤ Here's a RealAge kitchen tip: Buy the best knives you can afford! Using high-quality makes cooking easier. You'll use your knives every day, so don't skimp. Shop around before you purchase and make sure each knife feels comfortable and balanced in your hand. There are only a few that you absolutely must have: a great quality chef's knife (1 point), a paring knife (1 point), and a serrated knife (1 point). Select a chef's knife that's a little smaller than you think you need: shorter knives are easier to use than longer ones. Plastic handles are just fine; if left in water, wooden handles can crack. Unsheathed knives should not be stored in drawers with other knives, as contact with each other can dull the blades. Also, knives can be dangerous to pick up in such a setting. You can store your

Equipment	Description and Use
	knives in a butcher block or wall rack (1 point), or on a magnetic holder. Knives should not be washed in the dishwasher. That process dulls and nicks the blades.
Ladles (1 point)	➤ Many soups are RealAge-friendly, so having a way of serving them and of adding liquids to other dishes makes your kitchen smarter. Select a ladle that is made from one piece of dishwasher-safe stainless steel. A contoured grip that has a hole in it makes it easy to hold and store the ladle. Start with a 4-ounce ladle and move up from there.
Measuring cups (2 points)	➤ You'll need different measuring cups for dry and liquid ingredients. Glass is typically used for liquid measurements, and plastic or metal is used for dry ingredients. Buy a set with 1-, 2-, and 4-cup capacities. A useful feature on liquid measuring cups is a spout for easy pouring.
	Dry measuring cups are commonly available in sets of $1/4$, $1/3$, $1/2$, and 1 cup. Although a 2-cup measure is also available, the 1-cup set is sufficient. Dry measuring cups have a flat top so you can level off ingredients with a knife. There are also adjustable measuring cups that can be used for dry ingredients only. The sides of the measuring cup are marked with the different measurements. These are convenient because they save storage space.
Measuring spoons (1 point)	➤ I prefer metal sets to plastic sets. Both should be kept away from heat. Most sets are banded together at the handle so that they are easy to locate in your drawer, or can be hung on a hook. Adjustable measuring spoons are available, but we've found that these work well only with dry ingredients, not liquid ingredients.
Meat thermometer (1 point)	➤ A meat thermometer provides an instant read of the internal temperature of meat or poultry, letting you know the meat has reached the temperature necessary to kill harmful bacteria. Many thermometers have a scale on the face indicating what the internal temperature should be for a variety of foods. Digital thermometers are usually as accurate as the face thermometers.

Equipment	Description and Use
Mixer (1 point)	➤ Basic handheld mixers are used to combine and cream ingredients, and to aerate liquids. The more advanced stand mixers have attachments that knead dough and grind meats. Stand mixers are convenient because you can step away from the mixing process and work on something else. A stand mixer is a good investment in your kitchen.
Mixing bowls (4 points)	➤ Purchase bowls in small, medium, and large sizes: two of each, preferably 2-, 4-, 6- and 12-quart capacities. We prefer stainless steel mixing bowls because they don't break or react with food. Plastic bowls are not as durable, and warp easily. Some glass bowls are oven-safe and can be used for baking, but the larger ones are heavy and difficult to work with. The smaller glass bowls are great for serving and storage.
Mixing spoons (3 points)	➤ You'll need at least six wooden spoons of various sizes. Wooden spoons are preferable because they don't conduct heat and won't burn your hands. Also, they won't scratch nonstick surfaces. Wooden spoons are very inexpensive, so you can afford a variety of sizes. A slotted spoon, preferably of steel, is also useful. (If you have nonstick pans, such as those made of hard anodized aluminum—for example, Calphalon—you can use plastic or wooden spoons.)
Parchment paper (1 point)	➤ Keep a roll of parchment paper in your cabinet so you can provide cake pans and cookie sheets with a nonstick, easy-release surface. There's no added fat to your foods, and the cleanup is easy. The disadvantage of using parchment paper is that making the pan liners can be tedious if you're very precise or in a hurry. However, parchment paper can be used in baking, steaming, and roasting. It can also be rolled up to make a cone, filled with icing or mashed potatoes (among other things), and used to decorate cakes and various food dishes.
Pepper mill (1 point)	➤ All food that is RealAge-smart has to have great flavor; and freshly ground pepper can add great flavor. Get rid of all ground pepper and replace with a pepper mill and whole peppercorns. (Commercially ground pepper loses its flavor and aroma almost immediately after

Equipment	Description and Use
	the peppercorns are crushed. You'll get a lot more "bang" if you grind your pepper as needed.) Look for a mill that is small (so the peppercorns will be fresh), has an adjustable grind, and is easy to clean.
Potato masher (1 point)	➤ The long, slender shape of this utensil makes it easy to use in any bowl or pot. A masher makes mashed foods light and fluffy. It also does a good job of mashing other ingredients, such as beans for refried beans, bananas for banana bread, and sweet potatoes for sweet potato pie. Look for a masher that is sturdy, has a plastic handle, and is dishwasher-safe.
Rice cooker and steamer (1 point)	➤ This piece of equipment has gained popularity as Americans have discovered the flavor of rice and moved toward more whole grain in their diet. Rice cookers/steamers help cut calories and fat without destroying flavor and nutrients, making you (and all you share food with) younger. The steamer is also ideal for fish and vegetables. A built-in timer allows you to step out of the kitchen without overcooking the food. Look for cookers that can be easily cleaned and that can make a large quantity.
Salad spinner (3 points)	➤ Cleaning greens and herbs has never been easier. Wash the greens, place them in a salad spinner, and spin the water and debris off the greens, leaving them clean and crisp. Purchasing and preparing greens yourself may take a little more time than buying prepared salads from the store, but it's less expensive, the quality is under your control, and there are no additives. The salad spinner doubles as a storage container for greens in your refrigerator. If you can afford it, consider buying three: one for washing, one for rinsing, and one for all other uses. Consider this tool one of the most important and use it to clean vegetables and fruit as well as salad greens.
Scrapers and turners (spatulas) (3 points)	➤ You should have at least one small and one large scraper in your kitchen. Small scrapers work well to scrape food out of jars and cans. Large scrapers help scrape ingredients off the sides of bowls, pots, and pans. Look for heat-resistant scrapers—they're perfect when making sauces, puddings, and soups.

Equipment	Description and Use
	The turner has been referred to as a type of spatula, but they are two different tools. A turner usually has a wooden handle and a flat metal head that is bent where the metal meets the handle. A turner is useful for flipping foods, such as pancakes, French toast, and egg white omelets. You also need a turner for removing cookies and baked goods from sheet pans.
Tongs **(2 points)**	➤ If we could choose only one hand tool (excluding knives) in the kitchen, this would be it—that's why they make your kitchen 2 IQ points smarter. Tongs are perfect for grilling and turning foods, mixing, scraping, and gently inspecting the bottom of a halibut steak or portobello mushroom. Choose tongs that are strong, heavy, and durable. Stainless-steel tongs are superior to chromed steel tongs. Have two tongs; sometimes a pair is in the dishwasher, and sometimes you have several dishes going at once. You'll keep your RealAge younger with tongs that are about 10 inches long—just enough to keep you away from the heat. Longer tongs (about 18 inches) work well for outside grilling and help keep you a good distance from the surface.
Vegetable peeler and corer **(1 point)**	➤ The vegetable peeler and corer is an inexpensive but essential tool. It's great for peeling vegetables or for making chocolate curls from blocks of solid chocolate (use dark chocolate—only from cocoa—as that is a healthy fat that makes your RealAge younger). The curls give you the intense flavor and delight of chocolate with fewer fat calories, so it increases your Kitchen IQ. Buy one that has an easy grip, is dishwasher-safe, and is easy to use. Also, having a swivel head makes a peeler easier to handle.
Whisks **(1 point)**	➤ A whisk is very handy in a RealAge kitchen. A sauce whisk is the most common. Look for one that has lots of wires (at least 16) and a sturdy handle you can hold like a pencil. The joint where the handle meets the wires should be sealed with silicone to prevent food from getting caught, and decrease the risk of infection. We recommend stainless-steel whisks rather than plastic or plastic-

Equipment	Description and Use
	coated ones. Although plastic whisks have the advantage of not scratching nonstick cookware, they can put particles of plastic in your food. Your whisk should be dishwasher-safe.
Zester **(1 point)**	➤ We find a good zester infinitely useful in the RealAge kitchen. It can produce thin strips of citrus, curls of cucumber peel, or a squiggle of chocolate. Zest can be used in muffins and quickbreads and on top of fish. You can also zest carrots and radishes and use the colorful flavor on top of salads and as a garnish. Some zesters come with a scoring edge for decorating fruits and vegetables. Score citrus fruits and use the strips in drinks or tie the strips in knots or a bow for garnish.

A Word About Cast-Iron Cookware

Cast iron is terrific to cook with, but adds iron to the food (if the food is acidic), and extra iron makes your RealAge older. Because iron is stored in the body for long periods, over time, excess iron ingestion can lead to toxic levels of the mineral. Even a slightly elevated level of iron can be harmful. Early signs of iron overload are abdominal pain, fatigue, and loss of sex drive. Later symptoms include liver enlargement, diabetes, arthritis, and in severe cases, abnormal heartbeats and heart failure. Although the evidence is preliminary, it's cause for concern.

There are two ways that excess iron can lead to accelerated aging. First, excess iron may harm the arteries. One theory is that iron oxidizes bad (LDL) cholesterol (causes it to combine with oxygen), and the resulting *oxidized* cholesterol accumulates in arterial plaques in the lining of vessel walls. One Finnish study supports this theory. The study showed that the rate of heart attacks doubled when the concentration of iron in the blood was high. The risk quadrupled when this high iron level was coupled with high levels of bad cholesterol. Some data even suggest that donating blood regularly, and thus decreasing your iron, may result in a longer, healthier life. Giving blood also makes many people feel good (by doing good for others), so perhaps some of the RealAge benefit comes from that regardless of the iron-reducing benefit from blood donation.

The second way that excess iron accelerates aging involves, once again, its role as an oxidant. Acting as an oxidant, iron may increase the quantity of free radicals in the body. These free radicals cause DNA damage that can lead to cancer. Another theory is that cancer cells, which proliferate quickly, require more iron, so that having excess iron may actually stimulate cancer cell growth. Although neither of these theories has been proven, research in the United States and Finland indicates that increased iron levels may lead to a higher risk of cancer. The bottom line is that you should not get extra iron unless you are iron-deficient and are directed to do so by a physician.

With all this negative news about excessive iron, you may be wondering what good it can do. Although you want to avoid iron overload, iron is still an essential mineral. One of the primary functions of iron is to bind oxygen in red blood cells for the delivery of oxygen to body tissues. And lack of iron—or iron deficiency—is common in menstruating and pregnant females. Iron deficiency has been shown to cause oxidative damage to mitochondrial DNA. What does all this mean for our cookware choices? If you do cook with a cast-iron pot, just use it for nonacidic foods.

In addition, for many people, cast-iron pots are too heavy. Cast iron needs to be reseasoned periodically. This is easily done by wiping the pan with a few tablespoons of oil and then putting it in a 300-degree oven for over an hour. Copper pots and pans tend to tarnish easily, cost more, and require more upkeep than most cookware. Cast iron is heavier and less practical than cookware made of other materials.

Stovetops and Ovens: Gas or Electric?

For a cook, one ideal combination is a gas stovetop (4 Kitchen IQ points) and an electric oven (3 Kitchen IQ points), with the oven as a separate unit from the stove so you don't have to work over the heat. But if you don't have this setup, don't despair and don't feel you have to shell out several thousand dollars to replace your existing appliances. If you have an electric stovetop, you've probably been told that it's no good for cooking. Fortunately, this is not true.

The advantage of a gas stovetop is that you can alter heat immediately. With an electric stovetop, you simply have to learn to plan a little ahead. If a dish must go from high to low heat, for example, start two burners—one at high heat, one at low—several minutes before putting out the pan of food. Then, when you would turn down the flame on a gas stove, simply transfer the pan to the lower heat. Be sure you have hot mitts (2 Kitchen IQ points) on hand and plenty of free counter space with heavy trivets available (2 Kitchen IQ points) so you can take a pan completely off the heat when it is time to do so.

I discuss other appliances such as a microwave, refrigerator, and grill in Chapter 5. But one additional appliance deserves special mention here: the freezer and the equipment used to freeze food.

Freezing Your Assets

You get 5 Kitchen IQ points if you have a freezer, clear freezer containers, and marking pens (so you know what's in your container and when you made it), *and* if you know and use the "freeze-fast-and-thaw-slow" rule when freezing food. (We discuss this more in Chapter 5.) Knowing you have healthy food in the freezer any time you need an extra dish aids in RealAge living.

And that is the trick these few pieces of equipment provide: they allow you to cook RealAge-smart food more easily. They thus have a high Kitchen IQ that makes your RealAge younger, in more than one way. What a delight—to cook food that gives you the energy and physiology of youth, is fabulously tasty, and is quick and easy to prepare. And you don't have to tell anyone how easy it is. Why would you cook any other way?

4

The
RealAge Pantry

This chapter discusses the key principle of the RealAge pantry: "Easy Availability Begets Eating": that is, the first appealing thing you see is the first thing you'll eat. So, make the first appealing thing you see in your pantry a great-tasting healthy food. With a well-stocked RealAge pantry, you will always have a giant menu of delicious and healthy possibilities right at hand.

The secret to making your RealAge younger when you eat is to plan ahead. Have foods on hand that taste delicious and make you younger. If you don't have bad food choices on hand, you won't be tempted to eat them. So, go through your pantry and eliminate any food that doesn't fit a RealAge lifestyle. The more hydrogenated or saturated fat it has, the less healthy it is. *Easy availability begets eating.* The more fruits, vegetables, whole grains, legumes, fish, nuts, and seeds on hand, the better.

How you stock your pantry makes all the difference to your RealAge. Have you ever opened a cabinet door for a snack and found a PopTart staring at you? Or leftover holiday cookies? Chances are, you didn't close the door and grab a piece of fruit.

Simply put, if you keep RealAge smart food choices on hand, you'll choose to eat them. You can be tempted by such RealAge smart choices as dried fruit, Mexican salsa, whole wheat crackers, Kalamata olives, red peppers, or your favorite nuts.

Stock up on the items listed in this chapter. Most don't need refrigeration and usually aren't canned or processed (the key exceptions are beans, tofu, tomatoes, and chilies), so RealAge-smart foods also do not have a lot of unwanted preservatives. Start small. Add just one new item to your grocery cart the first week—one you know you'll like and use. Next week, add one or two more.

The Well-Stocked RealAge Pantry

(Figure ⅓ Kitchen IQ point for each of these items you have in your pantry. The Kitchen IQ points listed here are included in the quiz and calculations of your kitchen's IQ in Chapter 2.)

Food	Uses
Applesauce	➤ A good snack and a great replacement for fat in recipes for baked goods. To concentrate its goodness for baking, drain applesauce in a coffee filter or folded paper towel. To avoid added sugar and chemicals, select the unsweetened, organic kind.
Arrowroot	➤ A thickening agent used for sauces, puddings, and other foods. Like cornstarch, it should be mixed with a liquid before being added to foods. Mix the arrowroot with a little of the liquid you're thickening,

Food	Uses
	and then add this mixture a little later, when the soup, sauce, or stew is bubbling. As with cornstarch, the liquid must come to a boil for a few seconds for thickening to occur. We prefer arrowroot to cornstarch because arrowroot disappears into sauces and leaves nothing behind. However, cornstarch is more widely available and is much less expensive.
Artichoke hearts	➤ The tender center of the artichoke. Artichoke hearts are usually packed in an oil marinade or in water. Toss them with dried thyme and lemon juice for salads and pasta. They are delicious, low in calories, but rich in fiber, potassium, and calcium. Top pizzas with halved or quartered artichoke hearts straight from the jar.
Baking powder	➤ A leavening agent essential for making quickbreads (muffins, breads, scones). Always have a can in your pantry.
Baking soda	➤ A leavening agent for baked goods. Needs to be combined with an acid for the soda to work. As with baking powder, keep baking soda in your pantry, as some quickbread recipes will require it.
Beans and other legumes (black beans; garbanzo beans (chickpeas); kidney beans; lentils; pinto beans; pink,red, and white beans; split peas)	➤ Legumes include peas, lentils, and beans. Their high fiber and high protein content make them a healthy pleasure. They also come in a variety of beautiful colors. I especially love Anasazi beans, which cook faster than black beans and have a richer flavor and an interesting pink and white color. Include beans in soups and chili, blend them with garlic and chiles for dips, and combine them with tomatoes and peppers for a main course.
Broth or stock (beef, chicken, fish, and vegetable broth or stock; clam juice)	➤ Needed for many recipes, broth adds flavor without adding fat or (usually) salt. Two large cans or boxes of reduced-salt broth in the pantry will expand your flavor possibilities. When a recipe calls for water, try using broth instead. The flavor will be richer and more complex, and you'll also be getting more vitamins and minerals. Remember: you can't use broth or stock for sautéing, as steaming, poaching, or simmering results instead.

Food	Uses
Capers	➤ Little pickled flower buds from a shrub that grows only in the Mediterranean. Capers add a sharp, salty flavor to vinaigrettes, salads, pasta, and fish. For a tasty, healthy pâté, try puréeing capers with roasted red peppers, caramelized onions, and roasted garlic.
Cereal, dried	➤ Be sure to have oatmeal and whole rolled oats (not the instant, precooked kind) on hand. Then try corn flakes, raisin bran, Toasted O's, or even granolas that contain no hydrogenated fat (a granola made with olive oil is great). These are chock-full of healthy vitamins and fiber that make you younger. These can be used as toppings for yogurt and ice cream, as an easy snack, or for making cookies and breads. Experiment until you find a dried cereal you like—one that doesn't contain a lot of refined sugar and chemicals and *does* contain lots of fiber and vitamins.
Chiles (peppers)	➤ Available in many varieties, dried red peppers are all worth trying, as they taste great and are rich in flavonoids that make you younger. Try ancho chiles (dried poblano chiles that taste a little like oranges), chipotle chiles (dried, smoked jalapeño peppers), guajillo chiles (meaty), habanero chiles (extremely floral and fruity flavor, very hot, and often pickled), and pasilla chiles (long, thin, and fragrant). Look for chiles that are soft, not brittle. To decrease the heat and bring out the real flavor, discard the seeds and membranes, and then toast the chiles ever so slightly under a broiler. Or buy canned chipotles in a thick, spicy tomatoey adobo sauce, just to sample them.
Cooking oil spray	➤ Eliminates the need to pour oil in your pan to coat it. The spray helps control the amount of fat you're using. Use olive oil or infused, cold-pressed canola oil in a mister or spray bottle. To make the oil go further, spread it on the pan with a paper towel.
Cornmeal	➤ A "whole" grain that can be a main ingredient in breads, muffins, pancakes, polenta, tamales, and tortillas. Buy it coarsely ground for hearty polenta, and finely ground for mixing into pancakes. Cornmeal can also be sprinkled on the bottom of pans to prevent quickbreads and pizzas from sticking.

Food	Uses
Couscous	➤ Although couscous is just wheat, we've listed it separately from all the other grains because it's so easy to use. Still rolled by hand in many parts of Africa, couscous cooks instantly and takes on the flavor of whatever it's soaked or simmered in. We like it with spicy V8 juice, cilantro, and red onion. You might also like it with currants and dried cherries, simmered in white grape juice for just a minute, and topped with cracked macadamia nuts. Whatever you soak it in, couscous is a winner.
Dijon mustard	➤ Commercial yellow mustard is fine to have in your kitchen (I like the squeeze bottles), but if you want to add special flavor, use Dijon mustard, either smooth or whole-grain. Its tangy bite enlivens sandwiches and salad dressings and gives a kick to root vegetables, whole-grain breads, and hot dogs—tofu, turkey, or all beef!
Evaporated nonfat (skim) milk	➤ Has about 60 percent of the water removed and is a low-fat form of milk. You can use this product in baking and cream sauces, which will keep your RealAge younger.
Flour	➤ Used in baking and to coat pans or to prevent sticking when rolling out dough. For general cooking and baking, buy an all-purpose, unbleached, unbromated wheat flour—organic, if possible. (Check the label for those terms.) Avoid bromates! Bromates, a chemical group used to strengthen bread dough, can be toxic and cancer-promoting and can make you older. Add other varieties of flour (for example, whole wheat) for specific recipes.
Fruits, dried	➤ Have some dried fruit for a light snack, mixed with yogurt, or baked into healthier scones. Toss some in a salad and mix some into oatmeal. Be careful, however: fruit can be very caloric when dried— a little goes a long way. Try whole figs, dates, prunes, raisins (several kinds—golden, Thompson, red flame), cranberries, cherries, currants, blueberries, and strawberries. Select organic dried fruit whenever possible.

Food	Uses
Garlic	➤ Garlic is a joy because it complements almost anything. Gilroy, California, "The Garlic Capital of the World," even boasts a garlic ice cream. Garlic enhances fish and shellfish, pasta and grains, poultry and meats. Roast unpeeled foil-wrapped heads of garlic (45 minutes at 375 degrees is a starting point, as each oven is different) and squeeze out the pulp for a sweet spread for bread and crackers, a flavorful RealAge alternative to butter and margarine (maybe not right before you go to work!).
Ginger	➤ Fresh ginger can be sliced, diced, and chopped. It's great in marinades, stir-fried dishes, soups, vegetables, and gingerbread. Look for a smooth, papery skin. If the root is shriveled or sprouting, pass it up: it's drying out and may have lost most of its juice. Ginger will last about two weeks when stored in a cool, dark, airy place.
Grains, whole (arborio rice, barley, brown rice, bulgur, millet, oats, quinoa, wild rice)	➤ Having several types of grains on hand can simplify meal preparation. Grains are easy to prepare and can be eaten alone, mixed with seasoning, or cooked in combination with other foods. Arborio, a short-grain rice, is usually used for making risotto because it releases starch quickly and makes the dish extra creamy. Barley is used in breads, cereals, and soups. Brown rice, which is rice that has not had its husks removed, is rich in fiber and can be used in any dish calling for white rice. Bulgur is wheat that has been steamed and cracked into grits; it's commonly used for tabbouleh, a classic Mediterranean dish, but has many other uses. Try bulgur in mixed-grain salads or with lentils. Millet is a round nutty grain that resembles couscous; it can be used in salads or the stuffing for peppers, or mixed with corn. Oats are not just for breakfast anymore! Breads, cookies, and granola would not be the same without oats. Oats have lots of soluble fiber, which helps reduce the level of lousy (LDL) cholesterol. Quinoa is another whole grain that's gaining popularity; it's a light, high protein grain that's very versatile. Add it to muffins and breads or use it as a side dish. Wild rice, one of the most well-known grains on this list, isn't really a rice at all, but a long grass. Wild rice complements fish and poultry well.

Food	Uses
Herbs	➤ Herbs can give a bland dish a new flavor. Use the chart provided in Chapter 11 for pairing herbs with foods. Dried herbs stored in the pantry will last for about six months.
Honey	➤ Widely used as a spread for bread and as a sweetener and flavoring agent for baked goods, liquids (such as tea), desserts, and savory dishes such as honey-glazed ham or carrots. The darker the honey, the more intense the flavor. The flavor of a honey depends on the flower visited by the bee. For example, clover honey has a clean, light flavor, and orange blossom honey has a slightly citrusy flavor.
Hot pepper sauce	➤ The intense flavor of hot pepper sauce can turn dull vegetables into an exciting dish. The chiles used are often generic—usually arbol peppers, or whatever is available—and some hot sauces can be plain hot and salty. No matter. There are thousands of hot pepper sauces, and each is worth a try.
	To cut the heat of these hot pepper sauces, take a swig of skim milk, rather than a drink of water or beer. Only dairy protein works to bind the hot substance in peppers! (The hot stuff combines with the casein protein in milk. Cottage cheese and sour cream do not work, unfortunately.) This is another good reason to keep evaporated milk or powdered milk on hand; it will help cool your nerves if you've had too much hot pepper sauce.
Instant coffee, espresso	➤ Instant coffee can be used for making coffee if you don't have freshly ground beans in the house. It adds a bit of tantalizing bitterness, as chocolate does, and a lot of caffeine to whatever you want.
Ketchup	➤ In most homes, ketchup (catsup) is a staple condiment. However, it's also an ingredient in many recipes and sauces. Ketchup is incredibly high in lycopene (and, unfortunately, usually, sugar). Remember to eat it with a little fat first to facilitate absorption of the lycopene and decrease the peak level of sugar in your blood. Look for organic ketchup in the supermarket, with tomatoes or tomato paste (not water, sugar, or corn syrup) as the first ingredient.

Food	Uses
Nuts	➤ Almonds, walnuts, pine nuts, pecans, pistachios, Brazil nuts, soy nuts—I love them all. (Peanuts, which are really a legume, can rarely pose a hazard. The cancer-causing toxin called aflatoxin is produced by a mold that sometimes grows on peanuts. This is not much of a problem with modern growing processes; so peanuts are also lovable.) Buy nuts by the half pound and keep them tightly sealed in see-through glass containers. Toasting nuts brings out their flavor and reduces the amount needed in recipes. One of my favorite "fat-first" strategies is to eat just ½ ounce of mixed nuts before a meal, as it makes you as much as 4.4 years younger (6 walnuts, 9 cashews, or 12 almonds).
Oils, healthy	➤ Canola, sesame, and olive oils are mainly monounsaturated fats that help make your RealAge younger. These three oils are sufficient for most baking and cooking purposes (nut, fish, and peanut oils are healthy oils also). Cold-pressed canola oil has lots of omega-3 fatty acids, too. Extra-virgin olive oil works for general cooking and often has a fragrant, distinctive bouquet and flavor.
Olives	➤ Pitted canned black olives are what many of us grew up eating. While they have a place, there are many exciting, delicious multiflavored and textured choices just waiting for you. Look for Kalamata, Niçoise, and spicy green Sicilian olives. All of these olives have clear, distinct, wonderful flavors, sometimes redolent of herbs and spices like cumin, fennel, and bay leaf. All have healthy fat, too. Use them as a relish, on pizza, and in pasta dishes, stews, ragouts, and salads.
Onions	➤ Onions will last for a long time in a dry, dark place in the pantry. You never know when you'll need onions for a sauce, salad, rice dish, or main dish. Use white onions for a clear, clean flavor for Mexican dishes, for grilling, and for caramelizing; use yellow onions for Italian, French, and Spanish dishes; and use red onions for color and crunch. Look for cippolini onions (sweet, small, and flat), Vidalia and Walla Walla onions (sweet and huge), and shallots (sometimes

Food	Uses
	even mild enough to eat out of hand). Onions help keep your arteries and immune system young.
Pasta (whole-grain)	➤ Whole-grain pastas come in a variety of flavors and colors (for example, spinach pasta and jalapeño pepper pasta). Although we recommend whole wheat pasta as a staple because of its fiber content, selecting the right brand is important. Some pastas cook up so tough they're almost inedible. Don't give up! Try different brands until you find one that cooks up just the way you like it.
Pepper	➤ Pepper is a versatile spice that goes with almost any dish. For the best flavor, whole peppercorns should be kept in the pantry and ground as needed. You can use black, white, and even pink (!), or green peppercorns; look for grinders that easily can grind all four at once.
Potatoes	➤ Sweet, red, and baking or russet potatoes are the varieties you need. Potatoes, like beans and lentils, can take center stage in meals. Also, potatoes are rich in artery-protecting folate. Sweet potatoes are underappreciated, have twice as much folate for their weight as other types of potatoes, and roast beautifully. They also keep well. Look for Garnets, plus the usual Jewels and Beauregards; Garnets have darker skin and lighter flesh, and a sweeter roast. Red potatoes are good for salads because they hold their shape well; look for the smaller "creamers," or small, red potatoes of a waxy type. Specialty potatoes, such as Peruvian Blues and Fingerlings, are fun to experiment with and are delicious, as well.
Salsa	➤ Salsa has a variety of uses in the kitchen—as a topping for a Southwestern dish or a baked potato, or as a dip for chips. You can also cook with salsa: mix some into egg whites, blend some with an avocado, or pour some into a stew. Use salsa to top grilled fish. Look for salsa that is minimally processed and that is made from whole tomatoes or tomatillos, onions, garlic, and herbs.
Salt	➤ Salt brings out the flavor of foods. I use mainly sea salt and kosher salt. Sea salt is usually ground more finely and, gram for gram, is usually saltier than kosher salt, which has bigger crystals. Both taste

Food	Uses

richer and fuller, and not as sharp or as slightly bitter as iodized salt. (While too much salt—sodium—can increase blood pressure a little—systolic 1 to 4.7/diastolic 0.5 to 3 mmHg—in most people and a lot in some rare individuals with salt sensitive high blood pressure, a little salt adds great taste to many dishes. Use it judiciously if your blood pressure is around 115/75.)

Soy Sauce

➤ Soy sauce is used commonly in Asian recipes and is a component of marinades. It blends well with other strong flavors—garlic, chiles, ginger, and flavored oils. Flavored soy sauce is available in specialty markets; mushroom soy sauce is my current favorite. Look for low-sodium soy sauce; it often carries much of the flavor of regular soy sauce but not as much salt. Also try shoyu and tamari. Their flavor comes from fermented grains and is often rich and deep.

Spices, dried

➤ Spices are one of the most important ingredients in your RealAge kitchen. When you can, buy them whole, not ground. Here are some spices you should get to know: allspice, bay leaves, caraway seeds, cardamom, cayenne pepper, chili powder, cinnamon, cloves, coriander, cumin, curry powder, dill, epazote, fennel, garam masala (a traditional blend of ground spices), ginger, mace, marjoram, mustard, nutmeg, oregano, paprika, rosemary, saffron, sage, sesame seeds, tarragon, and turmeric. See our "RealAge Herbs and Spices" chart in Chapter 11 for suggested uses for these spices.

Sugar (brown, granulated, and powdered)

➤ Although there are four basic varieties of sugar, there're no nutritional differences among them. Common granulated sugar is a fine white sugar that's used for everything from coffee to cake. Brown sugar, colored with molasses, usually flavors candies, condiments, and baked goods. While sugar does not make you younger, a little can add intense flavor. Here's a RealAge kitchen tip: spice muffins (usually flavored with cinnamon, nutmeg, or other spices) made with brown sugar taste less "spicy" than those made with white sugar. Powdered sugar, or confectioners' sugar, is used in frostings and icings, or sprinkled on desserts for eye appeal. Unrefined cane

Food	Uses
	sugar has no more nutrients than the other types of sugar, but does have a more complex taste.
Sun-dried tomatoes	➤ Sun-dried tomatoes have an intense, sweet, slightly salty flavor; they're dense and delicious. You'll find them packed in oil or in cellophane. Stock up in the fall for the winter months ahead.
Tea	➤ Tea, especially green tea, should find its way into your RealAge pantry. Buy it in bags unless you're going to drink a lot. If so, you may want to buy half a pound of loose tea at a time. Green tea contains the most antioxidants. In green tea, the leaves are steamed and dried. In oolong tea, the leaves are steamed, dried, and partially fermented (here, fermented means oxidized). In black tea, the leaves are steamed, dried, and fully fermented. They're all the same leaf, just in different stages. All make your RealAge younger.
Tofu	➤ Tofu can be a great addition to your pantry. Because it accepts flavors readily, tofu can be made to taste like a great many other foods (including chocolate). Tofu is available in three forms: firm, soft, and silken. Firm tofu is solid and dense, and works well in stir-fried dishes and soups, and grilled. It holds its shape well, even after being pressed between blocks, or after freezing, which makes it slightly chewy, and much firmer. Firm tofu is also higher in protein, fat, and calcium than the other two types. Soft tofu is good for recipes that require blended tofu; it's also used in Asian soups. Silken tofu, the softest type, works well in dressings, dips, desserts, smoothies, puddings, guacamole, and cannoli and cream pies.
Tomato paste	➤ Tomato paste is used as the base for a variety of sauces or mixed in with grains. Tubes of tomato paste are especially convenient. Remember to add healthy fat such as olive or canola oil for better absorption of the age-reducing lycopene that is found in tomatoes, guava, watermelon, and pink grapefruit.
Tomatoes (canned)	➤ Canned tomatoes come in handy all the time. Use them in sauces, soups, and stews. Whenever you can, buy the organic varieties that are unpeeled (90 percent of the lycopene is within 1 millimeter of

Food	Uses

the skin). These cooked tomatoes may be even better than fresh, as they release age-reducing lycopene into your system. (Why lycopene is better released from cooked tomatoes than from raw tomatoes is unclear, but this is found consistently in studies.)

Tortillas (corn, flour, and whole wheat)

➤ Tortillas are used in or with chiles, casseroles, soups, refried beans, quesadillas, scrambled eggs, and tostadas. Corn tortillas tend to be the best choice for making your RealAge younger. Even though, traditionally, they consist of just corn, lime, and salt, you'd be amazingly lucky to find them fresh. If they're not fresh, it's easy to rejuvenate them. Roll them up and cover them with two paper towels. After sprinkling them lightly with water, microwave them for 15 to 45 seconds, just until they're soft and steaming. Flour tortillas are often loaded with chemicals and some hydrogenated fats. Colored flour tortillas (those made with spinach or tomatoes) are pretty but no different in flavor or nutrition. Whole wheat tortillas are increasingly available but may have suffered the same fate—added chemicals and hydrogenated fats. Look for those made with oils that are not hydrogenated, and have "whole wheat" as the first ingredient on the label.

Vanilla extract, pure

➤ A bottle of pure vanilla extract is a good substitute for the more expensive, more elusive, incredibly fragrant vanilla bean pods. The seed pods of a plant in the orchid family, vanilla is used commonly in desserts and sauces and also perks up soy milk and cereal in wonderful, fresh ways. Buy a vanilla bean just for the experience: it's long and dark and curled at the end, potent and seeded and just a little gooey in the middle.

Vinegar

➤ How do you know which of the great variety of flavored vinegars to use? It depends on what you're cooking. Buy one bottle at a time to see what you like and continue until you have tried all of these varieties: balsamic, cider, herb, raspberry, rice, sherry, tarragon flavored, white distilled, and wine (both red and white). Balsamic vinegar is dark and a bit sweet—just a little brings out the best in fruits, grains, and vegetables. Look for traditional balsamic; it's the

Food	Uses
	real stuff. Cider vinegar, which is made by fermenting apple cider, is light and a little sweet. Rinsing diced white onions in cider vinegar takes away their sting of taste. Raspberry vinegar (a favorite) has a fruity flavor and makes salad dressings tangy, dresses up grains, and goes well with tropical fruits. Rice vinegar is a pale, golden liquid that adds, when seasoned, a little salt and a light, lemony flavor. Tarragon flavored white wine vinegar is nice sprinkled over fish and chicken. White distilled vinegar is an all-purpose vinegar that does well in pickling, but is harsh in cooking except for an occasional chutney. Red wine vinegar goes well with Mediterranean dishes that are tomato-based, and white wine vinegar is gentler still. It can be combined with lighter oils and herbs for a dressing.
Wine	➤ White and red wines are used in our kitchen for poaching, and in soups, stews, and sauces. Avoid wines labeled "cooking wines," as these have added salt, and often their flavor may leave something to be desired: Here's a RealAge kitchen tip regarding wine used in cooking: If you wouldn't drink it, don't cook with it, either. The quality of wine used in cooking really does make a difference.
Worcestershire sauce	➤ Worcestershire sauce is one of the best-kept secrets of good home cooks—just a few drops will perk up meats, gravies, soups, and vegetable juices, or serve as a table condiment. Its ingredients include soy, vinegar, and garlic.

Stocking your pantry with these items makes it more likely you'll choose healthy foods that will make your RealAge younger. You'll enjoy these dishes more as they will taste better. So enjoy stocking your pantry with foods that increase your Kitchen IQ, and relish becoming younger.

5

Becoming a RealAge Chef

*Learn How to Cook for
the Health of It!*

This chapter helps you learn how to cook food that will delight your taste buds. Those who get to enjoy what you cook will be amazed—"I didn't know healthy food could taste this good!" But it can, and you'll soon find out how easy it is to become a RealAge chef by mastering these techniques.

People often worry that a healthy diet means bland food. Perhaps they're used to rich restaurant food that depends primarily on butter and cream for flavor. Fine dining restaurant food is often delicious (if you can stand the richness), but the effect of all that saturated fat on the coronary arteries, the brain, the reproductive organs, and the immune system is huge, and it is likely you will live a shorter life filled with more disability.

To understand how a RealAge kitchen can help you control your genes, it is important to realize that you can prepare very delicious meals without excessive use of either artery- or immune system–aging saturated or trans fats. These delicious meals omit ingredients that raise blood pressure and include ingredients that lower blood pressure. With just a little effort and practice, you can create RealAge-smart and energy-giving meals that are as delicious as a top chef's, but with ingredients that can help make you younger. Really, by eating to keep disability at bay, you can reverse the aging of your arteries and immune system—and enjoy some great-tasting meals at the same time.

Each of our recipes was created for great taste and to make your RealAge younger. Many of them use techniques that spare arterial-aging fat and, instead, rely on healthy fats.

This chapter explains how to use and adapt time-tested culinary methods to prepare healthy foods at home. We also show how you can make extra quantities of those healthful meals and freeze them to enjoy later, when you might be a little short of time. Lastly, we give some cooking tips to enhance the flavor of your meals in a healthy, RealAge-smart way.

RealAge Cooking Techniques

Grilling and Broiling

Both grilling and broiling involve cooking with dry, direct heat that is transferred across the surface of the food into its center. Grilling is done on a rack. Why don't cooks grill more often? They should, but most people can't use their porch, deck, or backyard grills year-round, and many people don't have indoor grills.

But the way foods are most commonly grilled in the U.S. can be bad for a

RealAge diet. The traditional Fourth of July barbecue, with hot dogs, hamburgers, and other meats coated with sodium- and sugar-rich barbecue sauce, is typical. Red meats are full of artery- and immune system–aging saturated fat. Every natural cut of meat has at least 29 percent fat to begin with, and sometimes it gains twice that much by the time it hits the grill. In addition, blackening meat on an outdoor grill produces heterocyclic amines (HCAs), chemicals that may promote or even cause cancer. Finally, fat dripping onto the coals below may produce polycyclic aromatic hydrocarbons (PAHs), which are carcinogenic molecules. Although their effect on humans is not known conclusively, PAHs have been found to be cancerous in animals.

This doesn't mean you can't or shouldn't grill food, however. An easier and healthier "grilling" method is to use a nonstick stovetop grill (such as one made by Le Creuset), which you set directly on the burner of your gas stove, above the flame (*2 Kitchen IQ points*). These stovetop grills offer the delicious taste of grilling and the grill marks you get from an outdoor grill, but there is a much healthier food result. If your stovetop is electric, you'll need a ridged grill pan that is flat bottomed instead.

Popular stand alone grills are RealAge-smart. George Foreman–type grills are relatively inexpensive and seem to work well. The fat, marinade, and other juices drip down away from the food and out of the front of this slightly sloped grill. These grills are nice because they cook fast—the top closes so that the top and bottom of what you are grilling are grilled at the same time. Some say, however, that these grills steam meat rather than grill it. (I have not found this true in my tests of one version of this grill.) Steaming toughens animal proteins, so meats—including chicken—may not be as great-tasting as if grilled over wood or even gas. But sandwiches and vegetables are great prepared on this grill, especially panini (Italian grilled sandwiches).

When grilling on the stovetop, do not use high heat. The flame should be low or, at most, medium—high heat can build up and damage the stove or the grill. As with a sauté pan, you know it's time to put the food on the grill when a drop of water skips and sizzles.

A piece of fresh fish, such as salmon, cooked on a stovetop grill that has been spritzed with olive or canola oil, or cooking spray, and then served with a salad or topped with mango salsa, makes a delicious dinner that is quick and easy at the end of a busy day. Grilling chicken is simple. You need to grill bone-in parts all the way to the center until its juices run clear. Do not mash or press the chicken—it will dry out, especially chicken breasts, which have less fat than the legs. Chicken thighs, legs, or drumsticks can be cooked to about 170°F internally. Use your meat thermometer to check. Boneless parts can be cooked to 165°F internally for at least 15 seconds.

USING MARINADES

Many restaurants use grills primarily to finish boiled or braised pork and beef ribs; to prepare steaks, leg, and shoulder cuts; and to cook ground meats, such as hamburgers. Grilling cuts of meat that don't have much visible fat—chicken breasts, shrimp, and pork tenderloin, for example—requires extra basting, barding (wrapping lean meat with fat), or larding to prevent burning and drying. Instead, use oil-based marinades to prevent this drying and burning, and to baste and coat meats, including poultry and fish. Marinades also reduce the amount of aging heterocyclic and polycyclic amines and hydrocarbons (HCAs and PAHs) in grilled food. In several studies, bathing food in a marinade—such as balsamic vinegar and a little olive oil as a marinade for chicken—for as little as 15 minutes makes the food taste better and reduces amines and hydrocarbons by more than 90 percent. Although we do not know why marinades work, they have a consistent, beneficial effect. Remember, however, to keep the coating of meats and poultry in extra fat to a minimum, as you can use your daily fat (20 to 30 percent of your diet) to better use. And do not reuse marinades, and keep them and your food cold to minimize the risk of food-borne illness.

GRILLING FRUITS AND VEGETABLES

Are there tricks to grilling fruits and vegetables? These foods are low in fat (most are less than 8 percent fat) and difficult to grill because they tend to stick to the grill and steam instead of grill. Sure, a few tricks are needed. Some chefs use a hinged wire basket to grill and turn slices of summer squash and sweet onion (especially Walla Wallas and Vidalias) so they don't stick. Other chefs precook vegetables that would otherwise take longer than other items being grilled; fennel, leeks, and sweet potatoes are often steamed or parboiled before going on the grill for example. Use a hot fire and bring vegetables to room temperature before grilling them—the fire's concentrated heat lessens the chance of sticking. Very few foods take more than 30 minutes on a hot grill, even when placed 6 inches from the coals, where my grate usually stays. Placing the grate closer just invites charring and undesirable changes in texture and color. Here's another RealAge kitchen tip: never salt food, especially vegetables, before grilling; it will dehydrate them and they'll cook unpredictably.

When time is short, you can speed the grilling process by microwaving sliced vegetables or fruits in a covered microwave-safe bowl for a few minutes, and finish them on the grill for better flavor. They'll pick up some smokiness in just 3 or 4 minutes.

EASY OUTDOOR GRILLING

There are easy ways to use the outdoor grill. "Foil grilling," for example, is actually steaming. Simply enclose some mushrooms and onions in a foil packet with a few sprigs of thyme and drops of white wine, and use the heat of the fire to cook them gently. What about that fire? Use hardwood briquettes instead of charcoal. (Briquettes have fewer chemicals, and impart more flavor.) Skip the lighter fluid and its carcinogens, and use dry kindling to start the fire. It takes only a moment longer and is a good investment in your health. Toss a handful of dried thyme, sage, oregano, or rosemary on the fire just before placing your food on the grill. Herbal touches linger on slabs of polenta, mustard pitas, and even slices of eggplant and whole pizzas.

You'll need to be a little creative to make food healthy when cooked on your outdoor grill. Marinate the vegetables and fruits before grilling. Peach halves and pineapple slices, for example, can absorb spice rubs and marinades, and with them, extra flavor. If the grill is hot enough, and the marinade oil-based and liquid enough, the food does not stick and the oil stays out of the fire. You can tell this as you'll have few flare-ups and little charring.

Roasting

Roasting involves cooking indirectly with dry heat, usually in an oven. The heat is reflected off the walls of the oven, and together with warmed air, creates a wonderful enzymatic reaction that transforms many foods into delicious fragrances, textures, and tastes. The browning process occurs at the surface of the food, caramelizing it to a crackling crust.

Roasting is a term traditionally applied to cooking animal protein. We roast joints of beef, pork and lamb, turkey, and chicken. In the nineteenth century, the term itself came to mean, as it still does, a chuck, rump, or shoulder piece.

Roasting lean meat and skinless poultry requires the addition of fats to prevent the cuts from becoming dry and leathery, yet your RealAge can become older if you baste often with fat. One conventional way to keep roasted meats moist is to lard or bard them. Larding and barding involve penetrating or wrapping meats, respectively, with fattier meats or fat itself so that those fats can saturate and baste the lean meat. You can also baste lean meats with meat juices or drippings, butter, or an oil-laden marinade (olive or canola oil, we hope). Alternatively, you can select cuts of meat with visible layers of fat, so that the meat bastes itself.

Similarly, when restaurant chefs roast vegetables, they usually brush them with a brush full of oil to prevent dehydration and to help brown or char the skin. So as you can see, traditional roasting is a great way to get a month's worth of saturated (aging) fat in one meal. Yet roasting is too good a technique to reject. You can keep its potential and make your RealAge younger by doing a few things differently.

OVEN-ROASTING

You can roast vegetables for extra flavor and sweetness, either slowly and patiently to preserve their shape and color (for example, to dry plum tomatoes) or quickly and blisteringly to concentrate their flavor, melt their texture, or char their skins (for example, to prepare tomatillos for salsa). High heat (about 450 degrees) gives vegetables a deep, smoky flavor and a silky texture that becomes even smoother when the vegetables are puréed and strained.

Roasting allows the natural juices of vegetables to concentrate; also, for some strongly flavored foods such as garlic, roasting produces an unexpected mellowness. Root vegetables (from parsnips to Jerusalem artichokes to potatoes, carrots, and every kind of onion) are wonderful when oven-roasted. Their natural sweetness is concentrated, and their skins become crisp and crunchy. A cooler 375-degree oven bakes most one-inch chunks of root vegetables (beets, celery root, leeks, onions, parsnips, potatoes) in about 45 minutes. They're done when they are tender but not singed.

Using juicy, healthy fats for moisture and not peeling vegetables (*2 Kitchen IQ points* for using these two techniques) can harness the benefits of roasting for a RealAge, flavor-intense cooking result. Instead of dousing vegetables with oil, paint them lightly, using olive oil from a mister. Keeping the skins on vegetables is another way to retain moisture while roasting. Use natural insulators, like the husks of corn, the jackets of potatoes, or skins of tomatoes, to minimize drying—you can always skin vegetables after they are cooked or incorporate the skins in a dish. Use a whole head of garlic, cut off just enough of the husk to admit a few drops of stock and olive oil, and put the head on a baking sheet in a 450-degree oven for 15 minutes. Or wrap the garlic in foil for softer cloves or separate and roast the cloves in their skins in a 450-degree toaster oven for 10 minutes. (Use a toaster oven if you want to contain the fragrance; if you roast garlic in your regular oven, it may give off a garlic fragrance for several days.)

Both electric and gas ovens are notoriously inaccurate in producing the temperature specified, so be sure to use an oven thermometer to check the *actual* temperature of your oven before adding food.

PAN-ROASTING VEGETABLES, NUTS, SPICES

Roasting in a hot pan produces great flavor without heating up the whole kitchen. In a way, pan-roasting is like sautéing without the oil but with very high heat. If you're roasting in a pan, you'll need a wooden spoon with a flat edge *(1 Kitchen IQ point)* and a heavy-bottomed skillet. (I use a 12-inch seasoned cast-iron skillet.) A heavy skillet of any kind—even a seasoned wok—will do. The pan must be very hot. The vegetables that take the longest to cook should be added first. Move cubes of onions, potatoes, and squash around the pan quickly, as their outer layers darken and their flesh softens, becoming sweeter and more supple.

Pan-roasting nuts is a wonderful way to add smokiness, toasty flavor, and richness to sauces and stews, and to create a contrasting garnish. The technique requires a moderately hot, very heavy skillet, a watchful eye, and either an able wrist to shake the pan back and forth or the wooden spoon mentioned earlier. Each nut is a little different, so you must carefully smell for the toasty aroma, listen for "pops," and watch for a change in color. Heat the pan first, then add, for example, a single layer of pistachios, pepitas, pine nuts, or pecans and observe for half a minute. If the nuts smoke, take the pan off the heat. Then, every half-minute for 2 or 3 minutes, shake the pan from side to side to move the nuts on the outside toward the middle. The colors are terrific: pistachios quickly char a little on one side; dull green pepitas deepen to dark olive; pine nuts start to tan a little; and pecans do, too. After they're toasted, turn them out of the pan and pound them into pesto or a nut butter, or sprinkle them on our frittata (page 154).

Roasting (or toasting) spices is usually done on a stovetop in a small, heavy-bottomed skillet. It's easy to move the spices around a nonstick skillet and hard to burn them. The roasting releases the oils and concentrates the flavors of the spices, from anise to sesame seeds, and takes no more than 5 minutes. The secret is to stay at the stove while the spices are roasting.

To pan-roast whole spices, preheat a very clean, dry pan over medium heat, add the whole spices, and shake the pan or stir to keep the spices from burning. When you smell their fragrance, pan-roast for just half a minute longer or until they begin to darken. Do not let them smoke. (They set off our smoke detector, so it's an extra incentive for us not to let them smoke.) Transfer them to a dry bowl to cool, then add to a spice grinder or mortar and crush. The aromatic oils that have been intensified by the heat will vaporize a little further, just before they become part of your dish. Toasting and seasoning in this way helps reduce the salt needed to flavor dishes, which in turn helps keep your blood pressure low and your arteries and immune system RealAge-young.

Dried chiles—for example, anchos, guajillos, pasillas, chipotles—are good choices for pan-roasting. A small flame under a very dry, very clean cast-iron skillet, griddle, or Mexican *comal* (a cast-iron grill) is ideal. Whatever you use, keep a very close eye on the chiles. The second they begin to blacken, flip them, watch for blackening again and a wisp of smoke, and they're done. They usually take 10 seconds or less, but yield excellent richness and spiciness.

Grains and legumes can also be pan-roasted if stirred or shaken vigilantly until their color begins to darken. You'll usually be rewarded with faster cooking, better individual grain separation, and a toasty or nutty flavor. Grains and legumes are really tasty, texture-rich ways to make your RealAge younger. Eating two small fistfuls of whole grains and another serving of legumes every day will make your RealAge 3.4 years younger.

OTHER ROASTING TECHNIQUES

You can also roast on a stovetop grill (see "Grilling") or in a toaster oven (*2 Kitchen IQ points*)—just about anywhere there's dry heat. Whole sweet peppers and chiles roast fastest over the open flame of a gas burner but also can be roasted in the oven, under the broiler whether your oven is gas or electric. In either place, keep turning them until their skins are completely blackened. When you're finished, put them in a paper bag for a few minutes until the steam loosens the skin and it peels off. Don't wash the skin off because you will wash away the smoky flavor, too.

Baking

Baking and roasting both mean cooking indirectly with dry heat that surrounds and cooks the food evenly on all sides. One difference is that baking is often done at a lower temperature than roasting. Another is that the term *baking* has traditionally referred to nearly every food, from fruits and vegetables to fish and chicken, not just meat. Baking is usually done in an oven, but can occur atop a stove or a griddle (pancakes), over a covered barbecue grill (skewered peppers, onions, and cherry tomatoes), in a crockpot or stockpot (baked beans), and on the rack of a toaster oven (nearly anything that will fit).

Bake foods uncovered when you want a crunchy surface. The outside will be crisp while the inside remains moist and supple. Baking gives a good crust to the humble baking potato. Bake foods covered when you want juiciness. Trapped moisture helps to steam the food, softening its texture and sometimes capturing aromas that might have wafted away. Covering whatever you're baking protects the food from drying out and adds steam to the process.

Baking is wonderful for making muffins and cookies, which usually have enough fat in their dough to ensure a tender texture. However, have you ever noticed the oily circle that a fresh-baked commercial muffin leaves behind when you lift it off the plate? That's usually a solid fat (an aging fat), soaked right through. Cookies sometimes leave the same blotch. Commercial cookies are baked in a very hot oven to allow them to spread out, and this spread is at least partially caused by the fat that's inside. On the other hand, most fat-free commercial muffins and cookies are either bouncy enough to use for tennis or very sugar-laden that the calorie count lets you eat very little at the next meal. The effect of their sugar content on blood vessels is greater aging. In addition, the sugar load and variation in blood-sugar levels they cause can induce cravings that make you want more simple carbohydrates, leading to further aging of the arteries.

REALAGE BAKING TIPS

Creative RealAge baking methods keep the taste and make food healthier than commercial baking. Drained applesauce or mashed banana or prune purée plus a little canola oil can replace the solid fat in muffins, retaining their texture and bulk but not their risk of heart disease or cancer. (Routinely using drained applesauce, mashed banana, or prune purée as a substitute for fat is worth *4 Kitchen IQ points.*) The same goes for cookies, which will come out soft and chewy, never brittle. Use nonstick baking sheets or muffin tins or, if necessary, mist the pan with cooking oil spray, spreading the oil over the pan with a paper towel. Parchment paper can also be used to line a pan, although it sometimes cannot endure high heat.

Basting baked goods can also help retain moisture. If you stuff apple pears with gorgonzola, for example, basting is unnecessary because the fat in the cheese should permeate the apple's moist flesh. If you stuffed apple pears with raisins and toasted pine nuts instead, you could baste them with apple juice infused with a dried persimmon slice and a cinnamon stick, and then reduce the basting liquid to a glaze. The glaze will penetrate, softening as it is absorbed. In baking as in roasting, basting with liquids that add body, flavor, and texture is an easy, RealAge-smart alternative to basting with a gob of butter or some other solid aging fat, such as in most stick margarines.

Grains and vegetables can also be baked. The steam of covered cooking that can toughen meat and chicken will soften otherwise-tough barley, bulgur, and rice. In addition, some vegetables are better baked or roasted than steamed. Whole artichokes with stuffing are best baked, as the stuffing becomes just a little crunchy and contrasts with the texture of the meaty leaves.

Reducing

Reducing is simply cooking a liquid over high heat (a usual but not necessary condition) in order to decrease its volume. Reducing has two purposes: to concentrate flavor and to thicken. (Knowing how to reduce a liquid is worth *3 Kitchen IQ points.*)

Reducing deserves special mention because it is so effective and so effortless, save for having a careful eye. Decreasing the volume of a sauce to half can more than double its flavor. Because reduction thickens as it goes, you don't have to use flour, which can produce a grainy texture if added improperly. As much as possible, sauces and glazes should taste of the food itself, not of additives, and especially not of fat, salt, or sugar.

Reducing the stocks derived from meat, poultry, and fish can yield rich flavors. In professional kitchens, stocks and broths are sometimes reduced drastically to provide lusciously dense sauces and glazes. If the aging fat is skimmed, reduced sauces can serve as warm accents to a dish, often making your RealAge significantly younger.

Classic Sauces vs. RealAge Sauces

In making most classic French sauces, which are high in saturated and trans fats, reduction is only one method of thickening used. In nearly all classic thickening methods, including reduction, butter or another fat is combined with a starch, which absorbs water and thickens the sauce. But these products are energy-sapping and aging. In some French cooking, for example, butter is cooked with flour to make a roux, or is kneaded (uncooked) with flour to make a beurre manié. Sauces made with these thickeners, often added at the beginning of cooking, can also be reduced. However, high-fat sauces scorch easily, have to be watched carefully, must be simmered gently, and don't give up their volume quickly. They are also usually "finished" with butter, meaning that a little butter is swirled in at the end. But a RealAge chef can make delicious sauces by reduction without adding extra aging fat. Remember, healthy fats like nut oils, peanut oil, canola oil, and olive oil are fine to add here. They add great taste and make your RealAge younger.

When reducing a liquid primarily to thicken it, use a microwaveable bowl in the microwave and a saucepan on the stovetop. When reducing a liquid primarily to concentrate its flavor, couple the step with deglazing, sometimes in an oven roaster pan and sometimes on the stovetop. Deglazing and reducing on the stovetop require an uncovered pan, a careful eye, and high heat. To deglaze, with the heat on, pour some liquid (water, wine, broth, or a combination) into the hot pan in which you have cooked the food. Using the same spoon or spatula that was used in cooking the food, gently scrape the sides and bottom—these stuck-on bits contain a lot of flavor. Let the liquid boil until it has reduced to several tablespoons. You may want to add lemon juice, herbs, or other flavorings. Thickening with butter, cream, or egg yolk is not necessary.

There are other ways to thicken a sauce in addition to reducing it. For instance, I remove a small amount of the sauce, stir cornstarch or arrowroot into it, and then stir this mixture into the pot or pan of sauce at the end of the cooking process, bringing the pot to a boil for a moment. Both starches will thicken almost anything and add a smooth sheen. Try using a baked potato, toasted corn niblets, winter squash, and caramelized onions, puréed either with water or stock to add body and volume to soups.

An almost complete reduction of pan juices can concentrate the flavor so much that you can compound and layer the tastes, deglazing if necessary to restore the sauce's volume. Start with a pan of dried-up (or almost dried-up) juices left by whatever has been sautéed, roasted, or grilled. Add a flavorful liquid, deglaze the pan, and let the two flavors mingle; boil the solution rapidly to produce a sauce. Fortified wines (sherry, Madeira, or port), fruit juices (apple, orange, and seasoned tomato juices), and flavored vinegars (Chinese black, red raspberry, sherry, or tarragon flavored white wine vinegar) are some of my favorite liquids for reviving a reduction taken all the way to the bottom of the pan. Instead of "finishing" with butter, try a sprinkling of a little fresh basil, cilantro, mint, or epazote (a pungent herb native to Mexican and South American cooking).

Sautéing

In French, *sauter* means "to jump." To sauté food is to make it really move over high heat, cooking it thoroughly yet quickly to retain its shape and nutritional value. Sautéing requires high heat, little time, fast action, an uncovered pan, and enough fat to coat the sauté pan. Traditionally, pure oil or clarified butter is used. (Clarified butter is used because the solids have been removed, which decreases smoking and burning). Before sautéing, food is cut into small pieces—dices, strips, or slices—to increase its surface area, which speeds the cooking process.

There are two secrets to sautéing well: cook just a small amount of food at a time, and use very high heat. If you sauté only small amounts at a time, each piece can be heated and cooked by the fat very quickly, and the moisture does not escape from the food. If there is too much food in the pan, the temperature in the pan drops too low to brown the food, moisture escapes, and the food steams rather than sautés.

CLASSIC SAUTÉING VS. REALAGE "SAUTÉING"

Although sautéing has a popular reputation as a healthful cooking technique, sadly this reputation in restaurants is too often undeserved. In restaurants, sautéing is really more like pan-frying, and sometimes close to deep-frying. Some professional cooking texts recommend using as much as ⅛ inch of oil in the pan, and at least one such text equates sautéing with pan-frying. Actually, with that much fat, they are indeed the same.

Many chefs like to sauté cutlets and fillets, and added fat, aging or not, is always part of the technique because the fat in the pan merges with the fat or seasoning of the cuts, making them easy to cook and turn out of the pan. In fact, sautéing tenderloin gently in butter, not at high heat, preserves its lean shape and juiciness. Sautéing in butter unfortunately also ages you. Why pay to get older? A misting of olive oil would make your RealAge younger. Even omelets (actually, a sauté of egg) made in nonstick skillets usually have fat added to the pan first because it's easier for the chef to flip the omelet.

Can you sauté without fat? It's difficult. You can, if the food contains a certain amount of fat, if you use very high heat, if the pan is not crowded, and if the food touches the bottom or sides of the pan at all times. Using a touch of fat spread over the pan with a paper towel, plus a lot of spatula-turning work, I am able to sauté egg white–vegetable omelets.

So, unless you use enough fat, sautéing just doesn't work very well. Take, for example, aromatics—garlic, onions, shallots, and leeks. Each adds a slightly different flavor component to any given dish. Even cooking just two aromatics together adds complexity and depth to a dish. But without fat, the flavors of these foods are often restrained or absent. Misting the heavy-bottomed skillet with oil will bring out some, maybe much, of these flavors. I usually do not use a nonstick pan because less caramelization and browning can occur than with other skillets. In addition, nonstick skillets often cannot take the heat as well as cast-iron or heavy-bottomed cookware. Some cooks use just a teaspoon of oil for a preheated, very hot pan of sliced onions and garlic, with great success. (Learning how to sauté is worth *1 Kitchen IQ point.*)

Sautéing grains such as millet, barley, quinoa, and rices, or legumes such as lentils and yellow peas, gives a subtly different toastiness to each. Here a nonstick skillet performs well. Try misting the pan with oil, or adding a teaspoon of oil to coat the grains or legumes before cooking. Turn the temperature up high and stir or shake briskly, reducing the heat if the food starts to burn. Use a wooden spoon to keep the grains moving and prevent sticking. Rubber scrapers are not recommended, as they eventually melt.

A technique called "water sautéing" or "liquid sautéing" allows us to cook on the stovetop and enjoy moving the food around without adding fat. Enough stock, wine, juice, or sherry to cover the bottom of the pan is brought to a simmer, and food is added, shaken, and turned out when cooked. (Mike uses Ravenswood Zinfandel when "sautéing" many green vegetables.) This is actually simmering, poaching, or steaming the food, depending on whether it's submerged in the liquid, partially submerged, or floating. Each of these techniques yields its own flavors, but none is really sautéing.

Using a bottle filled with an infused oil, you can add flavor to sautés in two ways: by using enough fat to bring out the flavor of accompanying aromatics, and by adding the flavors of spices or herbs that come with your oil. I use canola oil for infusions and for cooking, as it is mild and has the least saturated fat of any widely available cooking oil. You could also use peanut oil, with its very high smoking point, as long as you don't overdo it. A squeeze from a squirt bottle is just ¼ teaspoon. I occasionally use extra-virgin olive oil for sautéing. With its strong or delicate taste, I know that it will leave its own flavor in the dish, even at the high heat needed for sautéing.

Microwave Cooking

Cooking in a microwave oven is a nearly all-purpose technique that professional and home cooks alike seldom use. Indeed, some of the finest restaurants in America still do not have a microwave oven. Those that do try not to talk about it. Why? It is considered amateurish. The microwave oven cooks without fat or salt—ingredients without which most chefs do not cook well. However, this characteristic can make the microwave oven RealAge-smart.

Microwaving does not lend itself to high-fat cooking because of the way food is cooked. Microwaves—short electromagnetic waves—penetrate food from the outside in, vibrating water molecules and generating heat. As a result, the food doesn't get much hotter than the boiling point of water—212 degrees Fahrenheit. Unfortunately, this temperature is not high enough to brown the outside surface of food or to caramelize it (brown it by heating the sugar in it). Browning meat, for example, begins at 310°F! So microwaving, while not usually suitable for preparing complete dinners, is great when you need simplicity and speed. Microwave cooking does not require the careful monitoring necessary for broiling, grilling, or roasting, or the quick responses needed in sautéing and deglazing. All you need is the microwave oven and a large microwave-safe nonmetal bowl or plate.

The microwave takes on a whole new persona in RealAge cooking. You can simmer, steam, boil, reheat, reduce, infuse, poach, and braise in the microwave. (Learning how to use the microwave not only for steaming vegetables but also for poaching, braising, cooking grains, and reducing liquids is worth *1 Kitchen IQ point.*) Sounds like a technique to make your RealAge younger. *But,* of course, we want and will insist on great taste, too!

THE MICROWAVE AND VEGETABLES

The microwave oven was made for cooking specific foods, and for vegetables, it's the best. In fact, I use the microwave primarily to steam vegetables, and that can produce great taste. My own oven uses 800 watts, and many microwave recipes are written for just about that amount of power. I almost always microwave on high and just vary the time.

Almost all vegetables steam well in the microwave—the moisture in vegetables is usually enough to cook them. Steam whole asparagus upright in a Pyrex tumbler and watch the stalks deepen and brighten in color. Steam florets of broccoli or sliced or julienned carrots in a round covered microwaveable dish just until the broccoli is bright green and the carrots are a radiant orange. To ensure even cooking, halfway through the time, stir the outside pieces toward the center or use a turntable. Corn on the cob steams—and surprises when dabbed with chili powder and a squeeze of lime. (One key to great taste is adding stocks, juices, sauces, herbs, and flavorings.) Arrange the ears in a spoke-like pattern, with the tip toward the center of the hub, before microwaving. Arrange other whole vegetables (even potatoes) in a circle, piercing those with skins, so steam can escape.

You can also poach and braise in the microwave. Strongly-flavored greens and root vegetables cook perfectly in beef, chicken, or vegetable stock. Collard greens, chard, and beet greens become smooth and velvety. Kale softens and its hidden sweetness emerges. Celery root and parsnips both become scented and tender, especially when diced and mashed with a little roasted garlic, salt, and pepper. You can poach whole fruits—plums, pears, apricots, and figs—in sweet wine, apple cider, or even water; they keep their shape and retain their essential tastes. Just fill the microwaveable dish to the needed level and cover; uncover after 5 minutes, and let the steam escape. Fruits poached in the microwave are done when they're fragrant and just soft.

THE MICROWAVE AND GRAINS

You can use the microwave for some grains and the stovetop for others, when you can sauté or pan-roast first. Couscous cooks in the microwave in the time it takes the stock, V-8 juice, or broth to simmer, plus 5 minutes: just add and let the grain absorb the liquid. Polenta cooks in water, stock, milk, or juice in 10 minutes using ordinary cornmeal. Risotto cooks in 18 minutes in the microwave, without the endless standing at the stove, stirring, adding of stock, and paying attention to the possible burning, sticking, or drying out. To microwave risotto, add the cooking liquid to the rice and zap; there's no need for tablespoons of butter or cream. It's naturally creamy. Risotto is a great RealAge treat when microwaved.

THE MICROWAVE FOR INFUSING AND REDUCING

You can infuse oils and vinegars in the microwave. For oils in particular, however, the microwave is deceptively efficient, and hot oil looks much the same as oil that is only warm. Warm for only 10 seconds, and then infuse to your heart's content.

Reduction is a snap in the microwave. You can go from liquid to sauce to demi-glace to glaze in as little as 10 minutes, depending on the starting quantity. The secret? Reduce in a microwave-safe container, do not cover, and use your timer. Reducing in the microwave is efficient, easy, and saves on cleanup—no pan or pot is needed.

Steaming

Steaming is often (but not always) a technique used for food that cooks quickly (such as shrimp) or food that might fall apart on the grill or in the pan (such as delicate fish fillets). The food is cooked by hot steam that rises from boiling water below and the food never touches the water. Steaming is a particularly healthful and low-calorie way to cook, as no extra aging fats are used. Also, vitamins that would be lost if you boiled certain foods, such as vegetables, are retained when you steam. (Don't overcook vegetables in your steamer; when the colors turn bright, they're usually ready. Learning how to steam is worth *3 Kitchen IQ points.*)

As with many aspects of cooking, you can buy beautiful, expensive steaming equipment, or you can put something together that will work just as well. For example, you can set a plate or rack on top of inverted cups inside a pot. A glass lid is handy because you can see the food without having to release steam, but if you don't have one, don't worry. Briefly removing the lid to check on your food won't affect the progress of cooking.

Steaming is used very often in Chinese cuisine. Take a trip to the Chinatown in the city nearest you and pick up a multi-layered bamboo steamer. It's very inexpensive, is a beautiful object to have in your kitchen, and allows you to steam several dishes at once, while adding and taking away layers to vary the cooking times. Before you leave Chinatown, visit some produce stores or stands and buy something you haven't tried before, such as bok choy or fresh vegetable dumplings, and steam them in your new steamer when you get home. Chinese produce shops are a feast for the senses and can inspire you to try new dishes. They are chock-full of good new ingredients that make your RealAge younger deliciously.

Poaching

Poaching is similar to steaming in its methodology and age-reducing benefits but involves placing the food in, not above, gently simmering water. (With the exception of pasta, most foods are never cooked in water at a rolling boil.) For extra flavor, poach your food in wine or low-sodium broth and experiment with adding different herbs, such as thyme or bay leaves. (Learning how to poach is worth *1 Kitchen IQ point.*) You can control the temperature by covering, partially covering, or completely uncovering the pot. These cooking techniques, together with juicy marinades and lots of fresh herbs, add zest and zing to meals every time. Go ahead! Be intense! Be younger!

Always Having RealAge Food on Hand: Freezing

Understanding how to freeze food properly is a vital part of your repertoire as a RealAge cook. Freezing enables you to provide healthy, nutrient-rich food for your family, and to have it available on really short notice. Also, when food has been prepared in advance and frozen, having it so easily available decreases stress. For cost-conscious consumers, buying in bulk and freezing for later use can help keep you within budget. For gardeners, learning the best methods of freezing produce will dramatically lengthen the time that the garden's yield can be enjoyed. For busy working people, freezing is the ultimate time-saver and stress-reducer.

However, freezing is more than simply tossing anything and everything into the freezer and then taking it out to thaw. Although the process is relatively simple, certain procedures help ensure best results. Learning how to freeze and then freezing extra portions of dishes is worth *15 Kitchen IQ points.* (It is that important!) Here are the three most important principles of freezing:

1. Try to freeze only the freshest food. Food should be frozen as soon as possible after it is harvested from the garden, purchased from the store, or baked in the oven, once cooled (*3 Kitchen IQ points*).

2. Remove all excess air from the packaging. Excess air will draw moisture out of the food, which may compromise the taste and texture (*3 Kitchen IQ points*).

3. Use frozen foods in a timely manner. It's impossible to safeguard against *all* loss of taste, texture, or vitamins, but you can minimize such losses by labeling with the date, rotating the contents of the freezer, and then eating what's in the freezer so that nothing is frozen too long (*2 Kitchen IQ points*).

What You'll Need

• **A freezer in a convenient location.** The freezer in your refrigerator is a good start. It's handy, it's already there, and it may need to be cleaned out anyway. If you plan to freeze food regularly, invest in a separate freezer, either the upright or the chest style. It should maintain a constant temperature of zero degrees Fahrenheit or lower (monitor the temperature with a thermometer); keeping frozen food at 25 or 30 degrees Fahrenheit for just one day does more damage to its flavor and nutritional quality than keeping the food frozen at zero degrees for a year. For the sake of your utility bill, keep the unit in an area that averages 50 to 68 degrees Fahrenheit, slightly below normal (the lower, the better).

• **Clear storage containers.** Use either the disposable plastic kind or the more expensive glass Pyrex-type that can go from freezer to microwave to table. I use inexpensive ½- and ¾-liter glass tumblers from Crate and Barrel. Why clear? So you can see what's inside!

• **Plastic wrap and extra-heavy aluminum foil.** You need these for packaging food.

• **Masking tape and a felt-tip permanent pen** for marking food with "thaw-by" dates, a description of the contents, and any instructions (such as "thin with broth").

Use your own freezer and taste experience to help create your guide for "thaw-by" dates. Regular masking tape is as good as the more expensive freezer tape.

Remember: freeze fast, thaw slowly (*3 Kitchen IQ points*). Freezing food quickly helps prevent the formation of ice crystals between food fibers, which decreases food quality. Also, always separate food into individual serving sizes before freezing (*6 Kitchen IQ points*). It is vital that the packaging be airtight. One way to remove air is to plunge the bag into a bowl or pot of cool water, keeping the open end of the bag out of the water. The water pressure forces excess air out of the bag. Tie or seal the bag before removing it from the water.

Your freezer should be stocked gradually, to keep the temperature as constant as possible. When you do add new food to the freezer, place it near the wall of the freezer, shifting the already-frozen food to the center. The exception to this rule applies to bread or other fresh-baked goods, which tend to attract too much moisture next to the freezer wall. Place these items against already-frozen packages in the center.

In general, freezing can stop the development of molds and bacteria, but it does not eradicate them. Thawed food will spoil more quickly than if it hadn't been frozen, so be sure to use thawed food in a timely manner. Do not refreeze thawed food.

If you and your family are to enjoy once-frozen RealAge foods, they must taste as great as you prepared them. That means the freezer must be working properly. If you have a stand-alone freezer that is not self-defrosting, the freezer should be emptied completely and defrosted every six months, or when the frost on the walls is a ½ inch thick. This keeps your freezer working properly, ensuring that your "thaw-by" dates are valid, and that no food remains frozen for too long. Using pans of hot water can expedite defrosting of an emptied freezer; however, they should be placed on a cookie rack or some other device that keeps the pan from actually touching the freezer, as direct heat can damage the freezer floor and walls. Wipe down the inside of the defrosted freezer and make sure it is completely dry before you turn it on again.

What to Freeze

FRESH VEGETABLES

Vegetables are a staple of the RealAge diet. Learning how to prepare them deliciously and having the few pieces of equipment so great-tasting vegetables are available year-round increases your Kitchen IQ. Eating five servings (a serving is the size of a small fist) of vegetables a day can make your RealAge as much as five years younger. Because vegetables contain lots of fiber, they help fill you up fast. At only 20 to 50 calories a serving, vegetables help you feel full and keep your weight down. One patient I worked with, who periodically has a weight problem, loses weight on a diet that allows unlimited servings of vegetables. With that program she loses weight even though she averages over twenty-five (yes 25!) servings of vegetables a day. That, coupled with exercise, makes her one healthy woman because vegetables are also full of vitamins, carotenoids, and flavonoids. Many of these substances have antioxidant properties that will help keep you young. And freezing vegetables is a key to keeping your RealAge younger.

It may surprise you to know how many types of vegetables can be frozen successfully. Blanching and then freezing (5 Kitchen IQ points) your garden produce is a wonderful way to extend summer's pleasure well into autumn. If the vegetables are garden fresh and are blanched and frozen properly, their taste is close to that of freshly picked produce. Although you may not be familiar with the process of blanching, it's simple and well worth learning.

Simply stated, blanching slows or stops the enzymatic process that continues after a vegetable is harvested. Slowing down that process is vital for good taste of a vegetable that has been frozen. There are two methods by which you can blanch vegetables: by boiling or by steaming. Boiling takes longer, has a high risk of losing the vitamins and minerals from vegetables (since most of the vitamins are just under the skin), and requires a large pot or a powerful microwave oven. For a RealAge cook, steaming is a better option, since you won't lose vitamins or nutrients. Steaming, which starts when water begins to simmer, can be accomplished in a variety of containers—rice makers, wire baskets, actual steamers, and so on. Vegetables with high water content, such as squash or corn (cut from the cob), can be steamed easily.

How to Blanch Vegetables for Freezing. Blanching by steaming is the method I recommend. Special blanching equipment is available at cooking specialty stores, but you can probably put something together more economically that will work just fine. You'll need a large pot (minimum 6 quarts) with a tight-fitting lid and a wire basket that can fit inside.

The vegetables are kept above the water, not in it, and the pot is covered. Time the blanching from when the steam starts to escape from under the lid. While you are bringing the water to a boil in your large pot, you'll also want to set up an ice bath (ice cubes and water) for your vegetables, perhaps in the kitchen sink or in another large pot. Put about a pound of vegetables in a wire basket that will stay above the water, catching the steam. Make sure the vegetables are evenly exposed to the steam. When the blanching time is up, lift the basket out of the pot and immerse it in the ice bath. (Some vegetables are not immersed but simply cooled over the ice water—see chart.) Spread out plenty of paper towels for blotting and drying the vegetables after they have emerged from the ice bath. It's imperative that your vegetables be completely dry before packaging.

Timing is the key element in blanching vegetables. Here are blanching and chilling times for some of the most common garden vegetables:

Times for Blanching Vegetables

Vegetable	Blanching	Chilling
Beans, including lima, green, and wax beans	Steam for 1½ min.	Chill for 4 to 5 min. in ice water.
Broad beans	Steam for 5 min. in the pod.	Chill for 5 min. in ice water; shell.
Beets	Steam until tender.	Cool over, not in, the ice water.
Broccoli, washed and split	Steam for 3 to 5 min.	Chill for 5 min. in ice water.
Brussels sprouts	Steam for 6 or 7 min.	Chill for 10 min. in ice water.
Cabbage, leaves or shredded	Steam until tender.	Cool over, not in, the ice water.
Carrots, well scrubbed	Steam for 4 min.	Chill for 5 min. in the ice water.
Cauliflower, florets	Steam for 3 min.	Chill for 4 min. in the ice water.
Celery, chopped	Steam until tender.	Cool over, not in, the ice water.
Chard	Steam for 1½ min.	Chill for 5 min. in the ice water.
Green peas	Steam for 1 to 3½ min.	Chill for 3 to 5 min. in ice water.
Kale	Boil or steam for 5 to 7 min.	Chill for 5 min. in ice water.
Mushrooms	Steam for 4 min.	Chill for 5 min. in the ice water.

Vegetable	Blanching	Chilling
Mustard greens	Boil or steam until tender.	Cool over, not in, the ice water.
Parsnips	Steam for 3 min.	Chill for 5 min. in the ice water.
Peppers	Steam for 2½ min.	Chill for 4 or 5 min. in ice water.
Pumpkin, puréed	Boil or steam until tender.	Cool over, not in, the ice water.
Rutabaga	Steam for 2½ min.	Chill for 5 min. in the ice water.
Spinach	Steam for 3 min.	Chill for 3 min. in the ice water.
Squash, Winter	Steam until tender.	Cool over, not in, the ice water.
Turnips, peeled and sliced	Steam for 1½ min.	Chill for 5 min. in the ice water.
Turnip greens	Boil or steam for 2 to 2½ min.	Chill for 4 min. in the ice water.

In general, cook frozen vegetables straight from the freezer—don't thaw them first. When you use frozen blanched vegetables, they will need to be cooked only one-half to one-third the time required for fresh vegetables, as they got a jump-start on the cooking process when they were blanched.

Unfortunately, many typical salad ingredients (such as fresh lettuce, tomatoes, onions, and cucumber) do not freeze well. Don't attempt to freeze them, as you'll just waste food—they'll turn out mushy and dull. Instead, enjoy them as much as you can from your garden during summer months, and, at other times, depend on your local farmers' market or grocery store for your salads.

Like everything else, learning to blanch vegetables properly takes practice. If you have a friend or relative who has a garden and some experience blanching produce, ask him or her to oversee your first try.

Just because you hated vegetables as a kid doesn't mean you won't like them now. Try eating them cooked just a little but prepared and combined with other foods in as many ways as possible. This book will give you plenty of ideas. Once defrosted, try steaming them with a little lemon juice or sautéing them lightly. Cook most green vegetables just until they turn bright green. If they turn dull green or gray, you've cooked them way too long. Make vegetables your new snack food: purchase bags of precut or baby vegetables and keep them in the fridge.

How to Roast Vegetables for Freezing. Roasting vegetables is another excellent way to prepare them for freezing. (You can also roast and freeze some fruit in a similar way.) Roasting is an excellent choice for the RealAge cook, as the process intensifies the natural flavors of the food. Although fat is required to keep the vegetables from sticking to the pan, a couple of teaspoons of olive oil should suffice for a small pan (I use a paper towel to spread the oil and remove the excess), or you might try an olive or a canola oil cooking spray (Spectrum makes an excellent expeller cold-pressed canola oil spray). As with all foods in the RealAge Kitchen plan, the best-quality organic vegetables will yield the most delicious results.

Roasting is extremely easy. After washing and chopping the vegetables, put them in a roasting pan and toss them with a little olive oil. (The vegetables should be in a single layer; try to leave a little space between the vegetables. It is okay if they overlap a little, since vegetables will shrink as they cook.) The roasting pan should be large and not more than 2 inches deep, or the vegetables may simply steam. Use a heavy, flat pan (without grooves for draining fat and juices). Don't buy disposable aluminum pans, which are too flimsy. Roasting pans vary in size; a standard one is 18 × 13 × 2 inches. Usually you will not cover the pan. For a small quantity of vegetables, a sheet pan or a half-sheet pan or a glass pie dish may be sufficient. Toss the vegetable pieces with your hands so there's an even coating of oil.

Preheat the oven to 450 degrees, then put in the pan. A high temperature is necessary so that you don't just steam the vegetables in their own moisture. Use a clean oven to avoid generating smoke at such a high heat. Halfway through the roasting time, shake the pan gently to rotate the vegetables, or take it out to turn the vegetables over. When you open the oven, there will be a blast of hot, steamy air, so take care to avert your face.

You can cook individual vegetables separately, or you can combine different vegetables that have the same cooking time. Experiment with the addition of herbs, spices, and a small amount of vinegar, lemon juice, and other flavorings before and after roasting.

Here are some common vegetables and the time you'll need to roast them. Any longer time will caramelize some, such as beets, parsnips, and onions, and simply crisp and darken others, such as broccoli and potatoes. (As with most aspects of cooking, once you've roasted several times, you'll probably be able to gauge for yourself and won't need the chart, but do continue to experiment with herbs, vinegars, lemon juice, and other flavorings.)

Time for Roasting Vegetables

Vegetables	Time (minutes)
Beets, baby	30
Bell peppers and small poblano chiles, sliced	10
Broccoli florets	10
Fennel slices	20
Garlic head, unpeeled	20
Leeks, roughly chopped	20
Mushrooms, whole portabello	10
Onions, wedges	20
Parsnips, chunks	20
Potatoes, wedges	20
Shallots, large whole	20
Shallots, medium	10
Sweet potatoes, wedges	20
Tomatoes, wedges	5
Turnips, wedges	20

A RealAge kitchen tip: Roasting zucchini yields mush.

After the vegetables have cooled, pat them dry, wrap them tightly in clear plastic wrap, and freeze them.

POULTRY

Most cuts of poultry freeze well. Within two days of purchase, chicken should be frozen if it is not cooked. A slight discoloration of the bones can result, but this is harmless. Do not freeze stuffed poultry. Freeze stuffing separately, then stuff the bird after thawing. Poultry freezes best when patted dry before being wrapped in clear, air-tight wrapping. I try to cool the cooked bird in the refrigerator, often for a couple of hours, before wrapping very well and transferring it to the freezer. Wrapping well prevents freezer burn.

FISH AND SHELLFISH

As with all other foods, fish freezes best when fresh. Shellfish runs the risk of getting tough if frozen too long, so eat frozen shellfish within a month or so. Shrimp should be frozen uncooked, in their shells. Lobster and crab are best cooked, shelled, and then frozen. Fish freezes best when patted dry before being wrapped in clear, airtight plastic wrap.

SOUPS, BROTHS, AND STEWS

These dishes are all perfect candidates for freezing, and having them on hand to serve later on is an enormous time-saver. When making dishes such as Rich and Spicy Black Bean Soup (page 291) or Tortellini Stew with Fresh Soybeans (page 172), *always* double the recipe and freeze half. Here's another RealAge kitchen tip: use ice cubes to cool your soup before you freeze it. The process will happen more quickly, and the extra water from the ice cubes will evaporate when you reheat the soup.

Remember to freeze these foods in the amounts you intend to serve (worth up to 6 *Kitchen IQ points*). If you have a small family and make a big pot of soup, freeze the portions in several small containers. (You can always thaw more than one if you decide you won't have enough, or if you have guests.)

FRUIT JUICES

Fresh-squeezed fruit juices and fruit smoothies are excellent candidates for freezing. Remember that liquid expands by about 20 percent when frozen, so package accordingly. Leave at least ½ inch below the lip of a cup container.

SAUCES

Sauces, such as pesto sauce or pasta sauce, and chicken or vegetable stocks are great time-savers to have in the freezer. Sauces and stocks make your RealAge younger in two ways: they lessen the stress of food preparation and they provide great-tasting, RealAge-smart food whenever you want it. As with soups and stews, always double your recipe and freeze half. For strongly flavored, concentrated sauces, here's another RealAge kitchen tip: freeze these sauces in an ice cube tray so you can use small amounts each time.

CHEESE

Hard cheeses are excellent candidates for freezing. RealAge recipes call for just a pinch of a cheese such as Parmigiano-Reggiano (real Italian parmesan) for flavoring. Simply grate a little from the frozen block of cheese, then rewrap it and return the block to the freezer. Or unwrap the whole block, thaw, shave curls off the block, and sprinkle them on top of your salads. You can use a small amount because a small amount of an intense flavor is all that is needed. Although all cheese contains saturated fat, and saturated fat ages the arteries and immune system, all of us can live better with a shaving of cheese.

BREADS

For almost everyone—small households and large—freezing bread is a great way to justify buying an excellent, crusty loaf from a favorite bakery without worrying that it won't all be eaten before it goes stale. Simply cut the loaf in half as soon as you get it home (that way you won't eat too much because of the guilt or fear of wasting food). After cutting the loaf in half, wrap it securely in airtight packaging, and put it in the middle of the freezer.

NUTS

Nuts such as almonds, pecans, and pine nuts—all an important part of the RealAge diet—will keep in the freezer very successfully. They can be frozen either shelled or unshelled. Just make sure you have a clear, airtight container. An ounce of nuts, five days of the week, can make your RealAge more than 3.3 years younger.

PIZZA DOUGH

Freezing pizza dough that has been baked (but not enough to become thoroughly cooked) is a perfect way to ensure a quick, delicious, and healthful meal at the end of a busy day. (Generally, you don't want to freeze unbaked pizza dough, as the extremely low temperature may kill the yeast and the dough may not rise later.) See the recipes for great RealAge-smart pizza on pages 158 and 163.

COOKIES, CAKES, AND OTHER TREATS

As explained in my first book, eating the RealAge way is about having dessert first. It's not about self-denial, so why not keep treats in your freezer, too? Of course, we hope that these are real chocolate-covered strawberries or bananas, or cookies and cakes that you have made yourself, substituting drained applesauce for saturated fats in baking, using healthy oils like canola and olive oil, and avoiding, whenever possible, almost all simple, empty-calorie sugars.

An added benefit of freezing is that when you must defrost a cookie or a piece of banana bread before you can eat it, you will not be tempted by the always-available full cookie jar or whole loaf of banana bread. It's easier to control your portion sizes—out of sight, out of mind. We love to keep our freezers stocked with fat-free sorbets, zucchini bread made with applesauce instead of shortening, and frozen Twix bars (John only).

Thawing

Remember the RealAge kitchen tip and the rule for freezing: *freeze quickly, thaw slowly.* The more rapidly food is thawed, the more likely its quality will suffer. Frozen food should always be thawed slowly in its packaging, preferably in the refrigerator. In the refrigerator, a whole (4 pound) chicken takes about 24 hours to thaw; chicken breasts take 3 to 8 hours to thaw. Thawing at room temperature is the next best option. Never thaw food uncovered, as this invites harmful bacteria. If you are pressed for time and the packaging on the food is completely waterproof, you can immerse the package in cool (not warm or hot) water to expedite the process.

Once you've had time to retrain your family's taste buds, start cooking in quantity. Freeze a large portion that's been divided into convenient amounts—*and* get used to the extra time you'll have. Congratulations! You're well on your way to a new, healthier RealAge lifestyle that will help you and your family feel great and live longer.

By the way, for another *10 Kitchen IQ points,* keep a set of free weights next to the kitchen and use them often, while waiting. For more about exercise, see Chapter 9 in *The RealAge Diet* or the Web site www.RealAge.com (go to the RealAge Café site and click on "My Fitness Plan").

As you develop as a cook and learn the fundamental methods so that they become second nature, you can broaden your cooking repertoire. Here's a unique and innovative approach to adding flavor to food, the seven RealAge "Assists."

RealAge "ASSISTS" to Flavor

For a cooking demonstration before a medical audience at a San Diego hotel, John was forced to create several no-cook, no-fat ways to enhance flavor. These flavor-enhancing methods had to involve no cooking because the hotel would not allow the use of a heating element in the conference room. So, with just a blender and a paring knife, John showed the audience members how they could boost flavor in several ways, calling these methods "ASSIST." For RealAge methods, we add an S for ASSISTS. Here are the seven buzzwords that will help you remember how to make cooking food even more fun and pleasurable and make your RealAge younger:

- Acidification
- Smell
- Spices
- Infusions
- Symmetry
- Tubes
- Senses

(Using these seven methods to enhance flavor boosts your *Kitchen IQ by 1 point each.*)

Acidify Your Foods

Used sparingly, acids enliven and brighten many foods. For example, traditional vinaigrettes (three-to-one mixtures of oil and vinegar) and lemon juice enhance almost any kind of seafood. The trick is to choose an acid that is doubly flavorful, so you're adding not only the tingle of the acid but another taste element as well. Citrus fruits do this naturally: they have a sweetness that tempers their sourness. Infusing white distilled vinegar with another ingredient modifies its harshness and gives it another dimension. When cider and wine vinegars are infused with another ingredient, yet another dimension emerges: the fruitiness of the cider, the mellowed tannin of the wines, and the pucker power of the acid. This acidification epitomizes RealAge cooking and the RealAge kitchen: it produces great taste and nutrient-rich but calorie-poor creations.

Vinegars are the most common type of acid and most of us have them in our pantries. Distilled vinegar, fruit vinegar, rice vinegar, and herb vinegars all have special uses. Keeping a variety of vinegars in your pantry increases your kitchen's IQ. I use distilled vinegar primarily for pickling and sometimes for chutney. The tangy fruitiness of a good fruit vinegar really wakes up salads and salsas; it's also good on couscous, bulgur, and baby lettuces. Rice vinegar is often lightly seasoned and mild—just sharp enough to complement the bite of serrano peppers and to harmonize with napa cabbage (one of the Chinese cabbages) or green cabbage. Herb vinegars are multidimensional, often have wine or cider vinegar as a base, and are easy to make.

Our favorite vinegars that increase a kitchen's IQ are high-quality traditional balsamic vinegar and sherry vinegar. Both are aged and strong in flavor. Although they can be expensive, they last a long time and are worth the money. We usually use only a few drops at a time. Add them to the cooking liquids for grains and to tomato sauces for pasta, and sprinkle them on sautéed vegetables or fresh berries and fruits.

Smell Your Food

Your sense of smell is responsible for as much as 80 percent of what is known as taste. It had long been thought that aging destroys a person's sense of smell, but recent data indicate this is not part of normal aging. We should be able to enjoy great smells and tastes well into the triple digits. That enjoyment of smell can help you have a younger RealAge. When you eat, the aroma of the food in your mouth wafts toward your nose and throat; when this aroma and your nose, soft palate (roof of the mouth), and taste buds all work together, you "taste" the food. So, if you can't smell, it's hard to taste.

What can you do to get the full benefits of the wonderful aroma of food? One way is to inhale the aroma and focus on it. Is it floral? Fruity? Spicy? Concentrating on "smell" makes you appreciate the great tastes of RealAge food. Also, you can maximize the aroma of fresh herbs by crushing them. However, don't overdo it—just crush them enough to release their perfume. Toast grains to bring out their taste—a nuttiness for bulgur and a light perfume for jasmine rice. Toast and grind spices; all will produce a lot of taste with just a little effort.

Add Spices (and Herbs) to Your Foods

Because they're aromatic wonders, spices pack more wallop per gram than any other food. What is a spice? Herbs are leaves, and spices are everything else—buds, blossoms, stems and roots. Just crush the spice between your thumb and forefinger, or in a mortar and pestle, or in a spice grinder, and the whole kitchen fills with the scent. This increases your kitchen's IQ as it offers intensified flavor.

One secret to using spices is to roast them before grinding or crushing them, to release their oils. See "Pan Roasting," page 95, for tips on pan-roasting spices. If spices are over-roasted, they can become bitter. Even if they're not over-roasted, they can become bitter if they're cooked too long. That's why freshly ground pepper is added at the end of cooking, not earlier. Seeds toast best, and you can use your nose to tell when they're done. If they blacken or smoke, throw them out and start over.

Most spices last about six months in the cupboard, and lose their punch if not kept airtight. Should you throw spices out after a certain amount of time? If their aroma is musty, yes. But if it's just faint, sometimes you can rescue them and use them in the dish you're making by toasting the spices lightly, letting them cool, crushing them, and adding a little extra. Careful, though—taste the spice before cooling or adding to the dish to be cooked. (We believe in throwing the spices out after six months. Rarely can you prolong the life of dried herbs or spices by storing in the refrigerator or freezer; but this is not usually helpful as they seem not to age well in the refrigerator or freezer.)

We've included herbs with spices here because the two are related and because both are critically important in flavor-intense cooking. Herbs (leaves) have the brightest, most delicate taste when they're fresh, and are more concentrated and potent when they are dried. In general, a dried herb is three times more powerful in flavor than an equal amount of fresh herb. Dried herbs are usually added at the beginning of cooking; fresh herbs should be added at the end.

Herbs are rewarding culinary investments. Most are easy to grow and can survive droughts, neglect, and window-box culture. Growing fresh herbs is not only economical and easy but also a year-round joy in the kitchen (see Chapter 11).

Experiment with Infusions

Intensifying the flavor or adding flavor to plain vinegars and oils can produce fabulous tastes without added calories or saturated fats, making infusions RealAge-smart. The simplest way to infuse juices, vinegars, and oils is to submerge some gently bruised fresh herbs, dried spices, citrus zest, or crushed aromatics in the liquid, and pour the mixture into a clean bottle. Cover with a lid and let the bottle rest in a sunny window for a week. Then strain the flavoring agent out of the liquid and store the liquid in another clean, covered container, such as a wine bottle, in the refrigerator.

Another method is a little more elaborate, but yields more flavor. Place your favorite oil and the chosen flavoring in a blender, give it a brief whirl and, using cheesecloth or a fine filter, let the now infused oil slowly drip, drip, drip into another scrupulously clean container. This process takes time and patience, but it produces a depth of flavor that could otherwise be obtained only with mild heat and two weeks of incubation.

The incubation method is probably the most reliable way to infuse. Warming both oils and vinegars with the flavoring seems to add more tang. (But be careful to keep the solution acid—pH 4.0 or less for aficionados—with vinegars as warming can activate spores.) The stems of herbs contain more tannin than the leaves, so if you want pure herbal flavor, strip the leaves and put the stems aside for another purpose, such as making vegetable stock. Otherwise, just gently warm the liquid on the stove and add the herbs—stems and all—stewing them just until their color brightens. Do not simmer or bubble, just bathe the herbs. Pour the liquid-herb mixture through cheesecloth into a clean, dry bottle and set it aside in a cool, dark place.

Use the freshest herbs you can find for infusions and don't be afraid to use plenty—you'll get more flavor. When you use citrus zest, crush it gently between your fingers to release the oils. Strands of orange, lemon, lime, and grapefruit zest are also beautiful additions to infusions.

For vinegars, I like to use herbs, spices, and dried fruits. Raisins, figs, berries, dried mango, and dried papaya all add complexity and sweetness to an otherwise puckery vinegar taste. (Try the delicious combination of fig balsamic vinegar and lemon zest.) Fruit vinegars have the best flavor if the fruit and vinegar are simmered together for a few seconds. Try mixing a quart of good white wine vinegar, 2 cups or more of berries, and several sprigs of mint or dill. Let the berries steep (soak) in this mixture in a clean, covered jar in the refrigerator for two weeks before straining. Experiment to see what you like. For example, after infusing the vinegar, leave the berries in. (It's really worth the trouble to make raspberry white wine vinegar; it has a wonderful fruit flavor that's great on salads. In clear Bordeaux bottles, the color of red raspberries is a translucent cranberry.)

Here are some of our favorite vinegar-infusion combinations:

Blueberry-dill vinegar
Raspberry-mint vinegar
Parsley, sage, rosemary, and thyme vinegar
Fennel–opal basil vinegar
Cranberry-clove vinegar
Lemongrass-chile vinegar

Herbs, hot peppers, and aromatics also lend great flavor to oils. I like canola oil for infusing because it has a neutral flavor, packs plenty of omega-3 and monounsaturated fatty acids, and absorbs flavor well. To accentuate the color of herbs and the subsequent oil, microwave any green herb for just a few seconds. The green leaves of sweet basil brighten in an instant! Too much microwaving will dehydrate all herbs, so make it brief.

Here are some of my favorite oil-infusion combinations (remember to keep acid):

Roasted garlic–hazelnut oil

Rosemary–orange walnut oil

Garlic, oregano, bay olive oil

Lemon sesame oil

Black, white, pink, and green peppercorn olive oil

Habanero-cilantro canola oil

By the way, infused oils made by Consorzio and by Boyajian are carried by local markets, and have luscious flavor and deep color and are the next best thing to home-made. For juices, especially fruit juices, experiment with whole spices: cinnamon sticks, shaved nutmeg, whole cloves, allspice berries, and juniper berries are among our favorites.

Strive for Symmetry in Flavor Combinations

How do you decide which flavors go together? We try to balance something sharp with something smooth, and something sweet with something sour. We call this principle "symmetry." It relies on the use of the four types of taste buds—sweet, salt, sour, and bitter—and on playing one against the other.

The way to pair flavors successfully is first to identify what you already like. Decide whether it's a clear, single taste (such as straight black coffee, which is bitter) or more than one taste (such as coffee with sugar, which is both bitter and sweet). Fresh mango is sweet; fresh mango with lime is sweet and sour. Fresh jicama is sweet; fresh jicama with lime is sweet and sour; jicama with lime and salt is sweet, sour, and a little salty.

If you like more than one taste, adding another taste-bud dimension to dishes (for example, a little salt or ketchup to crisped potatoes and onions) can bring out both the essence of the vegetables and the mellowed tones produced by cooking. Over-whelming a dish with salt can make it taste just one way—salty—so you get only one flavor. Understanding and using symmetry in flavoring food requires both care and a light touch.

Use Tubes of Food

Use tubes of food—they're convenient and worth the cost. Tubes contain powerfully concentrated foods that are not meant to be eaten straight from the tube. They're usually combined with tiny amounts of olive oil and occasionally with salt. Anchovies, garlic, harissa (a gutsy Moroccan red pepper hot sauce), olives, onions, sun-dried tomatoes, puréed tomatoes, and wasabi (Japanese horseradish) are all available in toothpaste-like tubes that have screw tops. Keep them in the refrigerator once opened. Tubes are nutrient rich, calorie poor, and add fabulous flavor so they increase your kitchen's IQ and make you RealAge younger.

These concentrates add an instant boost to sauces, dressings, and marinades. They can also add zip to the liquid used for cooking grains (but not beans, as beans toughen if salt or acid is added to the cooking liquid), and they add depth to pizza bases or cracker spreads.

Tubes are economical but not inexpensive. Although a 5-ounce tube can be $4, it's worth the extra money if it keeps you from throwing out sprouted garlic and onions, or almost whole cans of tomato paste that are minus 2 tablespoons. Tubes are also space- and time-savers: they're smaller than a basket of tomatoes, packages of sun-dried tomatoes, or jars of sun-dried tomatoes packed in olive oil, and they are faster to use than opening cans or packages, or slicing fresh tomatoes.

Use Your Sense of Color and Beauty When Preparing Food

Do your best to make your meals a full sensory treat: a production of beautiful colors, seductive smells, great tastes, and pleasurable feelings. Your dinnerware should be a source of enjoyment. The more pride you can take and the more pleasure your cookware, cooking, and presentations can give, the more food enjoyment you will have. We all need these enjoyments to overwhelm the stresses of life. Making eating a joyful, sensuous experience with beautiful cookware, dishes, and pleasurable smells makes you younger. Cooking should even *sound* good. Blend the richest colors and enjoy *all* of the sensual aspects of food. Remember, food is a celebration—a daily celebration that can foster a more energetic, vital, and younger life.

6 RealAge Cooking and Your Family

Helping your family members achieve their youngest RealAges says you want them around for a long time. Here are some tips and tricks you can use to help your family enjoy RealAge cooking—fabulous-tasting food that is also healthy and easy to make. Even getting your teenagers into the act isn't that tough.

Our social supports definitely reduce the aging effects of stress, and one of the best social supports is family. Happily married couples live longer than single people and with a higher quality of life. Although few data exist for unmarried people in long-term, mutually monogamous relationships, the same is probably true. Thus, people who live together should care about one another, and about the food the partner consumes. If your spouse is as interested as you are in making your RealAge younger, and enthusiastically participates in the RealAge lifestyle, congratulations! He or she is showing love for you and will probably be around to share a vigorous and happy life.

People who say they're happily married have as much as a 6.5-year younger RealAge than their unmarried counterparts. Widowhood and divorce can have an even greater impact on aging than being single. Studies in three countries found that successfully married men were less likely to have cardiovascular disease than unmarried men, even if their bad (LDL) cholesterol levels were much higher.

In making your RealAge younger, marriage seems to be more important to men than to women. A 35-year-old man who is happily married has a 6.3 year younger RealAge than his single counterpart. Women who are under age 50 show a RealAge benefit of only 2.4 years for being married and little effect for being divorced. Why? The disparity may relate to underlying social differences between the genders. We don't know for sure, but we assume that contemporary American women are more likely than men to have strong social support outside marriage. As popular psychologists "Dr. Phil" and John Gray note, outside of marriage, women (from Venus) tend to befriend, while for men (from Mars), it's fight or flight. This difference means that the social support of marriage is much more key for men than for women. Also, women are more likely than men to suffer from abuse within their marriage. About half of the divorced women under age 50 seem to have an older RealAge, and about half have a younger one. Those who get younger may do so because of the benefits of leaving unhappy relationships. However, marriage becomes increasingly important to women as they get older. After age 50, women show a three-year benefit in RealAge from being married and 3.5 years of aging from being divorced.

What does all of this mean to you? If you are happily married or involved in a stable, long-term relationship, it is making your RealAge younger. When you cook healthy food for your spouse, you are extending that benefit. Rationalizing bad food choices—"Well, he likes ice cream, so I'll treat him to a quart"—is not the way to "treat" your spouse. Such food choices will age your partner, sap energy, and make impotence, heart disease, and memory loss more likely to occur. It's a true act of caring to take the extra time and make the extra effort to improve your partner's diet with great tasting RealAge-smart dishes.

Learning to shop and cook together in the RealAge kitchen way can strengthen your relationship and improve your health, so you'll have the energy and young arteries to share a vibrant and vigorous retirement (and sex, too). With that younger and healthier RealAge, you'll be able to enjoy your grandkids and reduce the likelihood that your kids will have to take care of you. So stocking a kitchen in a RealAge-smart way isn't selfish; making sure your kitchen has a high IQ is really showing love for those you care about most.

Training Taste Buds

Perhaps your spouse isn't as keen as you are about making healthy changes in diet. Maybe, in fact, he or she is resisting the idea, mistakenly believing that healthy eating will mean nothing but alfalfa sprouts and unflavored boiled broccoli, and feelings of deprivation. Perhaps you have children. As we all know, some children instinctively balk when they suspect that something might be good for them.

If this is the case with your family, try a subtle strategy. Lectures on the value of a healthy lifestyle never work, and once battle lines have been drawn on an issue, it's hard to get them erased. A much more successful approach is to start retraining the family's palate or taste buds. To win over a resistant family, *gradually* shift to a healthier diet.

The value of this low-key approach was demonstrated by one of the most successful restauranteurs in America. Lettuce Entertain You is a Chicago-based food group that has thirty-eight very successful restaurants in Chicago. Some have become popular franchises, such as Corner Bakery and Maggiano's. Although the restaurants range from inexpensive to quite expensive, all have wonderfully delicious food. I am privileged to give medical advice to some of the general partners, and I've made repeated suggestions that their menus contain dishes that make people's RealAges younger. I even pushed to start a RealAge café restaurant that would feature great, tasty food that would also give diners more energy and make them younger. In approximately 1987, Lettuce Entertain You put heart symbols next to its menu items that were "heart healthy." Sales of those items fell dramatically! They were the same items, but just identified as healthy. Then the hearts disappeared, and the sale of those healthy items rose. But now I've noticed that the hearts have reappeared and sales have increased—people are gradually making their own choices to eat RealAge-smart. The people running Lettuce Entertain You think that attitudes have changed—people want to be shown that tasty can be healthy, and it can be. A low-key gradual approach also seems to win over the taste buds as well as the hearts of family members. Plan to train your own and your family's taste buds gradually. Reducing unhealthy fats is the first step to ease your family into a younger RealAge.

The Healthy Fat Substitutes

We weren't born with a genetic predisposition to prefer unhealthy fats. We learned to like those things just by exposure to them. Likewise, we can retrain our taste buds to prefer healthy food choices that give more energy and a younger RealAge, such as healthy fats.

Yes, some fats are healthy, and a little fat in your diet is healthy. But the fat should be unsaturated (monounsaturated or polyunsaturated fat), as those fats make you younger. In contrast, saturated fat ("four-legged fat," or animal fat) and trans fat are unhealthy. Saturated fat is found in red meats, full-fat dairy products, palm and coconut oils, and, to a lesser extent, poultry and other animal products. Saturated fats do more than make the bad cholesterol increase in your bloodstream, which ages your arteries and promotes heart disease, stroke, memory loss, impotence, and even wrinkling of the skin. Saturated fats and trans fats also impede your immune system, which increases your risk of cancer and serious infections.

In contrast, polyunsaturated fats, such as corn oil, soybean oil, and most vegetable oils, and the fats in fish, avocados, and nuts will make your RealAge younger. Monounsaturated fats are even better. These latter fats are specifically found in olives, olive oil, cold-pressed canola oil, and flax seed. Just substituting healthy fat for unhealthy fat makes your RealAge 3.5 to 6 years younger, depending on your age and gender. Decreasing the total amount of fat in your diet, switching from unhealthy to healthy fats, and making healthy substitutions (such as avocado for butter; skim or soy milk for whole milk) are all good ways of decreasing the amount of aging fat in your diet. And that switch can be made easily by retraining your palate.

Retraining the palate takes about eight weeks. Make small, gradual substitutions that slowly retrain your family's taste buds. If you switch suddenly from whole milk to skim, or from Doritos to Baked Lays potato chips, the skim milk will probably taste watery and the Baked Lays might taste like cardboard at first. If you switch gradually, food will always taste good, with no period of watery or cardboard taste. Once you've retrained your palate, whole milk will taste too fatty and the skim milk will be delicious; the Doritos will taste too oily, while the Baked Lays will be crisp, crunchy, and less aging. (Retraining the palate is worth *10 Kitchen IQ points.*)

But don't abandon fat! Eating a little fat before a meal is beneficial. First, a small amount of fat slows digestion—more specifically, will slow emptying of stomach contents into the small intestines. Because your stomach stays full for longer, you *feel* full, your appetite decreases, and you eat less. Second, a little fat helps keep blood-sugar levels stable. Because sugars are largely absorbed in the intestine, the fat-induced delay in the movement of food into the intestine means that sugars are absorbed more slowly. As a result, the level of sugar in the blood rises more slowly and doesn't peak as high. Evening out the peaks in the levels of sugar in the blood retards some of the aging that arteries experience when blood sugar levels are high.

The third reason to eat a little fat first is that healthful fats help in the absorption of fat-soluble vitamins such as A, D, E, and K, and fat-soluble nutrients such as lycopene and lutein. And fourth, healthy fats help improve your blood cholesterol levels. Although the exact mechanism is not known, monounsaturated fats reduce the amount of bad or lousy (LDL) cholesterol in the blood. At the same time, people who include healthy fats in their diets are more likely to see an increase in their healthy (HDL) cholesterol levels.

The Benefits of Other Food Substitutions

A host of RealAge foods—such as granola made with olive or canola oil, wheat germ, nonfat yogurt, or bone-strengthening skim or soy milk—can often be added to or substituted for less healthy foods without changing the taste very much at all. (Send a list of your favorite substitutions to us at DrsMikeandJohn@RealAge.com.) For example, a patient told me he grinds granola or wheat germ very fine in a blender or food processor and adds it to cake mixes or bread dough to make the texture more enjoyable. (It's often the texture, and not the taste, of a specific food that people crave.) Nonfat yogurt can be stirred into sour cream or a sour cream–based dip to reduce the aging fat content while keeping the zing. Skim milk can be added to whole milk.

If you experiment, you'll be surprised to see how many RealAge food substitutions you can make in your family's normal diet without anyone even noticing. The key to success is to detect, by trial and error, how much you can substitute before your spouse or children object to the retraining efforts. For example, start by adding ½ cup of soy or skim milk to a quart of whole milk. Then slowly increase this amount until a comment is made about the taste of the milk. Once this happens, cut back the amount of soy or skim milk a little. At this point, you've established the best ratio of soy or skim milk to whole milk for your family. Eight weeks or so later, add more soy or skim milk to the mix.

Try to assess all of your meals in terms of how they could be made healthier (and tastier) through additions, subtractions, or substitutions. For example, if your children insist on hamburger, crumble in a veggie burger or mix in a little cooked brown rice. Remember, it's the texture—or even just the *idea*—and not the taste of certain foods that people often object to or, conversely, enjoy. Your kids probably won't even notice the difference and may even prefer the new version.

You may feel sneaky and have pangs of guilt when you put out a container of whole milk you know contains a significant amount of skim or soy milk. The guilt will fade when you see the results: the healthy glow that comes from eating food that tastes great and makes their RealAges younger. Chances are, your family (especially the adults) will feel better physically without knowing exactly why. Retraining their palates shows you love them and care about not only their enjoyment of food but also their health and vitality.

RealAge Food for Infants

Of course, you don't have to feel the least bit guilty when it comes to feeding the healthiest foods to your infant. Substitutions keep your baby healthier, and you are creating a healthy palate from the start. One important RealAge kitchen tip is that cooking at home is often better than eating out or buying prepackaged food, in part because you have complete control over the ingredients. This health tip is certainly true for the food you give your infant—not to lower her or his RealAge, obviously, but to start it off with healthy eating habits.

For example, giving a baby commercial baby food that is high in sodium may be predisposing him or her to a lifetime of hypertension. Another ingredient you don't need is any kind of starch that has been added as a filler. Babies have small stomachs and need great nutrition from their food. The filler in commercial food is replacing nutrient-rich food in your child's stomach.

A great alternative to buying commercial baby food is to make it yourself. Although many tired parents might consider making baby food as just one more chore, they find that making baby food in bulk and freezing it properly for future use actually takes *less* time, overall, than making several trips to the market to pick up commercial baby food. All you'll need is your blender or food processor and small containers in which to freeze individual portions. These containers could be very small Tupperware types, or if you've bought commercial baby food in the past, you can wash the jars thoroughly and reuse them. You can also freeze the baby food in an ice cube tray and then store the cubes in a larger container.

For vegetables, cook the vegetables as you normally would, then thin the mixture in the blender or food processor with either the water in which you boiled the vegetables, as it will contain some vitamins, or low-sodium vegetable juice or broth (homemade would really be great). Very lean meats can be lightly sautéed (above 165 degrees for 15 seconds) and blended with broth. Celery or other vegetables may be added for flavor and flavonoids. Very young infants need liquefied food. As the baby grows, you can reduce the blending time so that the food is a little chunkier; chunkier food will promote chewing. Check with your pediatrician.

You can be just as creative with your baby's food as you are with the rest of the family's food. Cook and blend fruits with liquid, then stir in yogurt for a calcium punch. Remember, it is smart to train the palate to prefer certain foods at a very early age.

On many occasions, you won't even have to make baby food specially or thaw what you have in the freezer. The food you prepare for the rest of the family will often be perfectly fine for baby if the food is run through the blender or food processor with a little liquid. Taste it first, of course. Giving a baby a taste of the grown-ups' healthy food can be a great first step in developing a younger, more vigorous lifetime.

RealAge Foods for Children

The sooner you start your children on the path to healthy eating, the better. Many parents serve their children "kiddie" food and then expect them, at about age 12, suddenly to enjoy grown-up food. Of course, the change hardly ever happens that way. Be creative about introducing kids to different foods at an early age so they can develop a well-rounded palate. They'll then discover that hot dogs and fried-chicken nuggets are not as tasty or as good for them as a grilled still-juicy chicken breast with salsa or a RealAge burrito (page 348 in *The RealAge Diet* or at www.RealAge.com).

Small children love to help, and that is the key to instilling a preference for RealAge-smart foods and a high-IQ kitchen. Once a week, encourage your children to help you prepare a dish or meal. When they play a part in the meal and feel needed, they get hooked on cooking and feel comfortable in the kitchen. Even if they simply make a mess and cause more work for you, your extra effort will be rewarded in later years, when they are able to lend a hand in food preparation, and perhaps even cook healthfully for you. And, yes, it will take extra time, but it is truly quality time.

You might try introducing children to new foods by relating the foods to what is happening in current events. If your kids love soccer and the World Cup is being held in Italy, make Tuscan Tuna (page 170). If their favorite pop band is touring the South, make Cajun Couscous-Crusted Monkfish (page 223). If the president is visiting China, make Rainbow Shrimp Moo Shu Roll-Ups (page 273). You'll be able to discuss geography and current events while making it fun to experience a wide range of foods.

Kids of all ages love games and challenges, and it's easy to increase your kitchen's IQ and make eating RealAge-smart fun. See who can use celery sticks and peanut butter to pick up the most raisins as a snack. Or, when you go shopping, play the game my daughter Jennifer and I used to play: see who can find the healthiest peanut butter (least trans and saturated fat—remember to check the label). The person who finds the peanut butter made only with peanuts, like Smucker's, wins. (When I started looking for peanut butter with my daughter, I was surprised to find that some chunky peanut butters are made with just peanuts; thus, the fat present is peanut oil, a healthy oil. Other chunky peanut butters contain trans fat (the peanuts are mixed with partially hydrogenated vegetable oil), and this makes you older. If you eat a lot (a lot!) of peanut butter, the difference in just having the wrong kind of chunky peanut butter can translate to being as much as 3.5 years older.)

Other choices of packaged and canned or jarred foods can be used in this game. For example, see who can find the healthiest mayonnaise (made with canola or olive oil), or where the whole wheat pitas are in the store. Just hunt for one or two new "best" items during a shopping trip, and you'll soon accumulate a roster of great-tasting choices that are the healthiest in that store. (Reading labels and choosing the best products is worth a whopping *10 Kitchen IQ points,* as your kitchen will be stocked with healthy items. You and your children will have fun together, too.)

RealAge Foods for Teenagers

t's ironic (and sad, from a physician's point of view) that when human beings go through their most accelerated period of growth—the teenage years—they often have the least nutritious diet. Teenage bodies desperately need healthy calories, calcium, and vitamins, but all too often teens subsist on soda pop, vending-machine corn chips, burgers, and fries. Each of these foods saps energy—energy needed in the teen years more than ever—and ages the arteries, leading later in life to impotence, decay in the quality of orgasm, and wrinkling of the skin, in addition to heart disease, stroke, and memory loss. The unhealthy food choices of young Americans also age the immune system (leading to many types of autoimmune disease, including many forms of arthritis and cancer). That change in diet to unhealthy foods for American girls is thought to be one reason breast cancer is occurring in woman substantially earlier than it did four decades ago.

Teenagers are keenly aware of their bodies. Partly because of the unrealistic body images projected by the media, teenagers (especially females) often strive for impossibly thin bodies. Endless dieting can keep them nutritionally deprived, especially if what they do eat are nutrient-poor, calorie-rich foods such as onion rings and cheesecake or carrot cake. Such choices can deprive teenagers of key nutrients required for body and brain development at a time when they need those nutrients most.

To help a teenager, eat with them, and teach him or her how to order healthy foods at fast-food and pizza places—a salad shaker, grilled chicken with a red or green salsa (and no mayo), cheeseless vegetarian pizza with extra vegetables, a vegetarian sub without cheese or oil but with double vegetables, plus olives and avocado. Hold the bagged cheese and commercial sour cream and substitute avocados on that taco salad. Even at typical fast-food chain eateries, it doesn't take much effort to make substitutions that taste great and give more energy. Doing so is worth *0 to 24 Kitchen IQ points,* depending on how often your family uses such eateries.

You can't control everything your teenagers do when out of sight, and this certainly applies to what they eat. However, you can make sure that the meals they have at home, both breakfast and dinner, pack the biggest nutritional punch possible. Make sure your children know that they can have great-tasting food that also gives energy, such as healthy peanut butter, fruit, nuts, and cocoa-based chocolate. Talk with your children about the importance of making time for breakfast—it's a key to staying slim and energetic. (Eating breakfast every day is worth up to *21 Kitchen IQ points.*) If you really can't pry your kids out of bed until the last minute, teach them how to make a fruit smoothie they can bolt down before leaving, and tuck an apple (cut up and sprinkled with lemon juice) or a banana into the backpack they take to school. Make dinner a sit-down fun event to which every member of the family is expected—and will want—to attend.

Being a teenager is hard enough without feeling weak, dizzy, or fatigued from eating food that saps energy. Although teenagers may appear not to hear a word you're saying, they really do look to parents for advice. If you are a great role model by providing delicious, nutrient-rich food, you are giving your teenagers their best chance of enjoying those all-important years as they pass into adulthood. Remember what Dr. Phil says, "Talk with them, don't preach to them." Even if they do not change their diets now, they will have heard you and maybe will change later. I know Jennifer, our daughter, never "heard" me during high school, but since she's in college, she seems to have used those talks to influence her choices for the better.

Mealtime as a (Family) Stress-Reducer

Stress causes aging in all three systems that we know age us (arterial aging, immune aging, and aging from environmental factors and accidents). Stress makes it more likely for heart disease, stroke and memory loss; stress increases the likelihood you'll have an older immune system and be prone to cancer, infections, and arthritis; and stress increases your risk of accidents. Having three or four major stressful events in one year can make your RealAge more than thirty years older. Cultivating lots of friends, developing strong social support networks, and learning strategies for coping with stress can minimize these effects.

One good way to minimize the effects of stress is to use mealtimes to reduce stress. Connect with friends and laugh—laughter is a whole-body stress reducer that makes your immune system younger. Laughter opens lines of communication with others and reduces anxiety, tension, and stress. Having a network of close friends or family can help prevent aging from excessive stress.

Making the place where you eat special is another way to reduce stress and avoid eating absentmindedly. Always sit down when you're eating, and decorate the special place with colors and furniture that are particularly pleasing to you and your family. Making mealtime a fun-loving family event can greatly reduce the aging of your arteries and immune system, and help you avoid the aging that comes as a result of accidents.

7

RealAge Meals
for Busy People

Whether Eating by Yourself
or Entertaining

earning how to make great-tasting RealAge foods in less time than is required for "convenience foods" is one important way to find enough energy for all the activities of a good life. Learning the principles that significantly increase your kitchen's IQ can make RealAge cooking even faster than driving to the take-out place. This chapter describes some general principles, tricks, and shortcuts that shorten your time in the kitchen while increasing your kitchen's IQ. Almost all of the recipes in this book you can prepare in half an hour or less.

And these meals and preparations can be easy whether cooking for yourself and your family, or entertaining big time. Doing all you can for the health of your friends is one of the best ways to show you care. And what better way to entertain than by serving RealAge-smart foods? If you entertain more than once a year, this chapter is for you. Entertaining need not be stressful. The key to reducing stress for you and your family is to increase your kitchen's IQ so that entertaining is fun to plan and carry out. This chapter shares the principles that I—and many e-mailers—have used to make cooking for yourself and the entire entertaining process so age-reducing you'll want to do both more often.

At Home, Meals for One

The twentieth century was a time of tremendous change in food preparation at home. More and more women began to work outside the home. Also, after World War II, the so-called convenience foods made their appearance. As a result, the way we feed our families has changed completely. In our grandparents' time, all cooking was done from scratch, and it was a never-ending, time-consuming daily grind.

Because of modern conveniences and the increasing number of two-career families, we've found ways to escape that grind and get dinner on the table faster. Unfortunately, these methods frequently involve adding certain ingredients to food—such as sodium and saturated fat—that can sap your energy and make your RealAge older. Members of busy two-career families are the very individuals who can most benefit from home-cooked meals shared with loved ones at the end of the workday.

Fortunately, the idea that preparing a home-cooked meal must be a complicated and time-consuming process is a myth. In truth, you can put together a home-cooked meal just as quickly (and almost as easily) as picking up so-called fast food. In the process, you'll help keep your family much healthier and more energetic, now and in the long run. The salt, trans fats, and other additives in many convenience foods make their purchase a quick way to accelerate aging. Like most of the principles of RealAge-smart eating, learning to make fast but nutritious meals from almost-scratch is easy (and gets easier) with practice. Start by keeping the following rules in mind:

- **Organize and prepare.** It's those trips to the grocery store for some forgotten item during the week that are the worst waste of time. Create a master grocery list tailored to your family's smart-eating habits and take it with you on a once-a-week stock-up trip. Any perishable items you might hesitate to buy days in advance can almost certainly be frozen and served later (organizing and planning your meals is worth up to 6 *Kitchen IQ points*).

- **Strive for simplicity, spend for quality.** The heart of quick and delicious RealAge-smart meals is simplicity. The fewer the ingredients, the better. However, the fewer the ingredients in a dish, the better each should taste. A fresh, high-quality grilled salmon steak, for example, needs only a squeeze of lemon for perfection. Because the true taste of your foods won't be masked by complicated additions, buy the best-quality ingredients you can find. Testing, and not necessarily high cost, is the best means of judging quality. (Using six or fewer ingredients in 70 percent of the dishes you make is worth *3 Kitchen IQ points.*)

- **Set up beforehand.** Whenever possible, set the table and prepare the kitchen the night before, or in the morning before you leave for work. Nothing is a more welcome sight when you arrive home than a nicely set table. If you've already set out dishes on the stove (and put water in the pasta pot, or brown or basmati rice in the rice cooker), the wait time for dinner can be substantially reduced. Cooking slowly seems to be better healthwise—in one study, a group of diabetic patients was given food cooked with either high heat for a short time or food cooked slower with lower heat. Markers of aging were 50 percent less with lower, slow temperature cooking. So a crock pot cooking method may be healthier *(2 Kitchen IQ points).*

- **Develop a few favorite dishes.** Develop a few fabulous-tasting favorites that are particularly easy to make, and then make them often. You'll become so adept that eventually they'll take *less* effort than a so-called time-saving but artery-aging option such as picking up a heavily cheese-laden pizza *(5 Kitchen IQ points).*

- **Give up on elaborate perfection.** Many people who learned to cook during the gourmet cooking craze of the seventies and eighties developed an all-or-nothing approach to cooking—either high-end, multitiered entrees, or a bowl of cereal. An agonizing, stress-laden approach to cooking can be unlearned. Enjoy every meal that simply does what it should—provides delicious RealAge-smart nutrition to you and your family—and save your epicurean extravaganzas for special occasions *(3 Kitchen IQ points).*

- **Target your serving time.** The time to create a dinner is always defined by the dish that takes longest to make. This dish is most often on the whole-grain side, such as rice. Hit the button on the rice cooker the moment you get home. Then prepare the other dishes at a more leisurely pace. The completion time for that first dish is your target serving time. Counting back from this target time tells you when to start the other dishes, depending on how long each will take.

Don't be concerned if you can't get all the dishes to finish cooking at exactly the same moment. Instead, plan your serving time according to your most delicate dish. For example, most soups, stews, hearty salads, and grilled dishes can sit for several minutes after cooking and still taste just as good—or better—a few degrees cooler. Many cooked vegetables, however, are best nice and hot, and lose appeal if they sit for too long. The same is true for green salads once they've been dressed.

When You Care Enough to Serve the Very Best

If you think that having a cocktail or dinner party at your home is too stressful, think again. Several key steps will ensure that the evening is just as enjoyable and relaxing for you as for the guests. After all, stress-free living is an important part of the RealAge lifestyle.

- **To the greatest extent possible, take care of your guests' needs in advance.** Guests are uncomfortable when their needs are troublesome to their hosts. For the sake of your guests, take care of their needs—where to put their coats, how to get Great Aunt Sally into the house in her wheelchair, what drinks to serve the guests who don't want alcohol—well *before* their arrival. That said, don't require perfection and don't blame yourself if something goes wrong during the party. It's the gracious handling of a mishap—or perhaps even finding humor in it—that can make an event truly memorable and fun (*2 Kitchen IQ points*).

- **Choose *one* specialty dish.** This is an old catering trick: have one truly wonderful dish for which you are known. Some people believe that the success of a party depends on turning out endless complicated, completely home-cooked dishes. This is not true. Choose one dish that's a crowd-pleaser, RealAge-smart, fabulous tasting, and that you genuinely enjoy making and love eating. Make that dish the centerpiece of your special occasion. The other dishes can be extremely simple, such as crusty, home-baked bread or a fresh garden salad, and should serve only to complement the focus dish, not compete with it.

  Don't worry if you're serving a dish you served at your last party. That's the point of a signature dish. In fact, your guests may very well be attending with the hope that you're going to make that same delicious Cioppino (page 299) you made before (*4 Kitchen IQ points*).

- **Prepare as much of the food as possible in advance.** Aside from your specialty dish, as much as possible, serve dishes that can be assembled in advance and frozen, dishes that can be assembled the day before and refrigerated, and items that can be picked up from a specialty store on the day of the event *(2 Kitchen IQ points)*.

- **Enjoy the all-important half hour.** Professional caterer and author Nicole Aloni believes it's vital to have a free half-hour after you're dressed and ready for your guests but before their arrival. In this free time, you can have a glass of wine or champagne, take a quiet moment with your family member co-hosts, and admire the fruits of your labor. The time helps you relax and be refreshed when you greet your guests, and this relaxed state will probably set the tone for the entire evening. Since stress is the greatest ager of all, planning to ensure you have this half-hour to enjoy is key to keeping your RealAge younger *(4 Kitchen IQ points)*.

- **Pick one passion and let others do the rest.** Just as you should select one dish you love to make, you should select one aspect of decorating or preparation you particularly enjoy. Perhaps you're great at arranging flowers, or have a gift for artfully assembling unusual objects for a centerpiece, or can create beautiful ambience through lighting. Spend most of your prep time on that project and farm out the other chores to family members and friends or, if possible, paid professionals *(2 Kitchen IQ points)*.

- **Feel good, not guilty, about serving RealAge-smart food.** It's easy to think that guests might arrive to a party expecting rich, fat-laden dishes that often accompany a special occasion. Don't feel pressure to veer off your path of RealAge-smart eating because of that expectation. Instead, take the event as an opportunity to show your guests that a bruschetta made with fresh basil and tomatoes from your garden (see page 208) can be more delicious than the saturated fat-laden pâté they might have been expecting. Feel good about this benefit—it shows that you truly care about your guests *(2 Kitchen IQ points)*.

  If you prefer not to serve alcohol but are unsure about hosting an alcohol-free event, consider having a brunch early in the day, so that smoothies and fresh-squeezed juices can be served. By the same token, you shouldn't feel guilty about not serving alcohol. It might be a good idea to mention the fact in your invitation, especially for dinner parties. Or you could invite guests to BYOB. *(Lack of guilt is worth 6 Kitchen IQ points!)*

Like so many of the activities described in this book, entertaining in a relaxed fashion with RealAge-smart foods is a skill that gets easier and easier with practice. We hope you'll keep up your friendships with those people you like best by opening your home to them, all the while helping to keep them healthy and young with the recipes in this book.

8

Eating Out
the RealAge Way

Some people think it's gauche to bring your own items to a restaurant. However, wine connoisseurs do it all the time: they bring their own bottle of wine whenever they have a special bottle.

Similarly, you can make a restaurant a better restaurant and more fun for you if you bring some items that improve the restaurant kitchen's IQ. Because of our efforts, some of our favorite restaurants now stock items that make many of its patrons younger and their meals RealAge-smart. This chapter shows you how to make bringing products to a restaurant painless and even enjoyable.

Making your RealAge younger when eating out is easier than you think. In fact, most restaurants will try to accommodate your needs. Call ahead and ask what is on the menu, and if substitutions are possible. Most chefs are willing, but you have to ask. Remember, chefs want you to enjoy the experience of dining at their restaurant, so you'll return often.

Sometimes a restaurant simply cannot accommodate all your needs. Or perhaps you weren't able to give advance notice of your needs. That's when we recommend bringing some of your favorite products into the restaurant with you. Please don't bring the whole pantry with you! Some foods, however, will go a long way toward ensuring that your meal is delicious and healthful, no matter where you are. The best way to keep your RealAge younger is to be prepared. It's not just about bringing in food—it is also about how to prepare before going and how to order.

Before You Go

Before you leave for the restaurant, make sure you're not ravenous. You'll eat more at the restaurant if you've skipped a meal that day. When hungry, you'll tend to make food choices that age you (such as snacking on the white bread put before you). We recommend having a small snack before you go out. A piece of fruit, a cup of yogurt, or a handful of nuts (six walnuts, twelve almonds, or twenty peanuts) should suffice. The nuts also provide a little healthy fat before the meal.

Consider taking a few items with you to prepare for the "wait" time. A package of whole wheat crackers or chocolate-covered graham crackers is easy to put in your purse, coat pocket, or briefcase. Also, a small bite of true (cocoa-based, without milk fat) chocolate can ease your appetite and give you something to eat while others are diving into the bread basket. Bread and butter can be hard to resist, especially if the bread is homemade and powder-puff soft. Unfortunately, bread doesn't get that soft if it's not made with a lot of butter or hydrogenated fats, both of which have an incredible ability to sap your energy and make you old. One ordinary sized croissant can contain four days' worth of saturated fat—80 grams—enough to make you more than four days older.

One alternative is to ask your server to bring only whole wheat bread, corn tortillas, or cut-up vegetables and a small dish of olive oil, balsalmic vinegar, salsa, or marinara sauce. (If you're dining with someone else, it might be wise to ask before trading in the white rolls for whole wheat rolls, tortillas, or cut-up vegetables.) If the bread stays on the table, munch on a few whole-grain crackers you've brought with you. We like Whole Foods' Woven Wheats (all wheat and delicious crunch; and no fat at all!).

You could also snack on some fresh-cut vegetables that you carried in your purse, backpack, fanny pack, or briefcase. (Often, especially if you call ahead, the restaurant may serve cut vegetables instead of, or in addition to, bread. Be a real CEO—chief executive officer—and get what you want by asking for cut vegetables ahead of time, when you make your reservation; this strategy obviously applies only to restaurants at which you make reservations, but it also gives you an extra reason to make a reservation—a call just 20 minutes in advance is all the time needed in a restaurant I frequent for the fresh-cut vegetables to appear).

Ordering

Now it's time to order. Do you order an appetizer or not? They sound so good and you're pretty hungry. We're in favor of making appetizers your entire meal, but we suggest you ask for changes if necessary. Ask for warm tortillas and salsa to replace the tortilla chips (too often, straight out of a 10-pound box, and loaded with preservatives as they are "designed" to stay "fresh" for weeks, but are loaded with aging fats and preservatives that have at best unknown effects on your health!). Ask for sautéed (instead of deep-fried) mushrooms and onions as a side dish or as an appetizer. I love appetizers, sometimes ordering one as a starter and another as a main course. If you do not wish an appetizer, you can snack on some of those fresh-cut vegetables that you arranged for the restaurant to serve when you made your reservation.

Next comes the salad. What kind of dressings do they have? So many choices! To avoid the usual high-calorie, often aging, dressing from the vats, especially high calorie in "family" and "fast-food" restaurants, you can ask for basic oil and vinegar or bring your own. (One statistic that always amazes me is that American women between ages 20 and 40 often get 50 percent of their total calories from fat and other components of salad dressings.) A small bottle of a favorite healthy-fat dressing may be a youth-gaining decision; try several to find one you like.

High-quality balsamic vinegar or rice wine vinegar (try seasoned rice wine vinegar) are great dressings all by themselves. So are lemon and lime juices. Some people use straight Tabasco sauce. You can also carry a small bottle (perhaps 2 ounces) of extra-virgin olive oil, best in a sealed baggie and kept in your purse or briefcase. High-quality, highly flavorful, extra-virgin olive oil is a much better choice than the generic vegetable oil (especially partially hydrogenated vegetable oil) that is too often provided. A restaurant I frequent saw me carrying in a bottle because they had only a generic vegetable blend; soon they started stocking high-quality olive oil instead. They won me over as a more frequent guest.

The entrée is the next challenge. Remember to be the CEO. For example, perhaps the menu lists chicken with cream sauce on white rice; however, you would rather have chicken sprinkled with herbs, or served with the roasted tomato and garlic sauce that comes with the sea bass. Ask your server if the chef would prepare your dish that way. The answer is usually yes, and now your food is delicious and RealAge-smart. Remember to reward good service very well.

Will the kitchen do all this? Yes it will, or it should. If it doesn't or won't, you could bring your own dried herb packets to sprinkle on your chicken. Or your own little bottle of dried seasonings, packed in small plastic baggies. We like McCormick's jerk seasoning, Mrs. Dash's Grilling Blends, Frontera Foods' Tropical Spice, and Eden Foods' Nori Shake to enliven almost all fish and chicken dishes. It is very easy to ask for meals without sauce and season them yourself—maybe even easier than choosing another restaurant. But you should not have to pay for food that ages you and zaps your energy.

Hot pepper sauce is a good seasoning to carry into family restaurants that don't stock the sauce. It tastes great on baked potatoes and sweet potatoes and can replace the mounds of butter and sour cream that make your RealAge older with every bite. Use hot pepper sauce on poultry and vegetables in place of cream sauces and butter, in beans, and on top of whole-grain and rice dishes. Hot pepper sauce seasons food without adding a lot of calories—only lots of flavor and a little salt and vinegar.

To the credit of Lettuce Entertain You mentioned in Chapter 6, you *can* act like a CEO at each of their restaurants. This strategy, which first appeared in *The RealAge Diet* and was first shown to work at the CHEF Clinic, helps you stick to your RealAge goals to train your taste buds or keep them trained even when eating out. And it's great for family restaurants, too—a great learning technique for the whole family.

Ordering in a restaurant can be intimidating, especially if you have not been to that restaurant before, or if you're trying a new dish. At most restaurants, the servers are trained to be familiar with how food is plated and served. Moreover, in many good restaurants, servers have learned how the food is prepared and what the options are.

Simply asking the server will probably give you all the facts you need. The server will probably describe the features most important for you to avoid—for example, "seared in butter" or "covered in a creamy white garlic sauce." And it may be less intimidating to try this technique first with your family.

I have found that cooks in restaurants want your business next week, too, and that means making you happy today by giving you exactly what you want. Thus, the number one strategy is *don't be shy when it comes to asking questions and specifying your needs*. Usually the servers don't have the power to change food preparation, but they can ask the chef if changes can be made. So the key is to ask your server how each dish you want is made, and if the chef can modify it to make it healthier. Virtually every time, your request will be honored.

As for the rest of the restaurant selections, we often carry a few green tea bags with us. Although better restaurants tend to have a nice selection of teas, which sometimes include green tea, you'll be prepared in case they don't. Green tea has antioxidant properties that make your RealAge younger, so you might as well drink something that is both delicious and age-reducing. (However, to gain all of these green tea advantages relative to regular tea, you'd need to drink about fifty cups a day [and a nearby bathroom], at least according to current scientific estimates.) Enjoy the tea selection you like most: they're all age-reducing.

These are just some of the products and techniques that work well for us—small packages of whole wheat crackers; small packages of fresh-cut vegetables; packets of dried herbs and spices; tiny bottles of extra-virgin olive oil, balsamic vinegar, and mixed dried seasonings; small bottles of hot pepper sauce; packets of green tea; and a great bottle of wine (for groups of more than six). It's up to you to decide what is most practical and what you feel comfortable bringing in. Or call ahead and ask the restaurant to have these items for you; most are accommodating. With a little planning, you can eat out deliciously and use food to make your RealAge younger. *Bon appétit!*

9

Cooking
by the Seasons

*More Than 80 Fabulous Recipes
That Make Your RealAge Younger*

One of the great treats of cooking RealAge-smart is to use local produce. Farm-fresh food tastes better than the more traveled variety. So, getting the best to and from your RealAge meals means using local produce. However, local produce varies by the season. Knowing what is harvested in each season can help you choose the freshest ingredients for the healthiest, most fabulous-tasting dishes.

RealAge cooks tailor their meals to what's in season in their area. Foods that are in season are at the peak of flavor, they're the least expensive, and they need the least cooking. Let your garden or a trip to a farmers' market be your inspiration for your meals. Pick the ripest fruit, the crispest vegetables, and the most aromatic herbs; then, let the food speak for itself. To please your eye, mix bright colors. "Food joy" engages all the senses: food should not only look, smell, and taste good but even sound and feel good.

Do you want to cook by the seasons but aren't sure when foods are at their prime? Or what to do with them once you have them? This chapter provides this information. While foods are harvested at different times in different regions of the country, the following list shows the *usual* peak season for fruits and vegetables; we bring some large regional differences to your attention. Within each season, we've provided groups of recipes that utilize the respective seasonal foods to make you younger. Your *Kitchen IQ increases by 10 points* if you always or almost always use seasonal fruit, vegetables, and herbs.

RealAge Kitchen Recipes

Included in this book are delicious RealAge recipes we know you'll enjoy. Think of them, and of your new, healthy lifestyle, as a giant menu of possibilities: choices for growing younger and staying young. They've been tested for taste and require less than 30 minutes to prepare, start to finish. It's a menu for a lifetime—a long and healthy lifetime—of great-tasting foods.

Each recipe in this book carries with it a RealAge effect. We tell you how much younger or older enjoying this recipe twelve times a year will make you. For example, enjoying Barbecued Red Snapper with Spicy Red Beans and Rice (page 297) twelve times a year will make you 11.4 days younger. Although these calculations are approximations, they clearly provide a direction and magnitude of health effect for each recipe.

The recipes are organized by (1) ingredients that are likely to be at peak flavor in season; and (2) by meal—but do not feel limited by the suggested meal. If you want to start with dessert, feel free to do so. If you want a breakfast meal for lunch or a dinner for lunch, feel free to enjoy it. And do not be limited by the choice of seasons.

Calculating the RealAge Effect of a Recipe

Calculation of the RealAge effect of each recipe is complex in math but straightforward in concept. We already know in detail what each nutrient does to your RealAge. The results of those calculations are provided in the first two *RealAge* books for each age and gender group, and on the Web site www.RealAge.com. Here's a short summary of a sample calculation of how a recipe affects your RealAge.

We know that consuming 10 tablespoons of tomato sauce a week makes the average 55-year-old man 1.9 years younger. Therefore, if a recipe calls for 3 tablespoons of tomato sauce per serving, each serving provides 30 percent of the weekly benefit. For our purposes in calculating a RealAge benefit, we assume that one serving of the recipe will be consumed twelve times a year. Thus, the 55-year-old man would receive 12/52nds of the benefit derived from 30 percent of the 1.9 year benefit. In addition, for accuracy's sake, we have to adjust the calculations to take into consideration certain mathematical factors—covariance and interactions. Specifically, in our example, the figure of 1.9 years assumes that our man eats an average amount of all the other nutrients that the average American eats. But no one eats this "average" amount. So we assumed, in our calculations, what is known as "the least effect." That is, we have assumed that our man was already eating an ideal diet *except* for the nutrients in our recipe. This factor is called a covariance factor and is, in our example, 0.25. Combining all of these elements, we compute the RealAge effect of our dish as follows: $12/52 \times 0.3 \times 1.9$ years $\times 365$ days per year $\times 0.25$, or 12 days younger! Because each of the recipes contains many ingredients, the mathematics become complex. Nevertheless, the concept is straightforward.

In addition, each recipe was selected for great taste and ease of preparation. All were tested repeatedly by several amateur as well as professional chefs and rated on a scale from 1 to 10. For inclusion in the book, a recipe had to receive a rating of at least 8 (scale shown below) from many different samplings and audiences, rendered by professionally trained chefs and home cooks alike.

The Rating Scale for the RealAge Recipes

Based on Taste, Color, and Texture	Rating
I wouldn't feed this to anyone.	0
I wouldn't make this again.	6
I'd make this again.	8
This is almost as good as great sex.	10

⁖ Spring Produce ⁖

Spring is an exciting time for the RealAge seasonal cook because it starts the culinary year. Vegetables push through the earth, nuts and fruits blossom, and the smell of flowers and fresh herbs fills the air. Here's the produce that's in season primarily in the spring.

Spring Produce Chart

Vegetable/Fruit	Buying and Using
Artichokes	➤ **When:** Artichokes, which are grown mainly on the West Coast, are at their peak from March through May. Although an artichoke has a rough appearance that's meant to discourage predators, the globe yields delicious leaves and a tender heart.
	➤ **What to Look For:** Artichokes should feel firm and heavy for their size; this indicates a good moisture content. Rub an artichoke leaf between your fingers; it will squeak if it's fresh. (This doesn't work with the thornless varieties.) The skin should be free of bruises, and the leaves should be tightly closed. The stem should look as if it's just been cut. The scent of an artichoke stays on your hands until you wash them.

Vegetable/Fruit	Buying and Using

➤ **Why:** The RealAge-smart nutrients in an artichoke are calcium, potassium, and fiber.

➤ **How to Use:** Artichokes store best in an open plastic bag in the refrigerator. They should be cooked before eating. You'll have a hard time trying to eat a raw artichoke—except the very small, baby artichokes, barely the size of your thumb. These can be julienned and tossed with small amounts of grated Parmesan or pecorino cheese, extra-virgin olive oil, and toasted walnuts. Their big brothers can be boiled, braised, grilled, marinated, roasted, sautéed, and steamed.

Cook the artichoke halved or whole, break off each leaf, and pull the inside of the leaf slowly over your bottom front teeth. Then cut the globe and cut away the prickly part (the choke) to reveal the tender heart. Eat this plain or with a little lemon, garlic, salt, and/or olive oil. Artichokes can also be stuffed, or added to soups, stews, pasta, and rice dishes.

Arugula

➤ **When:** Although it can be found fresh throughout the summer, arugula is at its peak in April and May. It grows quickly and takes just a few weeks to go from seed to table.

➤ **What to Look For:** Arugula is best with a deep, dark green color and a fresh, upright, not-a-bit-tired look. Avoid wilted or yellow leaves. Choose leaves based on use: big ones for cooking and small ones for salads or sandwiches.

➤ **Why:** The high potassium, folate, flavonoid, and lutein content of arugula means it's age-reducing for your arteries, immune system, and eyes.

➤ **How to Use:** The warm, nutty flavor of arugula makes it perfect for a spring salad. Smaller leaves go well with salads; the larger, more peppery leaves work well in other recipes, especially those calling for a cooking green such as Swiss chard or spinach. Arugula also adds flavor to oil, olive oil mayonnaise, and other sauces, and can be used as a sandwich ingredient and as a base for a pesto.

Vegetable/Fruit	Buying and Using
Asparagus	➤ **When:** The optimum season for asparagus is March through June. The early, tender stalks have a beautiful green color and purple tips. Asparagus eaten as soon as picked is sweetest, as the stalks start losing their sweetness once cut. ➤ **What to Look For:** The skin should be smooth, and the spears should be green with very little or no white. If the stem is shriveled, the asparagus is old; pass it up. Asparagus picked in the wild will often have an irregular base because the spears are snapped off by the person who harvests it from the plant so another can grow next year. Look for thicker asparagus rather than thinner ones; they will roast and grill more easily, and there's less risk of toughening. ➤ **Why:** Asparagus is rich in potassium and folate, and this makes it a RealAge-smart choice. ➤ **How to Use:** Enjoy asparagus cooked by roasting, sautéing, steaming, and, my favorite, grilling. Serve it hot or cold, tossed with sesame oil and sesame seeds, or with a squeeze of lemon, a dollop of yogurt, and a sprinkle of dill. Asparagus is good in salads, risotto, omelets, soufflés, and stir-fried dishes.
Avocados	➤ **When:** Avocados are available all year. (California produces most of the nation's crop.) Two types of avocados are widely available: Haas, which peaks in spring and summer; and Fuerte, which peaks in fall and winter. Many others exist. ➤ **What to Look For:** Avocados should be firm to the touch, unless you plan to eat them very soon. They should feel heavy for their size, as this indicates a high oil content. The darker the Hass avocado—all the way to black—the closer it is to being perfect to eat. The flavor is best when the avocado is ripe. To ripen an avocado, place it in a paper bag with an apple at room temperature for a few days. ➤ **Why:** Avocados contain healthy monounsaturated fat that makes your RealAge younger.

Vegetable/Fruit	Buying and Using

➤ **How to Use:** Avocados are usually eaten raw, mostly in salads, on sandwiches, or as the main ingredient in guacamole. Mike likes to combine guacamole with asparagus and peas or other vegetables (see page 217) to make a healthy, age-reducing, energy-giving taste treat. Avocados are a RealAge-smart substitute for mayonnaise or butter; they can also be a garnish for stews and soups, or eaten as a snack mashed with tortillas, lime, and chiles.

Avocados are packed with calories, so use sparingly. (Florida avocados—any variety that is not Haas—contain only two-thirds the fat of Haas avocados, also known as California avocados. Florida avocados have a much milder, lighter flavor.)

Carrots

➤ **When:** Although carrots are available year-round, baby carrots are at their prime in early spring. These are very tender but not as flavorful or nutritious as carrots that mature later in the summer.

➤ **What to Look For:** Carrots come in all shapes and sizes. Generally, the deeper the color, the deeper the flavor. The top of the carrot should be bright and green; at home, remove all of it except an inch or so. If the top has been removed, check that the carrot isn't turning dark, shriveling, or sprouting where it's been cut. Carrots that are ready to eat are very firm and do not bend without snapping; they have no nicks and should smell faintly sweet.

➤ **Why:** Carrots are rich in beta-carotene (a pigment that is convertible to vitamin A, but that is only converted when your body needs vitamin A), potassium, selenium, and some of each of the essential amino acids. Although vitamin A taken in supplements has been shown to age your immune system when the dose exceeds 8,000 IUs a day, the vitamin A in food as beta-carotene does not appear to accelerate aging. The potassium and selenium in carrots also make your RealAge younger and increase your Kitchen IQ.

➤ **How to Use:** Few carrots actually need to be peeled, although they should be scrubbed. Carrots can be eaten raw—all by themselves, in salads, or as scoops for guacamole or salsas. They can also be boiled, steamed, roasted, baked, or added to soups and stir-fries.

English peas

➤ **When:** English peas, also known as green peas, are at their peak of sweetness in May or June. The freshest ones are still in their pods.

➤ **What to Look For:** Look for pods that are plump but not split open; you shouldn't be able to see the peas. Harvesting English peas at the right time makes all the difference in taste. Snap off the stem end, pull down the string that runs down the side, and run your thumb under the peas. Sample them to see if you like the flavor.

➤ **Why:** English peas are a real treasure trove of age-reducing flavonoids and fiber.

➤ **How to Use:** Eat English peas raw, steamed, or stir-fried just enough to warm them. Try them mixed into casseroles or blended into an intensely flavored and colored soup.

Fava beans

➤ **When:** Fava beans are at their peak from May through July. They have a delicious flavor that can be missed if you don't get them when they're at their peak. Removing the bean's thick skin reveals a hearty, buttery bean. It's worth the extra effort to find fava beans that are in season.

➤ **What to Look For:** Although fava bean pods are naturally a little hairy and irregular, avoid the ones with blackened ends or wrinkled skin. The freshest pods are firm, bright looking, and velvety to the touch.

➤ **Why:** These beans are rich in soluble fiber and also have potassium, both of which make your RealAge younger.

➤ **How to Use:** Grill or broil the beans briefly and peel the skin. Or simmer them just a little and savor their meatiness. Use fava beans in tomato- or olive oil-based pasta sauces, rice pilafs, spring vegetable medleys, vegetable soups, and stews.

Cooking by the Seasons

Vegetable/Fruit	Buying and Using
Radishes	➤ **When:** Radishes are at their peak around April and May. The round, often oddly shaped radish infuses color into spring meals. Every color and shape has a different flavor: Try as many as you can find.
	➤ **What to Look For:** Radishes should be smooth, firm, and juicy, with no cracks. The stem should be fresh and firm. Generally, the larger the radish, the stronger the flavor.
	➤ **Why:** Although radishes do not have many nutrients that make your RealAge younger, they do contain some selenium and potassium, and I love their texture.
	➤ **How to Use:** Radishes are commonly used raw. This peppery vegetable needs cleaning if you're going to eat it raw. (Cut off the ends and sprinkle the whole radish with salt or lime.) Radishes are usually not cooked unless used in a sauce. They deserve a more active role in salads, and as scoops for dips, salsas, and guacamole.
Rhubarb	➤ **When:** This tart vegetable is at its peak from April to June. Its stalks regenerate from one year to the next, and it's only in season briefly, so take advantage of its presence.
	➤ **What to Look For:** Rhubarb comes in different colors. Stalks should be crisp and blemish-free; they can become stringy late in the season. Avoid the leaves, as they are poisonous, and avoid stalks that are yellowing or that bend easily.
	➤ **Why:** Rhubarb is rich in fiber that makes your RealAge younger.
	➤ **How to Use:** For most people, rhubarb is too tart to eat raw. Cooked rhubarb is delicious. It's often used with fruits, which balance its tartness. Use it in sauces, jams, and desserts such as cake, pudding, pie, and compote.
Salad greens	➤ **When:** Greens are in abundance in the spring. Because many varieties are too delicate to ship, the selection is often better at a farmers' market than at the supermarket.
	➤ **What to Look For:** Leafy greens should have bright colors and fresh, crisp leaves. Avoid leaves that are turning colors and decaying.

➤ **Why:** Most leafy greens have enough potassium, folate, flavonoids, and lutein to make your RealAge younger.

➤ **How to Use:** Sample as many kinds as you can: Leafy greens grow easily and quickly, and there are so many different varieties. Each has a slightly different flavor. When combining greens, you may find that you want more chicory than arugula, more red leaf than frisée (curly endive), or more baby beet greens than Lollo Rossa. You can enjoy greens every day, and in so many different ways. Salad greens can be piled onto sandwiches, mixed into hot pasta, or wilted for an entrée salad.

Scallions

➤ **When:** Scallions are available year-round but are at their peak during spring and summer.

➤ **What to Look For:** Mid-size scallions with long white stems usually have the best flavor. Look for crisp, bright green tops and a firm white or purple base. Ramps (wild leeks) are early spring favorites, if you can find them; they have a strong aroma that is mellowed by heat.

➤ **Why:** Scallions are rich in organic selenium, as well as potassium, calcium, essential amino acids, and flavonoids, all of which make you younger.

➤ **How to Use:** The mild onion flavor of scallions is good for fresh dishes calling for only a hint of onion. Cook scallions whole or chop the leaves for salads, soups, and other dishes, such as pasta. John grills them whole with olive oil over mesquite, chars the leaves and whites, and sprinkles them with sea salt.

Sorrel

➤ **When:** Fresh young sorrel is available in limited supply year-round, with the peak season in spring. At that time, the crop has a milder flavor than the later crop; sorrel tends to become more acidic as the plant gets older and the leaves get larger.

➤ **What to Look For:** The leaves of the plant should be bright green and crisp, with no signs of wilting or decay. Avoid woody-looking stems or leaves. At home, sorrel should be bunched loosely and kept in water, stems down. For use in salads, get the younger, less mature sorrel—about 4-inch leaves.

➤ **Why:** Sorrel contains two nutrients in quantity that make your RealAge younger, folate and potassium.

➤ **How to Use:** Use young sorrel in salads or sautéed, blended into a pesto, or tossed as a garnish around whole roasted fish. Older, more mature sorrel can be used in breads or as an accompaniment for meats, vegetables, and soups.

Spinach

➤ **When:** Spinach is bountiful starting in April; in cooler climates, it's usually harvested a second time, in the fall.

➤ **What to Look For:** Leaves should be crisp and intensely green. Avoid yellow or wilted leaves.

➤ **Why:** Spinach is loaded with folate, selenium, calcium, and potassium, which means you're getting younger every time you enjoy it.

➤ **How to Use:** Spinach is used raw in salads or cooked as a vegetable, as a filling for pasta and omelets, with hot grains, and as a sandwich filling. Freshly picked spinach, wilted in a pan with garlic and hot red pepper sauce, and doused with rice wine vinegar and sesame oil, is a year-round favorite. I like it sautéed in just a touch of olive oil—even as a snack before dinner. It takes 5 minutes to prepare, it tastes great, and it's filling.

Strawberries

➤ **When:** A plump, juicy strawberry is best from April to July.

➤ **What to Look For:** Strawberries should be plump and firm and have a shiny skin, which indicates freshness. Look for tiny wild strawberries in markets: small alpine berries are fabulously sweet and concentrated in flavor.

➤ **Why:** Strawberries are nutrient-rich and loaded with age-reducing flavonoids.

➤ **How to Use:** As with nearly all fruits and vegetables, wash strawberries well. Mold spreads quickly on berries, so toss those that become moldy. Strawberries are so sweet and tasty, they're good just as they are. They're also wonderful in jams, pies, sauces, salads, and desserts. They can be used as decorations for desserts, filled with almond paste, sliced and soaked in balsamic vinegar and sugar (a heavenly dessert), or coated with real (dark) chocolate—another heavenly dessert or appetizer that contains healthy fat.

Watercress

➤ **When:** The spiciness of good watercress is seductive. Especially good are bunches harvested from March through June.

➤ **What to Look For:** Small leaves, delicate stems, and a feathery feel indicate that the watercress is sweet and mild. Flowers and firm stalks indicate that the watercress has a little bite, like the hot, bitter, mustard family of which it is a member. Some other kinds of cress—upland cress or garden cress—are sold as a collection of leaves instead of a bunch.

➤ **Why:** Watercress is an excellent source of vitamin C, calcium, potassium, and magnesium. It also contains other phytochemicals that fight cancer.

➤ **How to Use:** Salads that use watercress, especially the leaves without the stems, often pair it with a citrus fruit. The zing of the cress combined with the pucker and sweetness of an orange, blood orange, or grapefruit makes an appealing lunch. Alice Waters of Chez Panisse restaurant in Berkeley makes an intensely flavored, brilliantly green soup by puréeing watercress with a little chicken stock, onion, and garlic.

Recipes Using Spring Produce

FOR BREAKFAST

Shiitake Mushroom and Asparagus Frittata with Smoked Salmon

Preparation time: 12 minutes	*4 servings*
Cooking time: 12 minutes	*108 calories per serving, 32% from fat*

RealAge effect if eaten 12 times a year:	**RealAge–effect ingredients:**
High in omega-3 fatty acids, this breakfast wonder makes your RealAge younger by 4.9 days.	Mushrooms, asparagus, egg whites, soy milk, salmon (healthy fat, healthy protein, B vitamins, including folate)

ingredients

Butter-flavored cooking oil spray

6 ounces shiitake mushrooms, stems discarded, caps sliced

6 ounces asparagus spears, trimmed and cut into 1-inch pieces

5 large egg whites

1 large egg

3 tablespoons fat-free soy milk or milk

2 tablespoons chopped fresh dill

¼ teaspoon salt

¼ teaspoon freshly ground black pepper

4 ounces smoked salmon, coarsely chopped

2 tablespoons reduced-fat sour cream

preparation

Heat an ovenproof, slope-sided, 10-inch skillet over medium heat. Coat with cooking oil spray. Add mushrooms and asparagus; cook 5 minutes, stirring occasionally.

Preheat broiler. In a medium bowl, beat together egg whites, egg, milk, 1 tablespoon of the dill, the salt, and pepper. Stir in smoked salmon; pour mixture into skillet over vegetables; mix well. Press vegetables down into an even layer under the egg mixture. Cook without stirring until eggs are set on bottom, about 4 minutes (center will be wet). Transfer to broiler; broil 4 to 5 inches from heat for 2 minutes or until eggs are set. Cut into wedges. Drop spoonfuls of sour cream on wedges, and sprinkle remaining 1 tablespoon dill over frittata before serving.

substitutions: Crimini mushrooms may replace the shiitake mushrooms, but with some loss of flavor; lox that is not salty may replace smoked salmon.

tips: This dish keeps well. If there is any left over, take it on a picnic or have it for a snack.

nutritional analysis

Total fat (g) 3.9	Sodium (mg) 805	Vitamin A (RE) 77
Fat calories (kc) 35	Calcium (mg) 33	Beta-carotene (RE) 41
Cholesterol (mg) 63	Magnesium (mg) 27	Vitamin C (mg) 13
Saturated fat (g) 1.3	Zinc (mg) 0.8	Vitamin E (mg) 1.4
Polyunsaturated fat (g) 0.7	Selenium (mcg) 36	Thiamin B$_1$ (mg) 0.1
Monounsaturated fat (g) 1.4	Potassium (mg) 439	Riboflavin B$_2$ (mg) 0.5
Fiber (g) 1.3	Flavonoids (mg) 0	Niacin B$_3$ (mg) 3.6
Carbohydrates (g) 5.0	Lycopene (mg) 0	Vitamin B$_6$ (mg) 0.20
Sugar (g) 1.3	Fish (oz) 1	Folic acid (mcg) 60
Protein (g) 13.7	Nuts (oz) 0	Vitamin B$_{12}$ (mcg) 1.2

FOR LUNCH

Light But Hearty Hummus Sandwiches

■ ■ ■ ■

Preparation time: 12 minutes	*4 servings* *353 calories per serving, 21% from fat*

RealAge effect if eaten 12 times a year:	**RealAge-effect ingredients:**
Silken tofu adds calcium and isoflavones; chickpeas add lots of fiber and very little fat. All of these combine to make you 5.2 days younger.	Chickpeas, lemon juice, garlic, tofu, salad greens, whole wheat, radishes, olive oil (calcium, isoflavones, potassium, flavonoids, healthy fats)

ingredients

1 large garlic clove, peeled

1 can (15 or 16 ounces) chickpeas (garbanzo beans), rinsed and drained

2 tablespoons lemon juice

1 tablespoon extra-virgin olive oil

1 teaspoon dark sesame oil

½ teaspoon ground cumin

¼ teaspoon salt

½ cup (4 ounces) low-fat silken tofu, such as Mori-Nu brand

3 tablespoons chopped fresh mint

4 whole wheat pita pocket bread loaves (the 6-inch size, not the little ones)

2 cups mesclun (assorted young salad greens)

½ cup thinly sliced radishes

preparation

To make hummus: With motor running, drop garlic clove through the tube of a food processor and process until minced. Add chickpeas; process until finely chopped. Add lemon juice, olive oil, sesame oil, cumin, and salt; process 30 seconds. Add tofu; process until smooth. Stir in mint.

Cut each pita in half; open pockets. Stuff pockets with half of salad greens and radishes; top with hummus, then remaining salad greens and radishes.

substitutions: Cilantro may replace the mint, torn romaine lettuce may replace the mesclun, and shredded daikon (a large white radish) may replace the familiar round red radishes. Although cilantro would add that mysterious oomph—a little bit of parsley, a little bit of spice, and little bit of grassy pungency—instead of the sweet brightness of mint, they both work.

tips: Dark or toasted sesame oil, found in the Asian section of the supermarket, replaces the traditional tahini (sesame seed paste) because the oil has a more intense flavor and fewer calories than tahini. Drizzle dark sesame oil over stir-fries or on top of veggie burgers. You'll get just enough hint of its perfume to underline the flavor of your food.

nutritional analysis

Total fat (g) 8.6
Fat calories (kc) 78
Cholesterol (mg) 0
Saturated fat (g) 1.1
Polyunsaturated fat (g) 2.6
Monounsaturated fat (g) 3.7
Fiber (g) 3.9
Carbohydrates (g) 82.4
Sugar (g) 1.6
Protein (g) 30.6

Sodium (mg) 526
Calcium (mg) 257
Magnesium (mg) 58
Zinc (mg) 1.0
Selenium (mcg) 14
Potassium (mg) 1093
Flavonoids (mg) 0.3
Lycopene (mg) 0
Fish (oz) 0
Nuts (oz) 0

Vitamin A (RE) 43
Beta-carotene (RE) 67
Vitamin C (mg) 14
Vitamin E (mg) 3.8
Thiamin B_1 (mg) 0.5
Riboflavin B_2 (mg) 0.3
Niacin B_3 (mg) 3.5
Vitamin B_6 (mg) 0.12
Folic acid (mcg) 38
Vitamin B_{12} (mcg) 0

Mandarin Chicken

■ ■ ■ ■

| *Preparation time: 20 minutes* | *4 servings* |
| | *184 calories per serving, 28% from fat* |

| **RealAge effect if eaten 12 times a year:** | **RealAge-effect ingredients:** |
| 9.7 days younger | Garlic, oranges, snow peas, bamboo shoots, lettuce, sesame oil, sesame seeds (flavonoids, folic acid, vitamin B_3, selenium, potassium, magnesium, calcium, healthy fat, fiber) |

ingredients

¼ cup rice wine vinegar

2 teaspoons dark sesame oil

1 tablespoon minced garlic

1¼ tablespoons julienned pickled ginger

2 tablespoons low-sodium soy sauce

½ pound cooked boneless, skinless chicken breast, chopped or julienned

1½ cups drained canned mandarin orange segments

½ cup blanched snow peas

½ cup drained canned bamboo shoots

½ cup drained canned water chestnuts

4 cups shredded lettuce

2 teaspoons toasted sesame seeds

preparation

Mix the vinegar, sesame oil, garlic, ginger, and soy sauce thoroughly. Add chicken and orange segments; marinate for approximately 10 minutes. Add snow peas, bamboo shoots, and water chestnuts. Distribute lettuce on four serving plates. Top with chicken mixture, sprinkle with sesame seeds, and serve.

substitutions: Fresh orange segments may substitute for canned mandarin oranges.

nutritional analysis

Total fat (g) 5.7	Sodium (mg) 485	Vitamin A (RE) 185
Fat calories (kc) 51	Calcium (mg) 107	Beta-carotene (RE) 147
Cholesterol (mg) 49.9	Magnesium (mg) 67	Vitamin C (mg) 77
Saturated fat (g) 1.6	Zinc (mg) 1.5	Vitamin E (mg) 1.0
Polyunsaturated fat (g) 2.2	Selenium (mcg) 57	Thiamin B_1 (mg) 0.3
Monounsaturated fat (g) 2.7	Potassium (mg) 850	Riboflavin B_2 (mg) 0.3
Fiber (g) 4.1	Flavonoids (mg) 2.3	Niacin B_3 (mg) 9.7
Carbohydrates (g) 26.3	Lycopene (mg) 0	Vitamin B_6 (mg) 0.6
Sugar (g) 10	Fish (oz) 0	Folic acid (mcg) 126
Protein (g) 23	Nuts (oz) 0	Vitamin B_{12} (mcg) 0.2

Watercress-Topped Leek and Feta Pizzas

Preparation time: 8 minutes *Cooking time: 15 minutes*	*4 servings* *450 calories per serving, 29% from fat*

RealAge effect if eaten 12 times a year:	**RealAge-effect ingredients:**
Packed with calcium and phytonutrients, each pizza makes your RealAge 8.7 days younger.	Leeks, tomatoes (calcium, phytonutrients, lycopene, folic acid)

ingredients

2 large leeks

Cooking oil spray

4 (6-inch) individual pizza crusts, such as Boboli brand

½ cup (4 ounces) prepared pizza sauce

4 large plum tomatoes, thinly sliced

½ teaspoon fennel seeds

¾ cup crumbled feta cheese with sun-dried tomatoes, such as Saladena brand

1 cup packed coarsely chopped watercress sprigs, stems included

1 tablespoon raspberry vinegar

preparation

Heat oven to 450 degrees. Cut white and light green part of leeks into thin slices. Heat a large nonstick skillet over medium-high heat. Coat with cooking oil spray; add leeks. Stir-fry 3 to 4 minutes or until edges begin to brown.

Arrange pizza crusts on a large baking sheet; top with pizza sauce, leeks, and tomatoes. Crush fennel seeds slightly between your fingers and sprinkle over pizzas. Top with ½ cup of the feta cheese. Bake 8 to 10 minutes, or until crust is golden brown and cheese begins to melt.

In a medium bowl, toss watercress with vinegar; sprinkle over pizzas. Broil 3 to 4 inches from heat source for 1 to 2 minutes or until wilted. Remove from oven and sprinkle with remaining ¼ cup feta cheese.

substitutions: One 12-inch pizza crust, such as Boboli Thin Crust brand, may replace the four individual crusts; and cider or sherry vinegar may replace raspberry vinegar.

tips: Fruit vinegar cuts the richness of the cheese and adds another element of sweetness. Adding layers of flavor is a way to make this pizza especially good. Make sure you sauté the leeks until the edges brown; this is the beginning of caramelization, which shows the natural sweetness of the leeks.

nutritional analysis

Total fat (g) 14.9	Sodium (mg) 1043	Vitamin A (RE) 173
Fat calories (kc) 134	Calcium (mg) 310	Beta-carotene (RE) 588
Cholesterol (mg) 33	Magnesium (mg) 36	Vitamin C (mg) 26.6
Saturated fat (g) 2.5	Zinc (mg) 1.2	Vitamin E (mg) 2.0
Polyunsaturated fat (g) 4	Selenium (mcg) 4	Thiamin B_1 (mg) 0.7
Monounsaturated fat (g) 7.2	Potassium (mg) 422	Riboflavin B_2 (mg) 0.8
Fiber (g) 6.5	Flavonoids (mg) 1.9	Niacin B_3 (mg) 6.0
Carbohydrates (g) 84	Lycopene (mg) 3.1	Vitamin B_6 (mg) 0.4
Sugar (g) 3.9	Fish (oz) 0	Folic acid (mcg) 63
Protein (g) 17	Nuts (oz) 0	Vitamin B_{12} (mcg) 0.6

Roasted Pepper and Fresh Mozzarella Panini (Sandwiches)

■ ■ ■ ■

Preparation time: 10 minutes

4 servings
252 calories per serving, 26% from fat

RealAge effect if eaten 12 times a year:	**RealAge-effect in ingredients:**
Because they stay on the bush a few weeks longer, red bell peppers have much more vitamin C than green peppers. Rich in calcium and beta-carotene, too, this easy-to-make lunch makes you 6 days younger.	Arugula, bell peppers, (calcium, selenium, lycopene, potassium, beta-carotene, vitamin C, folic acid)

ingredients

1 (8-inch) round tomato bread or focaccia

¼ cup olive relish, such as American Spoon brand

1 cup packed arugula

¼ cup packed sliced basil leaves

4 ounces fresh mozzarella cheese, well drained (see Substitutions)

½ teaspoon freshly ground black pepper

1 to 2 jars (7 ounces each) roasted red bell peppers, as desired

preparation

Using a long serrated knife, cut bread into two rounds. Spread olive relish on the cut sides of bread. Layer arugula and basil on bottom half of bread. Cut cheese into thin slices; arrange over basil. Sprinkle pepper over cheese. Drain bell peppers well. Tear into thick strips and arrange over cheese. Close sandwich with top of bread and cut into wedges.

substitutions: The best-quality mozzarella—fresh mozzarella—is always kept in a liquid bath. If unavailable, use the low-moisture form found in most supermarkets.

One to 2 cups roasted and peeled fresh bell pepper strips may replace the bottled peppers; chopped pitted Kalamata or Sicilian olives moistened with a bit of olive oil may replace the olive relish, and baby spinach leaves may replace the arugula, although the sandwich will taste less spicy. An added roasted, peeled red jalapeño, also available in jars, or an added roasted, peeled poblano pepper would add extra zing—quite a lot of extra zing—and would be truly delicious. Be sure to seed and stem both of these peppers.

tips: Toast the bread in a toaster oven for 2 minutes before slicing it open, just to crisp it. Toasting—especially of baked goods—almost always increases flavor. Microwaving warms bread but doesn't make it slightly crusty, as toasting does.

nutritional analysis

Total fat (g) 7.2	Sodium (mg) 588	Vitamin A (RE) 128
Fat calories (kc) 64.9	Calcium (mg) 253	Beta-carotene (RE) 228
Cholesterol (mg) 16.0	Magnesium (mg) 47	Vitamin C (mg) 79
Saturated fat (g) 3.01	Zinc (mg) 1.2	Vitamin E (mg) 1.8
Polyunsaturated fat (g) 0.8	Selenium (mcg) 26	Thiamin B_1 (mg) 0.3
Monounsaturated fat (g) 1.9	Potassium (mg) 527	Riboflavin B_2 (mg) 0.4
Fiber (g) 9.5	Flavonoids (mg) 0.1	Niacin B_3 (mg) 2.4
Carbohydrates (g) 65.8	Lycopene (mg) 1.8	Vitamin B_6 (mg) 0.3
Sugar (g) 25.0	Fish (oz) 0	Folic acid (mcg) 43
Protein (g) 13.0	Nuts (oz) 0	Vitamin B_{12} (mcg) 0.2

Ginger, Carrot, and Orange Cappuccino Cup Soup

THIS RECIPE WAS DESIGNED BY RICK TRAMONTO AND GALE GAND AT TRU RESTAURANT IN CHICAGO FOR REALAGE.

Preparation time: 10 minutes
Cooking time: 30 minutes

4 servings (approximately 5½ cups total)
83 calories per serving, 26% from fat

RealAge effect if eaten 12 times a year:

8.6 days younger

RealAge-effect ingredients:

Onion, carrots, celery, orange juice, olive oil (flavonoids, folic acid, calcium, potassium, healthy fat, fiber)

ingredients

Cooking oil spray

½ cup thinly sliced yellow onion

1 rib celery, thinly sliced (½ cup)

¾ pound carrots, very thinly sliced

3 cups low-salt vegetable broth or stock

1½ teaspoons finely grated fresh ginger

½ cup orange juice

½ teaspoon salt

2 teaspoons extra-virgin olive oil

preparation

Heat a large saucepan or Dutch oven over medium heat; coat with cooking oil spray. Add onion and celery; cook 5 minutes, stirring occasionally. Add carrots; continue to cook 5 minutes. Add broth and ginger; bring to a boil. Add orange juice and salt. Reduce heat; cover and simmer until vegetables are very tender, about 20 minutes. Transfer mixture (in batches, if necessary) to a blender or food processor; blend until smooth. Reheat, if necessary; ladle into shallow bowls. Drizzle oil over soup.

substitutions: White onion will work in this recipe, although the soup will be a little sharper tasting. Sliced leeks (the white part) or sliced shallots can easily substitute for yellow onion.

tips: Slicing the carrots thin allows them to spend less time simmering. Spend a minute to do this, as it will speed cooking. Save a few carrot slices if you would like to add them to the soup once it's finished. They add good texture and make the soup more interesting to eat. Also, you don't have to peel the ginger when you're grating it: it's going into the blender anyway!

nutritional analysis

Total fat (g) 2.5	Sodium (mg) 568	Vitamin A (RE) 2397
Fat calories (kc) 23	Calcium (mg) 43	Beta-carotene (RE) 14,382
Cholesterol (mg) 0.8	Magnesium (mg) 22	Vitamin C (mg) 26
Saturated fat (g) 0.35	Zinc (mg) 0.4	Vitamin E (mg) 0.8
Polyunsaturated fat (g) 0.4	Selenium (mcg) 9	Thiamin B_1 (mg) 0.1
Monounsaturated fat (g) 1.9	Potassium (mg) 573	Riboflavin B_2 (mg) 0.1
Fiber (g) 3.5	Flavonoids (mg) 1.3	Niacin B_3 (mg) 3.5
Carbohydrates (g) 14.9	Lycopene (mg) 0	Vitamin B_6 (mg) 0.2
Sugar (g) 9.4	Fish (oz) 0	Folic acid (mcg) 41
Protein (g) 5.2	Nuts (oz) 0	Vitamin B_{12} (mcg) 0.2

FOR DINNER

Smoked Mozzarella and Veggie-Stuffed Pizza

■ ■ ■ ■

Preparation time: 8 minutes *Cooking time: 14 minutes*	*4 servings* *297 calories per serving, 29% from fat*

RealAge effect if eaten 12 times a year:	**RealAge-effect ingredients:**
One huge slice has less than 300 calories but plenty of lycopene and potassium, making your RealAge younger by 10.0 days.	Vegetables, tomato paste (beta-carotene, potassium, fiber, healthy protein, flavonoids, lycopene)

ingredients

Cooking oil spray

1 pound fresh, cut stir-fry vegetables (packaged or from the salad bar), such as broccoli, zucchini, mushrooms, red onion, bell peppers, and julienned carrots

Salt and freshly ground black pepper

¼ cup tomato paste

2 tablespoons olive relish, such as American Spoon brand

2 tablespoons sun-dried tomato bits, such as Sonoma brand

1 (12-inch or 10-ounce) prepared thin pizza crust, such as Boboli brand

¼ cup chopped mixed green herbs such as chives, thyme, parsley, and basil

½ cup (2 ounces) finely shredded smoked mozzarella cheese

preparation

Heat oven to 425 degrees. Heat a large nonstick skillet over medium-high heat until hot. Coat with cooking oil spray; add vegetables. Stir-fry 3 to 4 minutes or until vegetables are crisp-tender. Salt and pepper to taste.

Combine tomato paste, olive relish, and sun-dried tomato bits. Spread over pizza crust; top with cooked vegetables, herbs, and cheese, in that order. Bake the pizza directly on the oven rack for approximately 10 minutes, or until crust is golden brown and cheese melts.

substitutions: Olive paste, tapenade (olive-caper paste), or olivada (olive paste without capers) may be substituted for the olive relish. Look for jars of this rich Mediterranean mixture in specialty food markets and many supermarkets. If you can't find olive relish, substitute 2 tablespoons of any available commercial mixture of finely diced olives, oil, and other ingredients—perhaps garlic, anchovies, lemon juice, capers, or carrots. Smoked Gouda or Lorraine cheese may replace the smoked mozzarella.

tips: Baking the pizza directly on the oven rack produces a very crisp crust. If you don't have a pizza paddle (a broad, flat wooden board that has a handle), use a large cookie sheet to remove the pizza from the oven. Or, try cooking the pizza over a low fire on an open grill. Here's another RealAge kitchen tip: you can more than double the flavor by using dried and canned tomatoes together.

nutritional analysis

Total fat (g) 9.5	Sodium (mg) 682	Vitamin A (RE) 362
Fat calories (kc) 85.5	Calcium (mg) 170	Beta-carotene (RE) 564
Cholesterol (mg) 8.0	Magnesium (mg) 47	Vitamin C (mg) 38
Saturated fat (g) 3.0	Zinc (mg) 1.2	Vitamin E (mg) 0.76
Polyunsaturated fat (g) 1.9	Selenium (mcg) 3	Thiamin B_1 (mg) 0.3
Monounsaturated fat (g) 3.5	Potassium (mg) 481	Riboflavin B_2 (mg) 0.3
Fiber (g) 5.3	Flavonoids (mg) 2.8	Niacin B_3 (mg) 3.3
Carbohydrates (g) 42.7	Lycopene (mg) 4.2	Vitamin B_6 (mg) 0.2
Sugar (g) 3.7	Fish (oz) 0	Folic acid (mcg) 64
Protein (g) 12.2	Nuts (oz) 0	Vitamin B_{12} (mcg) 0.12

Garlicky Orzo with Spinach, Fennel, and Orange Zest

■ ■ ■ ■

Preparation time: 5 minutes	4 servings
Cooking time: 12 minutes	218 calories per serving, 16% from fat

RealAge effect if eaten 12 times a year:	RealAge-effect ingredients:
3.1 days younger	Garlic, olive oil, spinach, orange zest (folic acid, beta-carotene, calcium, healthy fats, flavonoids)

ingredients

2 teaspoons garlic-infused or extra-virgin olive oil

6 garlic cloves, minced

1 cup (6 ounces) orzo (a rice-shaped pasta), uncooked

2 cups low-salt chicken broth

1 teaspoon dried marjoram

¾ teaspoon fennel seeds, slightly crushed

¼ teaspoon crushed red pepper flakes

1 package (10 ounces) spinach leaves, sliced, or baby spinach leaves

1¼ teaspoons salt

2 teaspoons freshly shredded orange peel

preparation

Heat a Dutch oven or large saucepan over medium-high heat. Add oil and garlic; cook 30 seconds. Stir in orzo; cook 30 seconds. Add broth, marjoram, fennel seeds, and pepper flakes. Simmer uncovered until orzo is tender, 7 to 8 minutes. Stir in spinach, tossing for 1 minute until wilted. Add salt; mix well and transfer to serving plates. Top with orange zest.

substitutions: Low-sodium beef or vegetable broth may replace chicken broth. Predictably, beef broth makes for a meatier-tasting side dish, and vegetable broth gives a cleaner flavor.

tips: Crushing fennel seeds (and, actually, almost any seed) brings the aromatic oils to the surface and provides extra flavors. Don't toast these seeds, however, as their delicate perfume will evaporate. Orange zest brightens the dish, adding color and a touch of sweet sourness. If you don't have an orange, don't fret; any citrus fruit will do. Use a low-sodium broth so *you* control the salt content. A touch of red pepper flakes adds zing. If the dish seems to be missing a little something, use ½ rather than ¼ teaspoon of flakes.

nutritional analysis

Total fat (g) 4.0	Sodium (mg) 841	Vitamin A (RE) 479
Fat calories (kc) 36	Calcium (mg) 86	Beta-carotene (RE) 2860
Cholesterol (mg) 14.7	Magnesium (mg) 66	Vitamin C (mg) 23
Saturated fat (g) 0.6	Zinc (mg) 0.80	Vitamin E (mg) 1.7
Polyunsaturated fat (g) 0.6	Selenium (mcg) 5	Thiamin B_1 (mg) 0.16
Monounsaturated fat (g) 2.0	Potassium (mg) 533	Riboflavin B_2 (mg) 0.24
Fiber (g) 2.4	Flavonoids (mg) 0.7	Niacin B_3 (mg) 2.7
Carbohydrates (g) 15.4	Lycopene (mg) 0	Vitamin B_6 (mg) 0.2
Sugar (g) 0.4	Fish (oz) 0	Folic acid (mcg) 144
Protein (g) 7.0	Nuts (oz) 0	Vitamin B_{12} (mcg) 0.2

Roasted Chicken with Pesto Gemelli and Roasted Asparagus

▪ ▪ ▪ ▪

Preparation time: 10 minutes	*4 servings*
Cooking time: 10 minutes	*439 calories per serving, 26% from fat*

RealAge effect if eaten 12 times a year:	RealAge-effect ingredients:
With a generous serving of heart-healthy monounsaturated fats, this dinner will make your RealAge 2.5 days younger.	Whole-grain pasta, asparagus, olive oil, tomatoes (healthy protein, healthy fats, potassium, lycopene)

ingredients

8 ounces whole-grain pesto gemelli pasta, such as Eden brand

12 ounces boneless, skinless chicken thighs

1 tablespoon olive oil

2 teaspoons dried *herbes d' Provence* or *fines herbes*

1 bunch (about 14 ounces) asparagus spears, cut into 1-inch pieces

½ cup low-salt chicken broth

¼ cup prepared reduced-fat basil pesto, such as Contadina Buitoni brand

1 teaspoon salt

½ teaspoon freshly ground black pepper

Optional toppings: chopped fresh basil or parsley, grated Asiago cheese, and toasted pine nuts

preparation

Heat broiler. Cook pasta according to package directions. Meanwhile, cut chicken into 1-inch chunks; toss with oil and dried herbs and spread out on a nonstick jelly-roll pan. Broil 5 to 6 inches from heat for 6 minutes. Add asparagus to chicken, stirring to coat lightly with oil. Continue broiling 4 minutes or until chicken is cooked through and asparagus is crisp-tender.

Transfer cooked pasta to a colander to drain. Add broth, pesto, salt, and pepper to pot; mix well. Add pasta and chicken mixture; toss well and transfer to shallow pasta bowls; top with basil, cheese, and pine nuts, if desired.

substitutions: Mediterranean or Greek leaf oregano may replace the *herbes d' Provence*; the flavor will be sharper and a little more aggressive. Pasta that is not flavored can also be used, but I suggest cooking it al dente and using a little more pesto, so the pasta can soak up the flavor.

tips: If you prefer, the chicken may be baked in a 450-degree oven for 8 minutes and the asparagus added to cook for another 6 to 8 or until the chicken is cooked through. Don't be put off by the oil in this dish: three-fourths is monounsaturated fat and healthy for the heart. Tossing the chicken with the dried herbs and then offering a blast of hot dry heat is a nice way to maximize the flavor—just toasty enough to boost it, but not enough to burn it.

nutritional analysis

Total fat (g) 12.5	Sodium (mg) 808	Vitamin A (RE) 102
Fat calories (kc) 112	Calcium (mg) 40	Beta-carotene (RE) 92
Cholesterol (mg) 98.8	Magnesium (mg) 50	Vitamin C (mg) 27
Saturated fat (g) 2.6	Zinc (mg) 3.3	Vitamin E (mg) 2.9
Polyunsaturated fat (g) 2.4	Selenium (mcg) 16	Thiamin B_1 (mg) 0.3
Monounsaturated fat (g) 5.2	Potassium (mg) 554	Riboflavin B_2 (mg) 0.4
Fiber (g) 1.8	Flavonoids (mg) 0	Niacin B_3 (mg) 7.4
Carbohydrates (g) 18.7	Lycopene (mg) 0	Vitamin B_6 (mg) 0.5
Sugar (g) 1.6	Fish (oz) 0	Folic acid (mcg) 109
Protein (g) 29	Nuts (oz) 0	Vitamin B_{12} (mcg) 0.4

Salmon with Spinach and Mustard Sauce

Preparation time: 10 minutes	*4 servings*
Cooking time: 10 minutes	*409 calories per serving, 28% from fat*

RealAge effect if eaten 12 times a year:	**RealAge-effect ingredients:**
5.1 days younger	Salmon, olive oil, lemon juice, spinach, wine (healthy protein, healthy fat, potassium, folate, alcohol, vitamins E, B_3, and B_{12}, flavonoids)

ingredients

4 (4- to 5-ounce) skinless salmon fillets

2 tablespoons soy sauce

1 tablespoon each dry white wine, lemon juice, Dijon mustard, and olive oil

1 package (10 ounces) fresh spinach, coarsely chopped

2 teaspoons finely shredded lemon peel (optional)

preparation

Rinse salmon in cold water; pat dry with paper towels. Place salmon on a shallow plate; top with soy sauce, turning to coat. Let stand 10 minutes.

Combine wine, lemon juice, mustard, and oil; set aside. Heat a large nonstick skillet over medium-high heat until hot. Add salmon; cook 3 minutes. Turn salmon gently; pour mustard mixture evenly over salmon. Immediately reduce heat to low; continue cooking until salmon is firm to the touch, 1 to 2 minutes. With a slotted spatula, transfer salmon to four serving plates; keep warm. Pour any mustard sauce from plates back into skillet. Increase heat to high. Add spinach to skillet (in two batches, if necessary); cook until wilted, turning spinach with tongs (about 1 minute). Spoon spinach and sauce over salmon. Garnish with lemon peel if desired.

substitutions: Any dry white wine will work here, as will reduced-sodium soy sauce.

tips: When you buy a salmon fillet, ask your grocer to skin it. To skin it yourself, slide a knife between the skin and the fillet. Although this takes some practice, you will be removing the fishiness of the salmon when you remove the skin.

nutritional analysis

Total fat (g) 12.4	Sodium (mg) 667	Vitamin A (RE) 501
Fat calories (kc) 112	Calcium (mg) 175	Beta-carotene (RE) 286
Cholesterol (mg) 82	Magnesium (mg) 105	Vitamin C (mg) 27
Saturated fat (g) 1.9	Zinc (mg) 1.5	Vitamin E (mg) 4.5
Polyunsaturated fat (g) 4.0	Selenium (mcg) 1	Thiamin B_1 (mg) 0.2
Monounsaturated fat (g) 6.3	Potassium (mg) 538	Riboflavin B_2 (mg) 0.4
Fiber (g) 3.2	Flavonoids (mg) 0.7	Niacin B_3 (mg) 5.9
Carbohydrates (g) 24.2	Lycopene (mg) 0	Vitamin B_6 (mg) 0.3
Sugar (g) 0.2	Fish (oz) 4.5	Folic acid (mcg) 155
Protein (g) 22.7	Nuts (oz) 0	Vitamin B_{12} (mcg) 3.8

Golden Saffron-Flavored Paella

■ ■ ■ ■

Preparation time: 5 minutes	*4 servings*
Cooking time: 25 minutes	*353 calories per serving, 15% from fat*

RealAge effect if eaten 12 times a year:	**RealAge-effect ingredients:**
Amazingly quick, this elegant dish still manages to make you 0.6 days younger.	Brown rice, garlic, olive oil, tomatoes, peas, parsley, mint (healthy protein, healthy fats, lycopene, potassium, magnesium, calcium, vitamin E, antioxidants)

ingredients

2 teaspoons olive oil

6 garlic cloves, minced

2 cups quick-cooking brown rice, preferably Uncle Ben's brand

2 cups reduced-sodium chicken or vegetable broth

1/2 teaspoon saffron threads, crushed

1/2 teaspoon hot pepper sauce

1/4 teaspoon salt

8 ounces (thawed if frozen) medium or large uncooked shelled and deveined shrimp

1 pound fresh farm-raised mussels, scrubbed (see Tips)

1 1/2 cups diced drained canned tomatoes

1 cup frozen baby peas, thawed

1/4 cup chopped Italian parsley or mint leaves

preparation

Heat a large, deep skillet over medium heat. Add oil, then garlic; sauté 2 minutes. Add rice, broth, saffron, hot pepper sauce, and salt; bring to a boil. Reduce heat; cover and simmer 8 minutes.

Stir in shrimp and mussels. Keep covered, simmering 8 to 10 minutes or until shrimp are opaque and mussels open. Stir in tomatoes and peas; heat thoroughly. Transfer to four warmed serving plates; top with parsley or mint.

substitutions: If fresh Littleneck clams are in season, you may substitute them for the mussels, or use 8 ounces of each for a dramatic appearance and extra flavor. Mix in 1/4 teaspoon cayenne pepper to replace the hot pepper sauce. You may substitute

1 teaspoon turmeric for the saffron. The color will be vibrant, but the flavor will not be as intense. Look for small vials of saffron in the spice section of your supermarket or in gourmet food stores. If the saffron you find is ground into a powder, use ¼ teaspoon.

tips: Unlike wild mussels, farm-raised mussels are free of sand and are usually free of "beards" as well. I've also made this dish with just mussels and no other seafood, and it works wonderfully. Use the mussel shells as scoops for the rice, peas, and tomatoes.

nutritional analysis

Total fat (g) 5.8	Sodium (mg) 884	Vitamin A (RE) 162
Fat calories (kc) 52.6	Calcium (mg) 123	Beta-carotene (RE) 467
Cholesterol (mg) 240.4	Magnesium (mg) 94	Vitamin C (mg) 44
Saturated fat (g) 1.1	Zinc (mg) 2.8	Vitamin E (mg) 5.3
Polyunsaturated fat (g) 1.4	Selenium (mcg) 149	Thiamin B_1 (mg) 0.2
Monounsaturated fat (g) 2.5	Potassium (mg) 890	Riboflavin B_2 (mg) 0.2
Fiber (g) 3.2	Flavonoids (mg) 2.1	Niacin B_3 (mg) 8.3
Carbohydrates (g) 33.4	Lycopene (mg) 2.9	Vitamin B_6 (mg) 0.4
Sugar (g) 3.3	Fish (oz) 0	Folic acid (mcg) 45
Protein (g) 40.4	Nuts (oz) 0	Vitamin B_{12} (mcg) 2.7

Tuscan Tuna with Grilled Tomato, Onion, and White Bean Salad

■ ■ ■ ■

Preparation time: 20 minutes	*4 servings*
Cooking time: 10 minutes	*314 calories per serving, 20% from fat*

RealAge effect if eaten 12 times a year:	RealAge-effect ingredients:
It makes your RealAge 11.4 days younger.	Tuna, tomatoes, onion, beans, arugula, olive oil (healthy protein, healthy fats, lycopene, fiber, potassium, B vitamins, flavonoids)

ingredients

3 tablespoons high-quality, aged balsamic vinegar

1½ tablespoons extra-virgin olive oil

2 teaspoons chopped fresh rosemary, crushed

½ teaspoon salt

½ teaspoon freshly ground black pepper

4 (4-ounce) fresh tuna steaks (ahi preferable) cut ½-inch thick

4 plum tomatoes, halved lengthwise

4 slices (¼-inch-thick) red or sweet onion

1 can (15 or 16 ounces) Great Northern beans, rinsed and drained

1 cup packed arugula leaves

preparation

Prepare a charcoal or gas grill (see tips). In a small bowl, combine vinegar, oil, rosemary, salt, and pepper; mix well. Set aside 2 tablespoons mixture. Brush remaining mixture over both sides of tuna, tomatoes, and onion slices.

Grill the tomatoes and onion slices 4 minutes per side or until tender. Grill the tuna 2 to 3 minutes per side for medium-rare. Do not overcook or tuna will become tough.

In a large bowl, combine beans and arugula. Cut the grilled tomatoes into chunks and separate the onions into rings; add to the bean mixture. Add reserved 2 tablespoons vinegar mixture; toss well. Arrange on four serving plates. Top with tuna; sprinkle with additional freshly ground black pepper, if desired.

substitutions: Three-quarter teaspoon dried rosemary may replace fresh rosemary; cannellini beans may replace Great Northerns; and baby spinach may replace arugula, with a less peppery flavor.

tips: A ridged grill pan may be used if a charcoal or gas grill is not available. Heat the pan over medium heat until hot. Cook the tomatoes and onions first, then the tuna. The rosemary scents the tuna just enough to give it a sharp, citrusy zing. To get extra flavor from the herb, crush it between your fingers before adding it to the marinade. Its aromatic oils will rise and meet your nose in a heavenly way. Consider using any leftover beans and tuna as a pizza topping. Sprinkle with a little grated Asiago or fresh mozzarella for a Tuscan treat.

nutritional analysis

Total fat (g) 7.2	Sodium (mg) 347	Vitamin A (RE) 1296
Fat calories (kc) 64	Calcium (mg) 125	Beta-carotene (RE) 2475
Cholesterol (mg) 56	Magnesium (mg) 161	Vitamin C (mg) 112
Saturated fat (g) 1.2	Zinc (mg) 2.3	Vitamin E (mg) 3.0
Polyunsaturated fat (g) 2.2	Selenium (mcg) 130	Thiamin B_1 (mg) 0.6
Monounsaturated fat (g) 3.8	Potassium (mg) 1466	Riboflavin B_2 (mg) 0.5
Fiber (g) 8.8	Flavonoids (mg) 2.4	Niacin B_3 (mg) 13.8
Carbohydrates (g) 46.6	Lycopene (mg) 3.1	Vitamin B_6 (mg) 1.4
Sugar (g) 16.1	Fish (oz) 4	Folic acid (mcg) 138
Protein (g) 44.7	Nuts (oz) 0	Vitamin B_{12} (mcg) 12

Tortellini Stew with Fresh Soybeans

■ ■ ■ ■

Preparation time: 6 minutes	*4 servings*
Cooking time: 14 minutes	*243 calories per serving, 27% from fat*

RealAge effect if eaten 12 times a year:	RealAge-effect ingredients:
A powerhouse of soy protein and isoflavones, this stew gives you energy to last all day— making you 2.5 days younger.	Carrots, soybeans, soy nuts, tortellini, parsley or basil (magnesium, potassium, folic acid, fiber, isoflavones, healthy protein, healthy fat)

ingredients

3 cups low-salt chicken or vegetable broth

1 package (9 or 10 ounces) refrigerated small cheese-filled tortellini

¼ teaspoon crushed red pepper flakes (optional)

½ package (16 ounces of a 32-ounce package) frozen soybeans in their pods, thawed

1 cup packaged julienned carrots or thinly sliced carrots

2 tablespoons chopped fresh basil or flat-leaf parsley

Freshly ground black pepper

4 teaspoons toasted soy nuts (optional)

preparation

In a large saucepan, combine broth, tortellini, and, if desired, red pepper flakes.
Bring to a boil over high heat. Reduce heat; simmer uncovered 2 minutes.
Meanwhile, shell the soybeans (approximately ⅔ cup shelled soybeans). Stir soybeans

and carrots into the tortellini mixture; return to a simmer. Simmer 6 to 8 minutes or until tortellini and vegetables are tender. Ladle into shallow bowls and sprinkle with basil (or parsley) and pepper, and with soy nuts, if desired.

substitutions: Refrigerated ravioli may replace tortellini, and 1½ cups packed baby spinach leaves may replace soybeans. Just before serving, stir in the spinach until it is wilted.

tips: Soybeans now come shelled! Look for them in your supermarket's freezer case. Even so, shelling beans is easy and quick: Just press on the seam and pop them out of their shells.

nutritional analysis

Total fat (g) 7.4	Sodium (mg) 764	Vitamin A (RE) 980
Fat calories (kc) 67	Calcium (mg) 131	Beta-carotene (RE) 5500
Cholesterol (mg) 3.8	Magnesium (mg) 20	Vitamin C (mg) 7
Saturated fat (g) 2.1	Zinc (mg) 0.7	Vitamin E (mg) 0.8
Polyunsaturated fat (g) 1.1	Selenium (mcg) 7	Thiamin B_1 (mg) 0.30
Monounsaturated fat (g) 1.9	Potassium (mg) 857	Riboflavin B_2 (mg) 0.3
Fiber (g) 1.9	Flavonoids (mg) 0	Niacin B_3 (mg) 4.2
Carbohydrates (g) 28.9	Lycopene (mg) 0	Vitamin B_6 (mg) 0.1
Sugar (g) 4.9	Fish (oz) 0	Folic acid (mcg) 24
Protein (g) 17.2	Nuts (oz) 0	Vitamin B_{12} (mcg) 0.3

As a Side Dish

Keith's Asparagus

■ ■ ■ ■

Preparation time: 5 minutes	4 servings
Cooking time: 15 to 18 minutes	38 calories per serving, 35% from fat

RealAge effect if eaten 12 times a year:	RealAge-effect ingredients:
3.1 days younger. It's so simple, it must make your RealAge younger because of that, too!	Asparagus, olive oil (potassium, healthy fats, folic acid)

ingredients

1 pound asparagus, rinsed, dried, and trimmed

1 teaspoon extra-virgin olive oil

Kosher salt, to taste

A pinch each thyme, oregano, basil, and black pepper

Diced tomato (optional)

preparation

Heat the oven to 350 degrees. Toss the asparagus in a 9 × 13-inch baking dish or a shallow 3-quart casserole with the olive oil, kosher salt, thyme, oregano, basil, and black pepper. Arrange asparagus in a single layer in the dish. Bake uncovered 12 to 13 minutes for thin asparagus or 15 to 18 minutes for thick asparagus, or until crisp-tender. Garnish with tomato, if desired.

tip: When adding the herbs, crush them between your fingers to increase their flavor.

nutritional analysis

Total fat (g) 1.5	Sodium (mg) 5	Vitamin A (RE) 94
Fat calories (kc) 13.3	Calcium (mg) 27	Beta-carotene (RE) 102
Cholesterol (mg) 0	Magnesium (mg) 22	Vitamin C (mg) 31
Saturated fat (g) 0.2	Zinc (mg) 0.5	Vitamin E (mg) 2.4
Polyunsaturated fat (g) 0.3	Selenium (mcg) 4	Thiamin B_1 (mg) 0.1
Monounsaturated fat (g) 0.8	Potassium (mg) 352	Riboflavin B_2 (mg) 0.1
Fiber (g) 1.4	Flavonoids (mg) 0	Niacin B_3 (mg) 1.2
Carbohydrates (g) 5.0	Lycopene (mg) 0	Vitamin B_6 (mg) 0.2
Sugar (g) 1.8	Fish (oz) 0	Folic acid (mcg) 112
Protein (g) 2.9	Nuts (oz) 0	Vitamin B_{12} (mcg) 0

Chocolate Strawberry Sundae

■ ■ ■ ■

Preparation time: 5 minutes	4 servings
	216 calories per serving, 10% from fat

RealAge effect if eaten 12 times a year:	RealAge-effect ingredients:
Berries of all kinds are powerhouses of fiber. That plus the flavonoids in chocolate make your RealAge 7.2 days younger.	Strawberries, whole-grain granola (fiber, flavonoids)

ingredients

4 (½-cup) scoops nonfat or low-fat chocolate frozen yogurt

1½ cups sliced strawberries

1 cup low-fat granola cereal, such as Quaker brand

2 teaspoons confectioners' sugar

preparation

Scoop yogurt into four serving bowls; top with strawberries and granola. Place confectioners' sugar in a strainer and shake over sundaes.

substitutions: One cup whole-grain cereal flakes may replace the granola. Coffee-flavored frozen yogurt may replace the chocolate frozen yogurt, and blueberries may replace the strawberries (a Chocolate Blueberry Sundae).

tips: For a special occasion, drizzle a bit of Baileys Irish Cream (a cream liqueur) or chocolate liqueur over the sundae just before serving. The confectioners' sugar brightens the color of the dessert; just ½ teaspoon per serving is all that's needed. For color, place all the strawberries on top. If you can find them, get the tiny alpine strawberries instead. Nuggets of berry goodness, they still grow wild, and can be found in farmers' markets.

nutritional analysis

Total fat (g) 2	Sodium (mg) 107	Vitamin A (RE) 299
Fat calories (kc) 87	Calcium (mg) 232	Beta-carotene (RE) 20
Cholesterol (mg) 1.4	Magnesium (mg) 115	Vitamin C (mg) 41
Saturated fat (g) 0.49	Zinc (mg) 3.9	Vitamin E (mg) 3.3
Polyunsaturated fat (g) 2.3	Selenium (mcg) 21	Thiamin B_1 (mg) 0.6
Monounsaturated fat (g) 5.0	Potassium (mg) 588	Riboflavin B_2 (mg) 0.8
Fiber (g) 8.4	Flavonoids (mg) 1.9	Niacin B_3 (mg) 5.3
Carbohydrates (g) 12.8	Lycopene (mg) 0	Vitamin B_6 (mg) 0.5
Sugar (g) 26.7	Fish (oz) 0	Folic acid (mcg) 94
Protein (g) 15.7	Nuts (oz) 0	Vitamin B_{12} (mcg) 0.9

⁂ Summer Produce ⁂

The warm weather of summer brings new fruits, vegetables, and herbs. The plants that grow well in summer seem to go well together in salads and ragouts, and on a plate. Tomatoes and basil, potatoes and rosemary, corn and beans, and cucumbers and onions are all perfect pairs of flavor.

Summer Produce Chart

Vegetable/Fruit	Buying and Using
Apricots	➤ **When:** Apricots are best in June and July. Tree-ripened apricots have the best flavor but are so delicate they don't seem to make it to the supermarket. However, a trip to your farmers' market should produce an abundance. Blenheim apricots are a favorite.
	➤ **What to Look For:** Apricots should have a sweet aroma, good color, and yield to gentle pressure, which indicates ripeness. Avoid apricots with a slightly green color, as they were picked too soon.
	➤ **Why:** Apricots contain age-reducing lycopene.
	➤ **How to Use:** Apricots can be dried and eaten as a snack or used in breads, salsas, and salads. They're also used in pies, other desserts, and blended drinks.
Beets	➤ **When:** Beets are available year-round, but in colder climates they are best in May or June. Look for golden beets (the color of saffron) and Chioggia beets (concentric, candy-striped purple circles appear when the beet is cut). Because the sugar in beets quickly turns to starch, they're best eaten soon after they've been plucked from the earth.
	➤ **What to Look For:** Inspect the greens for freshness. The tops should be a bright color with no yellowing or wilting. Also, the roots should have a firm, fine texture and a regular shape. The small, hairy roots can be easily brushed away.
	➤ **Why:** Beets are rich in RealAge-smart magnesium and potassium.

Vegetable/Fruit	Buying and Using
	➤ **How to Use:** The intense color of beets makes them a beautiful addition to salads. Beets are surprisingly sweet and work well with tangy or salty foods. For example, a tangy vinaigrette offsets the sweetness of beets; so does a crumble of feta or blue cheese. Beets are also used in rice dishes and soup. Try cutting them into cubes and tossing with olive oil, salt, and pepper; then roasting them at 400 degrees until crisp and tender (about 30 minutes).
Berries (blackberries, blueberries, boysenberries, raspberries)	➤ **When:** Berries are at their best from June to August; strawberries may appear a little earlier. In some climates, a second crop of raspberries appears in the fall. ➤ **What to Look For:** Berries should have a rich color and shiny surface. The sacs of the berry should be firm and plump. Inspect the bottom of the container to see if juice has soaked through. If so, the berries have been crushed. Blueberries are a little different from other berries. They don't have much of an aroma and should have a solid, dark blue color, a powdery skin, and a firm texture. ➤ **Why:** Berries are chock-full of antioxidants, which slow aging of the arteries and immune system. ➤ **How to Use:** Berries are delicious on their own. The variety of colors makes berries a vibrant addition to dishes—in a fruit salad; added with nuts to a green salad; or as a topping for pancakes, French toast, and waffles. They're used mostly in sweet dishes: pies, jams, sauces, breads, muffins, and cakes. Wonderful salsas, relishes, and chutneys can be made with berries as well. Berries taste great in many ways, including our Double Strawberry Blender Blast (page 192).
Cherries	➤ **When:** Sweet cherries are available starting in late May. Sour (tart) cherries ripen later and appear for just a few weeks in July. They're only a little less sweet than Bing or Rainier cherries and have a delightful, subtle tang. Rainier and Royal Anne cherries are sun-colored and blushed with flavor—buy them wherever you find them; they're special.

Vegetable/Fruit	Buying and Using

➤ **What to Look For:** Cherries should be firm and have a shiny surface. A green stem indicates they were just picked. In general, the darker the color, the longer the cherry's been on the tree, and the more flavorful it is.

➤ **Why:** Cherries are a rich source of antioxidants, which help fight cancer and heart disease.

➤ **How to Use:** Cherries can be pitted, dried, and eaten as a snack or used in breads and muffins. They are frequently used in desserts, such as cherry cobbler, or as a topping or sauce.

Chiles (peppers)

➤ **When:** Chiles are in season in summer: jalapeños and serranos in June, July, and August, and habaneros and poblanos in August, September, and October. Look for manzanos—they're apple shaped, easy to grow in filtered light, and sweeter than most chiles. And hot when roasted! Experiment with all of them.

➤ **What to Look For:** Almost always, fresh chiles are green, red, or orange: The red and orange chiles have stayed on the plant several weeks longer, becoming sweeter and more mature. A chile is fresh if the skin is unbroken, the flesh is unmarked (although a darkening of the flesh does not indicate a problem), and it's bright and crisp at both ends. The skin of a chile should be shiny, and its fragrance faint and a little floral.

➤ **Why:** Most of us would eat chiles just for their taste, but their potassium, flavonoids, and fiber also make them an anti-aging delight.

➤ **How to Use:** Poblano chiles are an interesting, flavorful substitute for green bell peppers, and an easy way to get started with chiles. The flavor of chiles is more important to many chile-lovers than their heat. Most of the heat is in the seeds and ribs, not in the flesh. Chiles are often seeded and chopped fresh for salsas. Roasting brings out their sweetness for soups, sauces, salsas, and stews. Drying preserves them for use in the fall and winter.

Vegetable/Fruit	Buying and Using
Corn	

Corn

➤ **When:** Even though corn that is knee high by the Fourth of July has often been genetically modified, the best time for sweet corn is still summer. Field corn is grown for animal feed. You may find ornamental (Indian) corn and even popcorn ears: whole dried ears that respond to a deep freeze, a quick shucking, and then, pop!

➤ **What to Look For:** White, yellow, or bicolor varieties abound, as do individual tastes. The husk should be closed around the ear. The tip should be filled out with niblets. The colored tassel should be dark and intact. Ears with smaller uniform kernels are desirable. If you find a dark fungus (now a gourmet item on some Mexican menus called *huitlacoche*), put it back—save the gourmet item for the restaurant.

➤ **Why:** The most important RealAge-smart nutrient in corn is potassium.

➤ **How to Use:** Sweet corn can be eaten without cooking, with a quick steam or brief boil. You can soak whole ears in water and then grill them, husk and all. Niblets shaved off ears can be tossed into cold salads or hot soups and stews, or combined with beans and squash for succotash.

Cucumbers

➤ **When:** Cucumbers are available year-round, the peak season being May to August.

➤ **What to Look For:** These vegetables should be firm and turgid. Make sure they aren't wrinkled because that means they aren't fresh. (The exception is the Kirby pickle, which is used for dill and sweet pickles and is naturally wrinkled.)

➤ **Why:** I used to think cucumbers were mostly water and ate them mainly for their crunchy texture. I've since learned that cucumbers contain calcium, which makes me younger whenever I eat them.

Vegetable/Fruit	Buying and Using

How to Use: Cucumbers are good raw, with dips, in salads, and on sandwiches. A cucumber salad—cucumbers marinated in your vinegar of choice with a little water—is light and refreshing. Cucumbers can also be used in sauces. Removing the peel is usually unnecessary for young cucumbers, which often have thin and delicate peels. However, in the supermarket (but not the farmers' market), some cucumbers are waxed to keep moisture in, and these you'll want to peel.

Eggplants

➤ **When:** The peak season for eggplant is August and September.

➤ **What to Look For:** Shininess is a good indication of freshness. Also, the eggplant should give only slightly to pressure; if it's mushy, it's overripe. The blossom end indicates whether it's male (fewer seeds) or female (lots of seeds).

➤ **Why:** Eggplant is rich in potassium, which makes it a RealAge-smart choice.

➤ **How to Use:** Eggplant is seldom eaten raw. Try eggplant broiled, fried, grilled, roasted, and sautéed. It's a very versatile vegetable. Its meatiness lends itself to many dishes—stews, moussaka, ratatouille, dips, and baba ghanoush. It can even be a stuffed dinner entrée in itself, perhaps loaded with chickpeas, tuna, roasted tomatoes, roasted garlic, and sweet onions. Be careful about adding oil (even healthy oil), however, as eggplant is an "oil sponge." Just a *little* oil makes eggplant great.

Figs

➤ **When:** Fresh figs are at their best in July and August. Eating a ripe fig, with its seedy and chewy sweetness, is for many people a rite of summer.

➤ **What to Look For:** Look for soft figs. If they're too firm, like golf balls, they won't ripen properly. Figs should also be free of bruises, nicks, and mold. Black Mission figs taste especially good when they're slightly shriveled.

181

Vegetable/Fruit	Buying and Using

➤ **Why:** The RealAge-smart nutrients in figs are fiber, calcium, and potassium.

➤ **How to Use:** Dried figs are often used in desserts but can be cooked with meats or added to salads. Chef Oscar of Emilio's Restaurant in Santa Barbara tosses golden figs with Gorgonzola and arugula to make a special pizza. Use figs in pudding, tarts, and sauces. Fresh figs make a wonderful dessert because they're sweet yet not too heavy. Serve them with dates, almonds, and rose water for a taste of Morocco. Dry any extra figs for use in the winter.

Garlic

➤ **When:** Garlic is available throughout the year, although it's usually planted in the fall and harvested in the summer. Garlic is used in so many dishes, a RealAge cook couldn't live without it. Look for elephant garlic, which is larger and milder than most other types.

➤ **What to Look For:** Always buy a whole, firm, tightly closed bulb. Watch out for black and brown spots, which indicate mold or bruising, and green sprouts, which indicate aging. Some varieties are purple at the top, and some are white; some bulbs are smaller, and some very large. Each has a slightly different garlicky flavor.

➤ **Why:** Garlic slows aging of both the arteries and immune system, thanks to its high content of selenium and potassium, and probably other phytonutrients as well.

➤ **How to Use:** Garlic usually isn't eaten raw but is cooked as a flavoring for grains, vegetables, and sauces. If you want to eat a clove or two raw, mince the garlic and enjoy its taste in a freshly made guacamole or a white wine vinaigrette. Roasting garlic (350 to 375 degrees for 30 to 45 minutes, or 500 degrees for 15 to 25 minutes) produces a sweet, buttery spread for crackers, breads, focaccias, and pizzas. Roasted garlic adds a wonderful roundness to soups, sauces, spreads, and stews and takes the place of extra oil. In addition, whole cloves often become sweet when simmered.

Vegetable/Fruit	Buying and Using
Green beans	➤ **When:** Green beans (string or snap beans) are at their peak in the early summer and, in warmer climates, even earlier. Green beans represent the young, tender stage (the first week) in a bean's life. Especially tender are Blue Lake or Kentucky Wonder green beans and nearly any filet bean, or *haricot vert*. (The second stage produces shell beans—for example, cannellini, lima, and cranberry beans. The third stage produces dried beans—for example, black beans, scarlet runner beans, and Anasazi beans. All, when properly cooked, are vastly superior in flavor to canned or frozen beans.) ➤ **What to Look For:** Green beans can be green, yellow, or purple. Look for pods of any size that are bright in color and snap easily when bent. A few may have the stems still attached—that's fine. Avoid soft beans that bend easily. The seeds inside should be tiny, soft, and hardly noticeable. ➤ **Why:** The RealAge-smart nutrients in green beans are calcium, folate, and potassium. ➤ **How to Use:** Green beans can be eaten raw. Just snap off the ends and eat, or use them for dipping. Cook green beans quickly, if at all. They can be boiled, sautéed, or stir-fried. Mix them with other seasonal vegetables or add to soups and stews at the end of the cooking process.
Herbs (basil, chervil, chives, cilantro, dill, marjoram, mint, oregano, parsley, rosemary, sage, tarragon)	➤ **When:** You know summer is here when herbs are abundant in the garden. Although herbs are available all year, the herbs noted here are outstanding during the summer. ➤ **What to Look For:** Leaves should be fresh, with no signs of wilting or decay. ➤ **Why:** Replacing salt and unhealthy fats with the great flavors herbs add makes your arteries younger. ➤ **How to Use:** Herbs can be added to nearly any dish; they bring out extraordinary flavor and create a light but concentrated essence that

Vegetable/Fruit	Buying and Using

enhances almost all foods. Mix more than one herb, just for fun. Use herbs generously in your recipes, especially to replace aging fats and oils as a source of flavor. Make pestos with any leftover herbs; chop milder herbs (in large quantity) as the base for tabbouleh; strew herbs over fish and under tomatoes. Use the stems, too: Chop some of the thinner ones together with the leaves.

Kohlrabi

➤ **When:** Kohlrabi is a member of the cabbage family that has a greatly enlarged, edible stem. It's available from midspring to midfall but is best in the summer.

➤ **What to Look For:** This vegetable looks like a spaceship from another planet, with its purple- and green-streaked leaves flying everywhere. A fresh kohlrabi feels heavy for its size and has firm (not floppy) dark leaves. Avoid any kohlrabies having soft spots on the bulb or yellowing of the leaf tips. The tenderest kohlrabies are less than 3 inches in diameter.

➤ **Why:** Kohlrabi is not only tasty but rich in folate, flavonoids, and potassium, making it an almost-ideal nutrient-rich, calorie-poor, RealAge choice.

➤ **How to Use:** Kohlrabi is commonly served as crudités: peeled, cut into wedges, or sliced thinly and served with sea salt. It's also eaten raw in salads, on a sandwich, or in soups.

Melons

➤ **When:** Summer would not be the same without melons. Enjoy all the different melons summer brings. Look specifically for Charentais, Galia, and Ambrosia; these varieties of muskmelon have a wonderful perfume.

➤ **What to Look For:** Not all melons are the same. A cantaloupe (a muskmelon) should have a tan or gold netting and be firm, fragrant, and heavy for its size. Honeydew should be creamy white, velvety, and slightly sticky on the surface. In general, melons are ripe if they are heavy for their size. For other hints of ripeness, sniff melons near the blossom end for sweetness, and press gently.

➤ **How to Use:** Melons are eaten raw or used in salads or as a topping for desserts. Blended with lime and sweetener, they make a refreshing drink.

Nectarines

➤ **When:** Although nectarines are available from midspring to late September, their peak months are July and August.

➤ **What to Look For:** For best flavor, look for tree-ripened nectarines at a farmers' market because they'll usually have a sweeter, juicier flavor than those in the store. Nectarines should have a sweet scent and yield to gentle pressure. Avoid nectarines having a green tinge; some will still have their stems attached.

➤ **Why:** Although desirable just for their taste, nectarines are also loaded with potassium and vitamins, making your RealAge younger.

➤ **How to Use:** Nectarines are versatile. Eat nectarines as a snack or bake them in a pie, compote, or cobbler. They can be used in salads and sweet sauces or as a dessert topping. Brush them with a bit of barbecue sauce and toss them on the grill. For a quick fruit salsa, chop nectarines with jalapeño peppers, green onions, lime, and a little sugar.

Okra

➤ **When:** Okra is available fresh year-round in the South and is a favorite in Southern cooking. The rest of the country enjoys okra from May through October.

➤ **What to Look For:** Find small okra, no more than 3 inches long. The pods should be tender yet crisp and have little or no damage to the surface; they do not have to be smooth.

➤ **Why:** Okra is loaded with potassium.

➤ **How to Use:** Okra needs to be properly cooked; it's great steamed, grilled, or fried. It's best known for its role in gumbo, and as a thickening agent for stews and soup. Okra is also delicious pickled.

Onions

➤ **When:** For most of the United States, the peak onion season is late summer and early fall. Look for cipollini onions (small, flat, and

Vegetable/Fruit	Buying and Using

very sweet) and torpedo onions (they're red!). Try new onions you've never tried; their flavors are all slightly different.

➤ **What to Look For:** Avoid onions that have sprouts, mold, or soft spots. Fresh onions will last two weeks before they begin to sprout: most of the available onions are storage onions, which have been dried and last for months. Buy white, yellow, and red. If you can buy only one, buy white: the flavor is clean and fresh.

➤ **Why:** Onions contain age-reducing flavonoids and selenium. Another age-reducing benefit is that certain substances (we do not know what substances) in onions inhibit the bacteria associated with stomach ulcers.

➤ **How to Use:** Many dishes could use an onion, so have them on hand at all times. Sauté, grill, roast, or simmer them. Add them to sauces or vegetable medleys. Caramelize onions as a topping for portobello mushrooms or tuna steak. For a pasta sauce with a twist, blend roasted onions with roasted serrano peppers, roasted garlic, and roasted tomatoes or tomatillos, oregano, and olive oil. To store, keep onions in a cool, dark, dry place.

Peaches

➤ **When:** Although peaches are available from May to October in most regions of the United States, they're sweetest in the summer.

➤ **What to Look For:** Look for white-flesh peaches: They're usually even sweeter and more honeyed than the yellow-flesh ones. Peaches should have a sweet scent and yield to gentle pressure. Avoid peaches with bruised, shriveled, or dented skin.

➤ **Why:** Because peaches are rich in potassium and flavonoids, they are a delicious way to stay healthy.

➤ **How to Use:** A ripe summer peach is so sweet and juicy it can be a dessert all by itself. However, peaches are commonly used in pies, nectars, cobblers, cakes, and soufflés. They also make great salsas, can be grilled with other fruits, and blend happily into drinks. Try a Bellini—fresh peach juice and champagne.

Vegetable/Fruit	Buying and Using

Peppers (green)

➤ **When:** Peppers are good to eat July through late summer.

➤ **What to Look For:** Green peppers are sweet peppers that are not ripe. They may be slightly bitter because their full flavor has not yet developed. The skin should be smooth and not shriveled. Avoid peppers with soft spots or cracks, or with tops that are moldy or turning colors.

➤ **Why:** Peppers are loaded with vitamin C, flavonoids, and fiber, giving them an age-reducing benefit.

➤ **How to Use:** Green peppers have a bright, fresh, slightly grassy flavor that many people love. They're not sweet like their more mature red and yellow counterparts, and they mix well with most summer vegetables and herbs. Green peppers can be grilled, roasted, sautéed, used in sandwiches, and diced to top salads, soups, stews, chili, and sauces. Also see CHILES.

Plums

➤ **When:** Fresh plums are at their peak ripeness in August and September. There are dozens of varieties; some have yellow flesh, some purple, and some green. Italian plums tend to be smaller and have green flesh, and make wonderful jams. Try as many varieties as you can find; you'll be rewarded with great color and flavor.

➤ **What to Look For:** Plums that are perfect have a uniform color and sweet scent and yield to gentle pressure with a taut skin. Avoid very firm or hard plums, because they've been picked too soon and won't ripen properly. Ask for a sample.

➤ **Why:** Because potassium and fiber are found in plums in abundance, eating this fruit is an age-reducing benefit.

➤ **How to Use:** Eat ripe plums plain or save them for sweet dishes such as jams, desserts, and sweet sauces. They can also be chopped to make a stuffing, diced to make a salsa, and grilled to make an accompaniment for chicken or fish. Plums are good poached in wine with peaches, or stewed with lemon and cinnamon.

Vegetable/Fruit	Buying and Using

In addition, plums can be dried to make prunes. Puréed prunes make a good replacement for solid, aging fat in quick-breads.

Potatoes, new

➤ **When:** New potatoes are baby potatoes that have been harvested young in their life. They're best in early summer, all the way till August. New potatoes have a thin skin and are great with little preparation. They may be pink, brown, yellow, red, or white; all are beautiful and delicious.

➤ **What to Look For:** Small new potatoes tend to have better flavor and softer texture than larger ones. Avoid those with sprouts, a green tint, or dry, chapped skin. The green tint on potatoes contains a substance—solanine—that can be poisonous, and that can be very aging. (So don't eat potatoes that have started to sprout or have green skin!)

➤ **Why:** The major age-reducing benefits of potatoes come from the potassium and fiber in the skin. Because potatoes have a lot of simple carbohydrates, eat a little healthy fat first to gain the most RealAge benefit.

➤ **How to Use:** New potatoes are wonderful in salads because they hold their shape well, and because their flavor combines with other ingredients so well. Steaming and roasting work best for new potatoes, although pan-frying, and grilling work as well. For hash browns, try shredded new potatoes tossed with garlic and thyme, or grated with onion and then tossed in a skillet with dried leaf oregano.

Summer squash (zucchini, lita, pattypan squash, crookneck squash)

➤ **When:** Summer squash is well named because it peaks in the summer. These beautiful, easy-to-grow vegetables come in a variety of colors and shapes.

➤ **What to Look For:** The skin should be smooth, with few marks, and tender enough to be pierced easily by a fingernail. (Don't do this in the market; just squeeze gently.) Squash should have a bright color and feel relatively heavy for its size. A bit of juice coming out of the stem means it's fresh; in fact, it was probably picked that morning.

Avoid squash that bend easily or have a wrinkled skin: They're old or drying out.

➤ **Why:** Squash are rich in potassium and fiber, both of which provide a RealAge benefit.

➤ **How to Use:** Summer squash can be grilled, sautéed, used in soups and stews, or mixed with whole grains and vegetables. Combine diced zucchini with fresh corn and red chile pepper, or stew a tomato, garlic, and onion ragout. Large zucchini (over 10 inches) are best for breads, muffins, and pancakes. Also, squash blossoms can be eaten. They're usually stuffed and baked or fried but can also garnish a soup or be shredded and mixed into a salad.

Tomatillos

➤ **When:** Tomatillos are small, green, yellow, or purple tomato-like jewels that have a parchment-paper husk and are related to the ground cherry. These vegetables are a staple in Mexican cuisine. Tomatillos are, like tomatoes, available all year. Their jacket helps preserve them and their bright, tangy, slightly grassy flavor. Tomatillos are nearly all flesh, with few seeds. In the United States, they're best in late summer and early fall. Look for specialty tomatillos; the purple ones are smoky in flavor and worth trying.

➤ **What to Look For:** Tomatillos are freshest when they have no punctures, worms, or blemishes. If you can't see part of the fruit and the jacket is closed all around it, pass it up; the fruit has not fully ripened. Smaller tomatillos tend to be sweeter, and larger ones tend to be easier to peel. In general, tomatillos that are lighter green and almost yellow have been left on the vine and are naturally sweet; they're coming out of their jackets and are usually not sour.

➤ **Why:** Tomatillos have a lot of RealAge-smart nutrients, including lycopene, potassium, vitamin C, vitamin K, folate, and flavonoids.

➤ **How to Use:** Peel away the jacket just before you use the tomatillo. Wash these vegetables especially well, as dirt hides beneath the jacket. Eat only the smallest ones raw—halved in salads, as a garnish, or in salsas. To maximize their sweetness, broil a whole tray at a time, flipping them to broil the other side, or blacken them in a skillet. Boil them with green herbs and onion for a hot salsa, or for the base of a sauce or soup.

Tomatoes

➤ **When:** Although tomatoes are available year-round, nothing says summer like the plump, juicy, vine-ripened tomatoes of July and August. Most of the tomatoes available in the United States from December through March have not been grown in the ground near you.

➤ **What to Look For:** A tomato with an aroma is a tomato with flavor. A tomato should be firm to the touch but not hard. It should feel heavy for its size. The color is not an indication of flavor, except that the tomato should not be green (a gourmet exception is the heirloom tomato Green Zebra); green means it's not ripe. If the tomatoes are very ripe and have been stacked, pick the ones on top because the ones on the bottom are likely to be damaged from the weight of the others. Pick the brightest, heaviest, most aromatic tomatoes you can find to eat tonight.

➤ **Why:** Not only do tomatoes taste great but also, when eaten with a little fat, they're one of the most age-reducing foods. Eating 10 cooked tomatoes a week (the equivalent of 10 tablespoons of tomato sauce) decreases the risk of prostate and breast cancer by over 40 percent. Tomatoes are rich in other age-reducing nutrients, including potassium, folate, flavonoids, and vitamin C.

➤ **How to Use:** Ripe tomatoes are good in almost everything—classic Italian summer salads (layered fresh basil, fresh mozzarella, and tomato dressed with olive oil and vinegar), and as the base for casseroles, soups, sauces, salsas, stews, and chilies. Fill scooped-out tomatoes with couscous mixed with diced zucchini, carrots, and sweet onion, topped with fresh tangy goat cheese and toasted pistachios. Tomatoes that are not at their peak can be roasted to intensify their sweetness and then cooled and frozen. Some cooks

Vegetable/Fruit	Buying and Using
	peel and seed their tomatoes, but we believe this is hardly ever necessary and eliminates a major RealAge effect. Ninety percent of the lycopene—the ingredient in the tomato thought to keep the arteries and immune system young—lies within 1 millimeter of the skin. Store tomatoes at room temperature, ideally in an open paper bag, to ripen further.

Recipes Using Summer Produce

FOR BREAKFAST

Double Strawberry Blender Blast

■ ■ ■ ■

Preparation time: 8 minutes

4 (1-cup) servings
103 calories per serving, 4% from fat

RealAge effect if eaten 12 times a year:

Strawberries are loaded with vitamin C. I could drink this smoothie all day and skip the vitamin C supplement. Each cup 12 times a year makes you 5.7 days younger.

RealAge-effect ingredients:

Berries, soy milk (vitamin C, flavonoids, folic acid, antioxidants, potassium)

ingredients

3 cups (12 ounces) hulled, halved fresh strawberries

1 cup fat-free or light soy milk

1 cup (6 ounces) strawberry sorbet, such as Häagen-Dazs brand

preparation

Combine strawberries and soy milk in blender container. Cover and blend until fairly smooth. Add sorbet; cover and blend until smooth and thick.

substitutions: Thawed frozen unsweetened strawberries may replace the fresh strawberries; skim milk or 1% milk may replace the soy milk.

tips: Other berries and sorbets will work with this, too: blueberries and lime sorbet, blackberries and chocolate sorbet, and raspberries and lemon sorbet. Experiment and enjoy!

nutritional analysis

Total fat (g) 0.5
Fat calories (kc) 4
Cholesterol (mg) 3.5
Saturated fat (g) 0.2
Polyunsaturated fat (g) 0.2
Monounsaturated fat (g) 0.2
Fiber (g) 5.3
Carbohydrates (g) 35.3
Sugar (g) 6.3
Protein (g) 5.4

Sodium (mg) 18
Calcium (mg) 70
Magnesium (mg) 39
Zinc (mg) 0.9
Selenium (mcg) 12
Potassium (mg) 374
Flavonoids (mg) 2.5
Lycopene (mg) 0
Fish (oz) 0
Nuts (oz) 0

Vitamin A (RE) 15
Beta-carotene (RE) 29
Vitamin C (mg) 64
Vitamin E (mg) 0.2
Thiamin B_1 (mg) 0.2
Riboflavin B_2 (mg) 0.2
Niacin B_3 (mg) 1.4
Vitamin B_6 (mg) 0.1
Folic acid (mcg) 41
Vitamin B_{12} (mcg) 0.04

Cheese Blintzes with Blueberry-Lime Sauce

Preparation time: 10 minutes
Cooking time: 10 minutes

4 servings
352 calories per serving, 14% from fat

RealAge effect if eaten 12 times a year:	RealAge-effect ingredients:
The rich load of fiber and antioxidants in blueberries plus the phytonutrients in tofu combine to make you more than 6 days younger.	Tofu, berries, lime juice, and zest (fiber, antioxidants, calcium, folic acid, phytonutrients)

ingredients

1½ cups light ricotta cheese, such as Sargento brand

1 package (10 ounces) light silken tofu, such as Mori-Nu brand

¼ teaspoon salt

1 pint (12 ounces, about 2¼ cups) fresh blueberries

8 prepared crepes, such as Frieda's or Melissa's brand (see Tips)

5 tablespoons whole-fruit blueberry preserves, such as Dickinson's brand

Cooking oil spray

1 lime

preparation

Heat oven to 400 degrees. In a medium bowl, whisk together ricotta cheese, tofu, and salt. Set aside 1½ cups blueberries for sauce; stir remaining blueberries into cheese mixture.

Spread 3 tablespoons of the preserves (about 1 teaspoon per crepe) thinly over bottom half of the crepes. Spread the cheese mixture over preserves. Fold both sides of crepe in 1 inch over filling, then roll up completely to enclose filling.

Coat a 9 × 13-inch baking or casserole dish with cooking oil spray. Arrange blintzes in dish, seam side down. Cover dish with foil; bake 10 minutes or until warm.

Meanwhile, finely grate or zest 2 teaspoons lime peel from the lime; set aside. Squeeze enough lime juice from the lime to measure 2 tablespoons. Combine reserved blueberries, lime juice, and remaining 2 tablespoons preserves in a medium saucepan. Bring to a simmer; simmer gently 3 to 4 minutes or until berries pop and mixture is slightly thickened, stirring occasionally. Transfer blintzes to four serving plates; top with blueberry sauce and sprinkle with lime zest.

substitutions: Silken tofu that is not low fat will also work in this dish, and will make it slightly rich.

tips: Prepared crepes are usually found in the produce section of the supermarket, near the fresh berries.

When fresh blueberries are in season, freeze extras to use in this dish. Do not thaw the berries before using them. For a firmer, denser filling, drain the ricotta cheese in a strainer lined with a double thickness of paper towels.

nutritional analysis

Total fat (g) 5.6	Sodium (mg) 401	Vitamin A (RE) 132
Fat calories (kc) 51	Calcium (mg) 484	Beta-carotene (RE) 124
Cholesterol (mg) 26	Magnesium (mg) 99	Vitamin C (mg) 18
Saturated fat (g) 0.6	Zinc (mg) 2.8	Vitamin E (mg) 1.6
Polyunsaturated fat (g) 1.3	Selenium (mcg) 12	Thiamin B_1 (mg) 0.2
Monounsaturated fat (g) 1.4	Potassium (mg) 446	Riboflavin B_2 (mg) 0.4
Fiber (g) 4.7	Flavonoids (mg) 0	Niacin B_3 (mg) 2.7
Carbohydrates (g) 63.3	Lycopene (mg) 0	Vitamin B_6 (mg) 0.2
Sugar (g) 7.5	Fish (oz) 0	Folic acid (mcg) 51
Protein (g) 26.6	Nuts (oz) 0	Vitamin B_{12} (mcg) 0.3

Frothy Raspberry-Orange Smoothie

■ ■ ■ ■

Preparation time: 5 minutes	*4 (8-ounce) servings*
	253 calories per serving, 1% from fat

RealAge effect if eaten 12 times a year:

Packed with vitamin C, this smoothie offers great possibilities: add a scoop of soy powder for extra isoflavones. Even without it, what a great way to get your antioxidants, as each drink makes you 6.8 days younger!

RealAge-effect ingredients:

Bananas, berries, orange juice, soy milk (vitamin C, isoflavones, potassium, antioxidants, flavonoids, folic acid, fiber)

ingredients

2 cups nonfat or 1% vanilla soy milk

2 ripe medium bananas

2 cups frozen raspberries

2 tablespoons frozen orange juice concentrate

preparation

Combine all ingredients in a blender container. Cover; blend until smooth.

substitutions: Two cups skim or 1% milk plus ½ teaspoon vanilla may replace the vanilla soy milk. Frozen strawberries or mixed berries may replace the raspberries. If fruit is fresh rather than frozen, add two or three ice cubes.

tips: For a delicious, appetite-suppressing, RealAge-smart breakfast, serve this frosty fiber-packed breakfast shake with a toasted whole wheat English muffin spread with peanut butter.

nutritional analysis

Total fat (g) 0.2	Sodium (mg) 15	Vitamin A (RE) 20
Fat calories (kc) 2	Calcium (mg) 26	Beta-carotene (RE) 121
Cholesterol (mg) 0	Magnesium (mg) 55	Vitamin C (mg) 40
Saturated fat (g) 0.1	Zinc (mg) 0.7	Vitamin E (mg) 0.4
Polyunsaturated fat (g) 0.3	Selenium (mcg) 1	Thiamin B_1 (mg) 0.3
Monounsaturated fat (g) 0.1	Potassium (mg) 584	Riboflavin B_2 (mg) 0.2
Fiber (g) 5.3	Flavonoids (mg) 0.2	Niacin B_3 (mg) 1.1
Carbohydrates (g) 28	Lycopene (mg) 0	Vitamin B_6 (mg) 0.4
Sugar (g) 13.2	Fish (oz) 0	Folic acid (mcg) 51
Protein (g) 4.8	Nuts (oz) 0	Vitamin B_{12} (mcg) 0

Double Peach Parfait with Gingersnaps

■ ■ ■ ■

Preparation time: 10 minutes	*4 servings*
	351 calories per serving, 25% from fat

RealAge effect if eaten 12 times a year:	RealAge-effect ingredients:
6.3 days younger—low fat and low calorie, breakfast was never so much like a dessert.	Pecans, peaches (healthy fats, fiber, calcium, potassium, antioxidants)

ingredients

½ cup coarsely crushed gingersnap cookies

¼ cup chopped pecans, toasted

2 cups low-fat peach yogurt

2 cups sliced or diced fresh or thawed frozen peaches

preparation

Combine gingersnaps and pecans. Spoon 1 tablespoon of the mixture into each of four parfait or wine glasses. Layer each parfait as follows: ¼ cup yogurt, ¼ cup peaches, 1 tablespoon gingersnap mixture, ¼ cup yogurt, ¼ cup peaches, and 1 tablespoon gingersnap mixture. Serve immediately or chill up to 2 hours before serving.

substitutions: Toasted walnuts may replace the pecans. Look for peach soy yogurt, and try it instead of the dairy yogurt. Soy yogurt will work beautifully, for both breakfast and dessert. Add a teaspoon of maple syrup for extra sweetness, drizzled right on top.

tips: A drizzle of peach liqueur will turn this breakfast into an evening dessert. A little minced crystallized ginger will add spice. Look for chocolate-covered ginger in specialty shops and health food markets: diced into little nuggets of sweet spice, it adds a whole new dessert dimension to this dish.

nutritional analysis

Total fat (g) 9.6	Sodium (mg) 216	Vitamin A (RE) 216
Fat calories (kc) 86.4	Calcium (mg) 214	Beta-carotene (RE) 300
Cholesterol (mg) 5.0	Magnesium (mg) 76	Vitamin C (mg) 13
Saturated fat (g) 1.6	Zinc (mg) 2.0	Vitamin E (mg) 0.6
Polyunsaturated fat (g) 2.5	Selenium (mcg) 12	Thiamin B_1 (mg) 0.5
Monounsaturated fat (g) 3.7	Potassium (mg) 766	Riboflavin B_2 (mg) 0.5
Fiber (g) 5.3	Flavonoids (mg) 0	Niacin B_3 (mg) 3.4
Carbohydrates (g) 59.9	Lycopene (mg) 0	Vitamin B_6 (mg) 0.4
Sugar (g) 38.3	Fish (oz) 0	Folic acid (mcg) 21
Protein (g) 11.8	Nuts (oz) 0.3	Vitamin B_{12} (mcg) 1.1

Linda D's Orange Fruit Smoothie

Preparation time: 5 minutes	*4 (8-ounce) servings*
	200 calories per serving, 1% from fat

RealAge effect if eaten 12 times a year:	**RealAge-effect ingredients:**
Packed with vitamin C, this smoothie offers great possibilities and other great phytochemicals. It's been known to make your total cholesterol level fall. This makes you 6.8 days younger!	Bananas, berries, orange juice, soy milk (vitamin C, isoflavones, potassium, antioxidants, flavonoids, folic acid, fiber)

ingredients

2 cups cut-up honeydew melon

2 cups frozen or fresh hulled, halved strawberries

2 cups frozen raspberries or other berries

2 tablespoons frozen orange juice concentrate

4 ice cubes or 1 cup crushed ice

1 large tablespoon quick oats

preparation

Combine all ingredients in a blender container. Cover; blend until smooth.

substitutions: One glass of orange juice can replace the tablespoon of orange juice concentrate. Frozen blueberries or mixed berries may replace raspberries. If fruit is fresh rather than frozen, add 2 more ice cubes.

tips: This frosty fiber-packed breakfast shake must be served cold. With a few nuts, this works as a great afternoon snack or as a quick breakfast. A tip of the chef's hat to Linda DeFrancisco for this. She has a friend who had high blood pressure and high total cholesterol. Since substituting this drink for her normal saturated-fat breakfast, her blood pressure and total cholesterol have marched toward normality.

nutritional analysis

Total fat (g) 0.2	Sodium (mg) 15	Vitamin A (RE) 20
Fat calories (kc) 2	Calcium (mg) 26	Beta-carotene (RE) 120
Cholesterol (mg) 0	Magnesium (mg) 55	Vitamin C (mg) 40
Saturated fat (g) 0.1	Zinc (mg) 0.7	Vitamin E (mg) 0.4
Polyunsaturated fat (g) 0.1	Selenium (mcg) 1	Thiamin B_1 (mg) 0.3
Monounsaturated fat (g) 0.1	Potassium (mg) 600	Riboflavin B_2 (mg) 0.2
Fiber (g) 6	Flavonoids (mg) 0.2	Niacin B_3 (mg) 1
Carbohydrates (g) 28	Lycopene (mg) 0	Vitamin B_6 (mg) 0.4
Sugar (g) 13	Fish (oz) 0	Folic acid (mcg) 51
Protein (g) 4.8	Nuts (oz) 0	Vitamin B_{12} (mcg) 0

Pineapple-Banana Frappe

Preparation time: 5 minutes	*4 (8-ounce) servings*
	175 calories per serving, 4% from fat

RealAge effect if eaten 12 times a year:	**RealAge-effect ingredients:**
Chock-full of potassium and loaded with isoflavones, every glassful makes your RealAge 3 days younger.	Bananas, soy milk, pineapple (potassium, isoflavones, antioxidants)

ingredients

2 large ripe bananas

1 cup low-fat (1%) soy milk

1 can (8 ounces) crushed pineapple in juice, undrained

1 cup "pineapple-passion" sorbet, such as Select brand (a Safeway brand)

preparation

Peel bananas; break into chunks. Combine all ingredients in blender container. Cover; blend until fairly smooth.

substitutions: Low-fat (1%) milk may replace the soy milk; 1 cup chopped fresh pineapple with its juice may replace the canned pineapple; and lemon sorbet may replace the pineapple-passion sorbet (for extra mouth-puckering tanginess).

tips: This is one time you won't want to use fat-free milk. The light 1% milk gives a soft, roll-around-your-mouth feel that you'll welcome. Add some soy protein powder or silken tofu for extra endurance until lunch.

nutritional analysis

Total fat (g) 0.8	Sodium (mg) 31	Vitamin A (RE) 18
Fat calories (kc) 7	Calcium (mg) 39	Beta-carotene (RE) 41
Cholesterol (mg) 3.5	Magnesium (mg) 40	Vitamin C (mg) 12
Saturated fat (g) 0.5	Zinc (mg) 0.6	Vitamin E (mg) 0.22
Polyunsaturated fat (g) 0.2	Selenium (mcg) 1	Thiamin B_1 (mg) 0.2
Monounsaturated fat (g) 0.1	Potassium (mg) 428	Riboflavin B_2 (mg) 0.1
Fiber (g) 2.1	Flavonoids (mg) 0	Niacin B_3 (mg) 0.6
Carbohydrates (g) 38	Lycopene (mg) 0	Vitamin B_6 (mg) 0.4
Sugar (g) 17.0	Fish (oz) 0	Folic acid (mcg) 18
Protein (g) 3.0	Nuts (oz) 0	Vitamin B_{12} (mcg) 0.04

FOR BRUNCH

Creamy Goat Cheese Omelet with Chives and Corn

Preparation time: 8 minutes	*2 servings*
Cooking time: 5 minutes	*140 calories per serving, 36% from fat*

RealAge effect if eaten 12 times a year:	**RealAge-effect ingredients:**
Replacing egg yolks with egg whites and replacing fat and cholesterol with protein help you become 0.1 day younger.	Corn, egg whites, soy milk (antioxidants, healthy protein, calcium)

ingredients

Cooking oil spray

½ cup fresh or thawed frozen corn kernels

3 large egg whites

1 large egg

2 tablespoons nonfat soy milk or skim milk

¼ teaspoon salt

¼ teaspoon freshly ground black pepper

4 tablespoons (1 ounce) crumbled goat cheese or herbed goat cheese

1 tablespoon plus 1 teaspoon chopped fresh chives

preparation

Heat a large nonstick skillet over medium heat until hot. Coat lightly with cooking oil spray and add corn; cook 2 to 3 minutes or until corn begins to brown, stirring occasionally.

In a medium bowl, beat together egg whites, egg, soy milk, salt, and pepper. Add to skillet and cook for 2 minutes or until eggs begin to set on bottom. Gently lift edges of omelet with a spatula to allow uncooked portion of eggs to flow to edges and set. Continue cooking for 2 minutes or until center is almost set.

Reserve 1 tablespoon cheese and 1 teaspoon chives for garnish. Scatter remaining 3 tablespoons cheese and 1 tablespoon chives over the egg mixture. Using a large spatula, fold one half of omelet over the filling; cook 1 minute or until cheese is melted. Cut in half; transfer to serving dishes and garnish with remaining cheese and chives.

substitutions: Feta cheese or herbed feta cheese may replace goat cheese. Chopped dill or basil may replace chives.

tips: Using a 10-inch, nonstick, sloped-sided skillet makes it easy to fold the cooked omelet in half. For a family of four, double the ingredients and use two skillets.

nutritional analysis

Total fat (g) 5.6
Fat calories (kc) 50.3
Cholesterol (mg) 119.2
Saturated fat (g) 2.9
Polyunsaturated fat (g) 0.4
Monounsaturated fat (g) 1.6
Fiber (g) 0.9
Carbohydrates (g) 10.6
Sugar (g) 1.4
Protein (g) 12.2

Sodium (mg) 462
Calcium (mg) 107
Magnesium (mg) 21
Zinc (mg) 0.9
Selenium (mcg) 19
Potassium (mg) 198
Flavonoids (mg) 0
Lycopene (mg) 0
Fish (oz) 0
Nuts (oz) 0

Vitamin A (RE) 98
Beta-carotene (RE) 138
Vitamin C (mg) 3
Vitamin E (mg) 0.29
Thiamin B_1 (mg) 0.08
Riboflavin B_2 (mg) 0.5
Niacin B_3 (mg) 0.8
Vitamin B_6 (mg) 0.15
Folic acid (mcg) 27
Vitamin B_{12} (mcg) 0.65

Golden Banana Pancakes with Fresh Raspberries

■ ■ ■ ■ ■

Preparation time: 5 minutes
Cooking time: 10 minutes

4 servings (12 4-inch pancakes total)
315 calories per serving, 20% from fat

RealAge effect if eaten 12 times a year:	RealAge-effect ingredients:
0.7 days younger.	Banana, whole grain, fiber, soy milk, egg whites, berries (fiber, calcium, healthy fats, antioxidants, potassium, flavonoids, healthy protein)

ingredients

1 cup whole wheat pancake mix, such as Aunt Jemima brand

⅓ cup mashed ripe banana

¾ cup reduced-fat soy milk

2 egg whites, beaten

1 tablespoon canola oil

Butter-flavored cooking oil spray

⅔ cup pure maple syrup

1⅓ cups fresh raspberries or blackberries or a combination

1 tablespoon thinly sliced mint leaves (optional)

preparation

In a large bowl, combine pancake mix, banana, soy milk, egg whites, and oil; mix just until large lumps disappear. (Do not overmix or pancakes will be tough.)

Heat a large nonstick griddle or two nonstick skillets over medium heat until hot. Coat with cooking oil spray. Drop pancake batter by scant ¼ cupfuls onto hot griddle. Turn when pancakes begin to bubble and bottoms are golden brown. Turn and continue to cook until the other side is golden brown, 30 seconds to 1 minute.

Combine syrup and berries. Transfer pancakes to serving plates; top with berry mixture and garnish with mint, if desired.

substitutions: Fat-free or 1% low-fat milk may replace soy milk, and blueberries may replace raspberries or blackberries. The dish will not be quite as pretty, but a sprinkle of fresh ground nutmeg or cinnamon can substitute for the mint; both are wonderful with banana and berries.

tips: Drop a berry or two on the uncooked side of each pancake as it cooks. The heat will gently cook the berries, and the pan will bubble and smear the berries after you flip each pancake. When the warm berries are flooded with syrup, covered with more berries, and sprinkled with mint, you may want to make another batch. Give in and go for it.

nutritional analysis

Total fat (g) 6.9
Fat calories (kc) 62
Cholesterol (mg) 22.5
Saturated fat (g) 1.5
Polyunsaturated fat (g) 1.3
Monounsaturated fat (g) 3.7
Fiber (g) 3.4
Carbohydrates (g) 57
Sugar (g) 36
Protein (g) 5.9

Sodium (mg) 309
Calcium (mg) 104
Magnesium (mg) 30
Zinc (mg) 0.6
Selenium (mcg) 5
Potassium (mg) 300
Flavonoids (mg) 1.5
Lycopene (mg) 0
Fish (oz) 0
Nuts (oz) 0

Vitamin A (RE) 22
Beta-carotene (RE) 48
Vitamin C (mg) 11
Vitamin E (mg) 0.6
Thiamin B_1 (mg) 0.14
Riboflavin B_2 (mg) 0.2
Niacin B_3 (mg) 0.8
Vitamin B_6 (mg) 0.2
Folic acid (mcg) 18
Vitamin B_{12} (mcg) 0.4

Quinoa-Stuffed Chayote (or Zucchini) Squash

■ ■ ■ ■

Preparation time: 10 minutes	*4 servings*
Cooking time: 20 minutes	*319 calories per serving, 26% from fat*

RealAge effect if eaten 12 times a year:	**RealAge-effect ingredients:**
An excellent source of age-lowering calcium and filling fiber, one serving of stuffed squash will make you 1.4 days younger.	Lima beans, squash, salsa, quinoa, olive oil, cheese, cilantro (healthy protein, calcium, magnesium, potassium, zinc, selenium, antioxidants, vitamin B$_3$, folic acid, whole grains, fiber)

ingredients

1 cup quinoa (see tips)

2 cups low-salt chicken broth

1 cup frozen baby lima beans

2 large chayote squash (about 1½ pounds)

1½ teaspoons garlic-infused olive oil

1 cup tomatillo salsa or salsa verde, such as Frontera or Arriba brands

1 teaspoon salt

½ cup (2 ounces) crumbled farmer cheese

3 tablespoons minced cilantro

¼ cup toasted pumpkin seeds or sunflower seeds (optional)

preparation

Combine quinoa and broth in a medium saucepan. Bring to a boil over high heat. Reduce heat; simmer gently 10 minutes. Stir in lima beans; continue to simmer 5 to 6 minutes or until liquid is absorbed.

Meanwhile, cut chayote lengthwise in half. Cut out and discard pit. Using a sharp paring knife, cut out flesh leaving a ⅓-inch-thick shell. Chop flesh and set aside. Place hollowed chayote halves in a microwave-safe dish. Cover with vented plastic wrap and cook at high power 5 to 8 minutes or until crisp-tender.

Heat a large nonstick skillet over medium-high heat. Add oil, then chopped squash pulp; stir-fry 2 minutes. Add salsa; simmer 3 minutes or until squash is tender. Stir ½ cup of salsa mixture into quinoa mixture. Arrange cooked squash halves, cut side up on four serving plates; sprinkle with salt. Mound remaining salsa mixture into the squash halves. Spoon quinoa mixture onto and around squash; top with cheese and cilantro. Sprinkle 1 tablespoon of pumpkin or sunflower seeds over each serving, if desired.

substitutions: This is an easily adaptable recipe that works well with whatever you have in the kitchen. Vegetable broth may replace chicken broth, and flat-leaf parsley may replace cilantro. Shelled soy beans (edamame) may replace lima beans, and extra-virgin olive oil may replace garlic-infused olive oil.

Two large zucchini or yellow squash (about 1¼ pounds) may be substituted for chayote. Cut each squash in half lengthwise. Use a paring knife to cut out squash pulp, leaving a ¼-inch shell. Proceed as recipe directs, reducing microwave cooking time to 3 to 4 minutes or until squash is crisp and tender.

tips: Quinoa (pronounced KEEN-*wa*) is a weed from the high Andes. For all practical purposes, however, it is treated as a grain. Do not rinse the quinoa or rinse very quickly. Rinsing washes away the naturally occurring saponins, slightly bitter substances that ward off the plant's would-be predators and that may have beneficial nutritional effects for humans.

nutritional analysis

Total fat (g) 9.2	Sodium (mg) 944	Vitamin A (RE) 90
Fat calories (kc) 49	Calcium (mg) 118	Beta-carotene (RE) 454
Cholesterol (mg) 0.5	Magnesium (mg) 188	Vitamin C (mg) 23
Saturated fat (g) 3.9	Zinc (mg) 2.1	Vitamin E (mg) 0.4
Polyunsaturated fat (g) 1.5	Selenium (mcg) 6	Thiamin B_1 (mg) 0.4
Monounsaturated fat (g) 2.2	Potassium (mg) 1369	Riboflavin B_2 (mg) 0.3
Fiber (g) 9.0	Flavonoids (mg) 0.9	Niacin B_3 (mg) 4.8
Carbohydrates (g) 64	Lycopene (mg) 16.8	Vitamin B_6 (mg) 0.5
Sugar (g) 7.8	Fish (oz) 0	Folic acid (mcg) 62
Protein (g) 13.0	Nuts (oz) 0	Vitamin B_{12} (mcg) 0.1

Grilled Summer Vegetable Sandwiches
with Fresh Goat Cheese

■ ■ ■ ■

Preparation time: 10 minutes	*4 servings*
Cooking time: 10 minutes	*245 calories per serving, 33% from fat*

RealAge effect if eaten 12 times a year:	**RealAge-effect ingredients:**
This dense and satisfying sandwich makes your RealAge 3.0 days younger.	Vegetables, garlic, olive oil, dark bread (vitamin C, fiber, potassium, calcium, magnesium, zinc, selenium, vitamin B_3, folic acid, healthy fats, antioxidants)

ingredients

1 large yellow summer squash

1 large zucchini squash

1 small eggplant or white eggplant, about 8 ounces

1 large red or orange bell pepper

1½ tablespoons garlic-infused olive oil

1 teaspoon dried thyme leaves

¼ teaspoon each salt and freshly ground black pepper

8 slices dark rye or pumpernickel bread, such as Baltic Bakery brand

Cooking oil spray

¼ cup (1 ounce) crumbled goat or feta cheese

2 teaspoons chopped fresh thyme (optional)

preparation

Trim ends and cut yellow and zucchini squash lengthwise into ¼-inch-thick slices. Trim end and cut eggplant lengthwise into four ½-inch-thick slices (reserve any remaining eggplant for another use). Cut bell pepper lengthwise into quarters; discard stem and seeds. Combine oil and dried thyme leaves; brush lightly over both sides of vegetables and sprinkle with salt and pepper.

Grill vegetables over medium-hot coals or in a ridged grill pan (in batches) over medium-high heat 4 to 5 minutes per side or until vegetables are tender. During the last 2 minutes of cooking, coat bread lightly with cooking oil spray and place around outer edges of the grill to toast (or grill in the ridged grill pan after the vegetables cook).

Top four slices of the bread with the vegetables; sprinkle with cheese and, if desired, fresh thyme. Close sandwiches.

substitutions: Extra-virgin olive oil may replace garlic-infused olive oil.

tips: The bell pepper will take longer to grill than the other vegetables. Place over the hottest coals or leave in the grill pan 1 to 2 minutes longer than the other vegetables.

nutritional analysis

Total fat (g) 9.0	Sodium (mg) 427	Vitamin A (RE) 37
Fat calories (kc) 80.6	Calcium (mg) 92	Beta-carotene (RE) 61
Cholesterol (mg) 6.2	Magnesium (mg) 59	Vitamin C (mg) 22
Saturated fat (g) 1.8	Zinc (mg) 1.1	Vitamin E (mg) 0.9
Polyunsaturated fat (g) 0.6	Selenium (mcg) 29	Thiamin B_1 (mg) 0.3
Monounsaturated fat (g) 4.1	Potassium (mg) 464	Riboflavin B_2 (mg) 0.4
Fiber (g) 5.3	Flavonoids (mg) 0	Niacin B_3 (mg) 2.6
Carbohydrates (g) 35	Lycopene (mg) 0.7	Vitamin B_6 (mg) 0.2
Sugar (g) 1.9	Fish (oz) 0	Folic acid (mcg) 19
Protein (g) 7.7	Nuts (oz) 0	Vitamin B_{12} (mcg) 0.1

Roasted Red Pepper and Kalamata Olive Sicilian Salad

■ ■ ■ ■

Preparation time: 12 minutes	4 servings
	140 calories per serving, 46% from fat

RealAge effect if eaten 12 times a year:	RealAge-effect ingredients:
The age-reducing quality of olives, filling your stomach quickly with their monounsaturated fat, is a special feature of this dish. Its RA benefit is 3.4 days younger.	Lettuce, escarole, bell peppers, tomatoes, olives, olive oil (healthy fats, vitamin C, lycopene, folate, fiber, flavonoids)

ingredients

3 cups each packed torn romaine lettuce and escarole or curly endive

1 jar (7 ounces) roasted red bell peppers, drained, cut into short, thin strips

1 cup yellow tomatoes

8 pitted Kalamata olives, halved

¼ cup golden raisins

3 tablespoons white balsamic vinegar

1½ tablespoons extra-virgin olive oil

Salt and freshly ground black pepper, to taste

2 tablespoons crumbled feta or goat cheese (optional)

preparation

In a large bowl, combine lettuce, escarole, bell peppers, tomatoes, olives, and raisins. Combine vinegar and oil; add to lettuce mixture. Toss well and season with salt and pepper to taste. Transfer to four serving plates. Top with cheese, if desired.

substitutions: Dry-cured olives or Niçoise olives may be substituted for the Kalamata olives. Yellow tomatoes are small, pear-shaped tomatoes that have a sweet flavor. If they are not available, substitute cherry tomatoes. One-fourth cup bottled Italian dressing may be substituted for the vinegar and oil. Mesclun (assorted salad greens) may replace escarole.

tips: Bottled roasted red bell peppers make this dish a cinch to put together, but if you prefer a sweeter flavor, use fresh red bell peppers that have been broiled until the skin blackens; peel, seed, and cut them into strips.

nutritional analysis

Total fat (g) 7.6	Sodium (mg) 322	Vitamin A (RE) 188
Fat calories (kc) 67	Calcium (mg) 81	Beta-carotene (RE) 257
Cholesterol (mg) 6.2	Magnesium (mg) 23	Vitamin C (mg) 64
Saturated fat (g) 2.0	Zinc (mg) 0.5	Vitamin E (mg) 1.53
Polyunsaturated fat (g) 0.7	Selenium (mcg) 10	Thiamin B_1 (mg) 0.13
Monounsaturated fat (g) 4.9	Potassium (mg) 424	Riboflavin B_2 (mg) 0.14
Fiber (g) 2.6	Flavonoids (mg) 2	Niacin B_3 (mg) 1.0
Carbohydrates (g) 14.9	Lycopene (mg) 1	Vitamin B_6 (mg) 0.25
Sugar (g) 8.8	Fish (oz) 0	Folic acid (mcg) 75
Protein (g) 3.1	Nuts (oz) 0.21	Vitamin B_{12} (mcg) 0.12

Tomato Bruschetta

■ ■ ■ ■

Preparation time: 10 minutes	*4 servings (16 crostini)*
Cooking time: 8 minutes	*210 calories per serving, 25% from fat*

RealAge effect if eaten 12 times a year:	RealAge-effect ingredients:
2.5 days younger	Tomatoes, olive oil, garlic (antioxidants, flavonoids, calcium, potassium, lycopene)

ingredients

1 small whole wheat or French bread baguette (8 ounces)

Olive oil cooking spray

1 tablespoon extra-virgin olive oil

3 large garlic cloves, unpeeled

2 medium tomatoes (about 12 ounces), chopped (about 2 cups)

1 tablespoon chopped fresh basil

¼ teaspoon salt

⅛ teaspoon freshly ground black pepper

preparation

Heat oven to 450 degrees. Cut bread crosswise into sixteen ½-inch-thick slices. Spray cooking oil spray lightly over each slice and arrange on a baking sheet. Bake 6 to 8 minutes or until lightly toasted. Cool at room temperature.

Meanwhile, heat a small skillet over medium heat until hot. Add garlic cloves; cook until the skin is slightly charred, about 5 minutes, turning garlic occasionally. Cool, peel, and chop garlic. Use the back of a large knife to mash garlic to a paste. Combine tomatoes, garlic, basil, salt, and pepper. Spoon mixture over toasted bread.

substitutions: You can use canned, drained whole plum tomatoes for a slightly more acidic, cooked flavor. You don't have to roast the garlic, but it makes the flavor more sweet and subtle if you do. Instead of three roasted cloves, one clove of minced fresh garlic is plenty.

tips: For an extra rustic, smoky flavor, grill the bread briefly on both sides on a wood-burning outdoor grill!

nutritional analysis

Total fat (g) 5.9	Sodium (mg) 321	Vitamin A (RE) 53
Fat calories (kc) 53	Calcium (mg) 71	Beta-carotene (RE) 96
Cholesterol (mg) 0	Magnesium (mg) 21	Vitamin C (mg) 17
Saturated fat (g) 0.8	Zinc (mg) 0.5	Vitamin E (mg) 0.8
Polyunsaturated fat (g) 1.1	Selenium (mcg) 17	Thiamin B_1 (mg) 0.3
Monounsaturated fat (g) 3.2	Potassium (mg) 247	Riboflavin B_2 (mg) 0.2
Fiber (g) 2.5	Flavonoids (mg) 2.5	Niacin B_3 (mg) 2.8
Carbohydrates (g) 33	Lycopene (mg) 4.2	Vitamin B_6 (mg) 0.1
Sugar (g) 4.6	Fish (oz) 0	Folic acid (mcg) 34
Protein (g) 6.3	Nuts (oz) 0	Vitamin B_{12} (mcg) 0

Tomato Potato Salad with Canola Oil Mayonnaise

■ ■ ■ ■

Preparation time: 10 minutes
Cooking time: 12 minutes

4 servings (approximately 5½ cups total)
190 calories per serving, 4% from fat

RealAge effect if eaten 12 times a year:	**RealAge-effect ingredients:**
4.3 days younger	Tomatoes, onion, basil, canola oil (antioxidants, lycopene, potassium, flavonoids, healthy fat)

ingredients

2 pounds red potatoes, unpeeled, cut into 1-inch pieces

2 tablespoons water

2 large plum tomatoes, diced (1 cup)

¼ cup finely chopped white or red onion

¼ cup canola oil mayonnaise (see Substitutions)

1½ tablespoons white balsamic vinegar or white wine vinegar

¾ teaspoon salt

¼ teaspoon freshly ground black pepper

¼ cup packed thinly sliced basil leaves

preparation

Place potatoes and water in a large microwave-safe casserole dish. Cover; cook at high power 10 to 12 minutes or until potatoes are tender. Drain; cool to room temperature.

Cook tomatoes and onion in a large nonstick skillet over medium-high heat 3 to 4 minutes or until thick, stirring occasionally. Let cool briefly. Add mayonnaise, vinegar, salt, and pepper to a large bowl. Add potatoes; mix well. Add tomato mixture; mix well. Set aside 1 tablespoon of the basil. Add remaining basil to potato mixture; mix well. Transfer to serving plates; top with reserved basil.

substitutions: If canola oil mayonnaise is not available, prepare the following. Place ¼ cup egg substitute, 2 tablespoons lemon juice, 1½ teaspoons dry mustard, ½ teaspoon each of sugar and salt, and ¼ teaspoon cayenne pepper in a blender container. Cover; blend well. With motor running, add 1 cup canola oil in a thin stream. Continue blending until thick. Cover and refrigerate up to two weeks. Makes about 1⅓ cups.

For a more intense potato flavor, roast the potatoes instead of steaming them. Then dice them into small to medium pieces (maximum, ½-inch pieces). Toss with 1 teaspoon olive oil and ½ teaspoon salt. Bake at 425 degrees for approximately 15 minutes or until soft. Then combine with the other ingredients, as above. You could also boil the potatoes instead of steaming them. Be sure to save the water (and all the potato vitamins) for making rice, beans, or stock.

tips: Cooking the tomatoes and onion until thick concentrates their flavors, and is simple and quick to do.

nutritional analysis

Total fat (g) 0.9	Sodium (mg) 455	Vitamin A (RE) 20
Fat calories (kc) 8	Calcium (mg) 20	Beta-carotene (RE) 41
Cholesterol (mg) 4.8	Magnesium (mg) 49	Vitamin C (mg) 23
Saturated fat (g) 0.2	Zinc (mg) 0.7	Vitamin E (mg) 2.9
Polyunsaturated fat (g) 0.5	Selenium (mcg) 7	Thiamin B_1 (mg) 0.2
Monounsaturated fat (g) 0.2	Potassium (mg) 832	Riboflavin B_2 (mg) 0.1
Fiber (g) 3.0	Flavonoids (mg) 4.0	Niacin B_3 (mg) 3.2
Carbohydrates (g) 48.8	Lycopene (mg) 6.1	Vitamin B_6 (mg) 0.64
Sugar (g) 4.8	Fish (oz) 0	Follic acid (mcg) 26
Protein (g) 4.2	Nuts (oz) 0	Vitamin B_{12} (mcg) 0.01

Canola Double Corn Cakes

■ ■ ■ ■

Preparation time: 20 minutes	*4 servings (12 4-inch corn cakes total)*
Cooking time: 5 minutes	*208 calories per serving, 24% from fat*

RealAge effect if eaten 12 times a year:	**RealAge-effect ingredients:**
1.2 days younger	Bell pepper, corn, onions, cornmeal, canola oil (folic acid, healthy fats)

ingredients

1 teaspoon butter

1 teaspoon canola oil

¼ cup minced red bell pepper

2 cups corn kernels

¼ cup thinly sliced green onions or scallions

½ cup cornmeal

½ cup unbleached whole wheat flour

½ teaspoon baking powder

½ teaspoon baking soda

½ teaspoon salt

2 large eggs (or ½ cup egg substitute)

1 cup 1% buttermilk

Cooking oil spray

Optional toppings: minced cilantro leaves, guacamole

preparation

Melt butter in a small skillet. Add the canola oil, bell pepper, and corn and sauté over medium heat for approximately 5 minutes. Remove from heat, stir in the green onions, and set aside.

Combine cornmeal, flour, baking powder, baking soda, and salt in a medium bowl. Make a well in the center. Combine eggs and buttermilk and beat until frothy. Pour this mixture and the corn mixture into the well in the center of the dry ingredients, stirring briefly until everything is combined. Do not overmix.

Coat a griddle or two skillets with cooking oil spray. Use a ¼-cup measuring cup to pour a scant ¼ cup of batter for each corn cake. Cook the corn cakes for approximately 2 minutes on each side or until golden. Serve hot, topped with a few cilantro leaves or a dollop of guacamole, if desired.

substitutions: Three egg whites (½ cup) can replace the two whole eggs for a lighter, less rich canola cake; another teaspoon of canola oil can replace the butter for the same effect.

tips: A little heat often brightens the green of the scallions just enough to accentuate color and flavor. Just use enough heat to show that they've been cooked.

nutritional analysis

Total fat (g) 5.90	Sodium (mg) 263	Vitamin A (RE) 59
Fat calories (kc) 54	Calcium (mg) 50	Beta-carotene (RE) 80
Cholesterol (mg) 86	Magnesium (mg) 19	Vitamin C (mg) 23
Saturated fat (g) 2.4	Zinc (mg) 0.562	Vitamin E (mg) 0.7
Polyunsaturated fat (g) 0.3	Selenium (mcg) 18	Thiamin B_1 (mg) 0.2
Monounsaturated fat (g) 1.1	Potassium (mg) 175	Riboflavin B_2 (mg) 0.2
Fiber (g) 0.8	Flavonoids (mg) 0	Niacin B_3 (mg) 3.2
Carbohydrates (g) 20	Lycopene (mg) 0.23	Vitamin B_6 (mg) 0.2
Sugar (g) 2.8	Fish (oz) 0	Folic acid (mcg) 63
Protein (g) 5.4	Nuts (oz) 0	Vitamin B_{12} (mcg) 0.3

Dijon Chicken

■ ■ ■ ■

Preparation time: 10 minutes	*4 servings*
Cooking time: 10 minutes	*174 calories per serving, 17% from fat*

RealAge effect if eaten 12 times a year:	**RealAge-effect ingredients:**
0.5 days younger	Shallots, wine, chicken (potassium, alcohol, flavonoids, healthy protein)

ingredients

¼ cup and 1 tablespoon Dijon mustard

2 tablespoons white wine (such as a Chardonnay or Sauvignon Blanc)

¼ teaspoon Worcestershire sauce

Black pepper to taste (ground)

2 tablespoons finely minced shallot

3 tablespoons pure maple syrup

4 (4-ounce) boneless, skinless chicken breast halves or fillets, trimmed of all visible fat

preparation

Combine ¼ cup mustard, the wine, Worcestershire sauce, pepper, 1 tablespoon shallot, and 1 tablespoon maple syrup in a shallow dish for a marinade. Add chicken and turn to coat thoroughly; let stand for 5 minutes. Preheat charcoal or gas grill or heat a ridged grill pan. Remove chicken from marinade; discard marinade. Grill or pan-grill chicken 3 to 5 minutes per side or until chicken is no longer pink in the center.

Meanwhile, in a small bowl, combine the remaining 2 tablespoons maple syrup, 1 tablespoon mustard, and 1 tablespoon shallot. Mix well and serve as a dipping sauce for the chicken.

substitutions: Chicken breasts with the skin on can be used; just take the skin off before serving.

tips: Grade B (the darker) maple syrup adds complexity to the dish; it is a stronger flavor than the lighter, more expensive Grade A.

nutritional analysis

Total fat (g) 3.2
Fat calories (kc) 29
Cholesterol (mg) 65.8
Saturated fat (g) 0.2
Polyunsaturated fat (g) 1.1
Monounsaturated fat (g) 1.2
Fiber (g) 0.2
Carbohydrates (g) 6.9
Sugar (g) 4.3
Protein (g) 35

Sodium (mg) 582
Calcium (mg) 46
Magnesium (mg) 36
Zinc (mg) 1.2
Selenium (mcg) 31
Potassium (mg) 314
Flavonoids (mg) 0.09
Lycopene (mg) 0.01
Fish (oz) 0
Nuts (oz) 0

Vitamin A (RE) 32
Beta-carotene (RE) 0
Vitamin C (mg) 0.4
Vitamin E (mg) 0.8
Thiamin B_1 (mg) 0.8
Riboflavin B_2 (mg) 0.1
Niacin B_3 (mg) 15
Vitamin B_6 (mg) 0.4
Folic acid (mcg) 4.1
Vitamin B_{12} (mcg) 0.4

Smoky Posole with Chipotle Chiles and Avocado
(Hominy Stew)

■ ■ ■ ■ ■

Preparation time: 5 minutes	*4 servings (approximately 5 cups total)*
Cooking time: 15 minutes	*182 calories per serving, 29% from fat*

RealAge effect if eaten 12 times a year:	**RealAge-effect ingredients:**
No wonder so many of us love a fiesta! With fiber like this and the monounsaturated goodness of avocados, your RealAge drops by 3.2 days with every serving.	Spinach, carrots, onion, avocados (fiber, healthy fats, antioxidants, potassium, magnesium, carotenoids, flavonoids, calcium, folate)

ingredients

1 teaspoon canola oil

1 small white onion, cut into slivers

1 cup thinly sliced carrots

3 cups low-salt beef or chicken broth

1 tablespoon puréed canned chipotle chiles in adobo sauce (see Tips)

1 can (15½ ounces) white hominy, drained

¼ teaspoon salt, or to taste

3 cups packed baby or torn spinach leaves

½ ripe medium avocado, diced

¼ cup chopped cilantro

Optional toppings: lime wedges, shredded cabbage, and slivered radishes

preparation

Heat a large saucepan over medium-high heat. Add oil, then onion and carrots; cook 4 minutes, stirring occasionally, or until the onion starts to darken. Add broth and chiles; bring to a simmer. Stir in hominy and salt; simmer uncovered 8 minutes. Stir in spinach; simmer 1 minute or until spinach wilts. Ladle into shallow bowls; top with avocado and cilantro. Serve with desired toppings.

substitutions: One tablespoon of the adobo sauce from the canned chipotle chiles may replace the puréed chiles. Vegetable broth may replace the beef or chicken broth.

tips: Look for cans of these spicy smoked jalapeño chiles in a spicy tomato sauce in the ethnic section of your supermarket. Purée the contents of the can, portion it into small amounts, and freeze it up to 3 months.

For a rich broth instead of a clear one, scoop out 1 cup of the soup just before adding the spinach, purée it, and add it with the spinach to the soup. It will thicken the soup and distribute the flavor throughout.

nutritional analysis

Total fat (g) 6.2	Sodium (mg) 562	Vitamin A (RE) 1074
Fat calories (kc) 56	Calcium (mg) 79	Beta-carotene (RE) 6503
Cholesterol (mg) 0.8	Magnesium (mg) 70	Vitamin C (mg) 28
Saturated fat (g) 0.8	Zinc (mg) 1.8	Vitamin E (mg) 2.6
Polyunsaturated fat (g) 1.4	Selenium (mcg) 8	Thiamin B_1 (mg) 0.1
Monounsaturated fat (g) 4.8	Potassium (mg) 696	Riboflavin B_2 (mg) 0.2
Fiber (g) 6.5	Flavonoids (mg) 0.9	Niacin B_3 (mg) 3.7
Carbohydrates (g) 26.4	Lycopene (mg) 0	Vitamin B_6 (mg) 0.3
Sugar (g) 2.8	Fish (oz) 0	Folic acid (mcg) 110
Protein (g) 7.7	Nuts (oz) 0	Vitamin B_{12} (mcg) 0.2

FOR HORS D'OEUVRES/STARTERS

Donna's Basic Guacamole

Preparation time: 15 minutes	4 servings (approximately 1½ cups total) 178 calories per serving, 69% from fat

RealAge effect if eaten 12 times a year:	RealAge-effect ingredients:
7.4 days younger	Avocados, tomatoes, garlic, onion, lemon juice, chile pepper (lycopene, flavonoids, potassium, folate, vitamin B_3, vitamin C, healthy fats)

ingredients

2 ripe medium avocados, Hass preferred

1 large plum tomato, diced (½ cup)

1 tablespoon minced white or yellow onion

1 tablespoon lime or lemon juice

2 teaspoons minced, seeded serrano or jalapeño chile

1 small garlic clove, minced

½ teaspoon salt

preparation

Peel and seed avocados. Scoop avocado flesh into a medium bowl; coarsely mash with a fork. Add remaining ingredients; mix well. Serve immediately with fresh vegetable dippers, baked tortilla chips, or fresh corn tortillas.

substitutions: If you use white onion, serrano, and lime (instead of yellow onion, jalapeño, and lemon), you'll get a punchier, more robust dip.

tips: If you're not going to eat this right away, squeeze the lemon or lime over the top of the guacamole rather than mixing it in. This keeps the guacamole from oxidizing and browning. If you do have to refrigerate the guacamole, put a sheet of plastic wrap directly on the surface, for the same reason. Stir well before serving. A few sprigs of cilantro, bunched together like a small bouquet and placed right in the middle, is a nice garnish.

nutritional analysis

Total fat (g) 13.6
Fat calories (kc) 122
Cholesterol (mg) 0
Saturated fat (g) 2.7
Polyunsaturated fat (g) 2.3
Monounsaturated fat (g) 7.4
Fiber (g) 4.5
Carbohydrates (g) 15.5
Sugar (g) 2.1
Protein (g) 2.7

Sodium (mg) 10
Calcium (mg) 20
Magnesium (mg) 55
Zinc (mg) 0.7
Selenium (mcg) 0
Potassium (mg) 805
Flavonoids (mg) 0.7
Lycopene (mg) 1.0
Fish (oz) 0
Nuts (oz) 0

Vitamin A (RE) 107
Beta-carotene (RE) 599
Vitamin C (mg) 22
Vitamin E (mg) 1.7
Thiamin B_1 (mg) 0.18
Riboflavin B_2 (mg) 0.2
Niacin B_3 (mg) 3
Vitamin B_6 (mg) 0.5
Folic acid (mcg) 85
Vitamin B_{12} (mcg) 0

RealAge Guacamole

| Preparation time: 5 minutes | 10 (½-cup) servings |
| Cooking time: 10 minutes | 41 calories per serving, 47% from fat |

| RealAge effect if eaten 12 times a year: | RealAge-effect ingredients: |
| 3.2 days younger | Zucchini, onion, tomatoes, lemon, avocados, garlic, peppers (lycopene, flavonoids, potassium, folate, vitamin B_3, vitamin C, healthy fats) |

ingredients

1 pound zucchini squash, chopped

1 envelope unflavored gelatin

2 tablespoons cool water

½ cup boiling water

⅓ cup chopped white or yellow onion

1 large tomato, seeded and chopped

½ cup reduced-fat sour cream

2 tablespoons lemon juice

1 teaspoon salt

½ teaspoon each chili powder and ground cumin

¼ teaspoon each freshly ground black pepper and garlic powder

⅛ teaspoon hot pepper sauce

1 recipe Donna's Basic Guacamole (page 215)

preparation

For Mike's Veggie Boost for Guacamole: Steam zucchini until tender; set aside to cool. Soften gelatin in cool water. Add boiling water and stir until gelatin dissolves completely. Combine zucchini and gelatin mixture in blender container. Cover; blend until smooth. Add remaining ingredients except guacamole; blend until well mixed. Mix two parts of this mixture with one part of Donna's Basic Guacamole. Cover and chill before serving.

substitutions: *For Mike's Quick Veggie Boost for Guacamole (to be added to Donna's Basic Guacamole in the same way):* Prepare the zucchini, gelatin, and cool and boiling water as described above. However, for the remaining ingredients, substitute your favorite salsa plus 1 tablespoon lemon juice, so that the total is approximately 5 cups. You can also use peas or asparagus to substitute for the squash.

tips: Although RealAge Guacamole represents a two-to-one ratio of Mike's Veggie Boost to Donna's Basic Guacamole, feel free to add the vegetable mixture to Donna's Basic Guacamole in whatever ratio tastes best to you.

nutritional analysis

Total fat (g) 5.7	Sodium (mg) 176	Vitamin A (RE) 108
Fat calories (kc) 51	Calcium (mg) 43	Beta-carotene (RE) 387
Cholesterol (mg) 8.0	Magnesium (mg) 42	Vitamin C (mg) 25
Saturated fat (g) 2.4	Zinc (mg) 0.5	Vitamin E (mg) 0.7
Polyunsaturated fat (g) 1	Selenium (mcg) 4	Thiamin B_1 (mg) 0.14
Monounsaturated fat (g) 3.2	Potassium (mg) 598	Riboflavin B_2 (mg) 0.1
Fiber (g) 3.2	Flavonoids (mg) 1.5	Niacin B_3 (mg) 1.5
Carbohydrates (g) 10.8	Lycopene (mg) 1.8	Vitamin B_6 (mg) 0.3
Sugar (g) 2.8	Fish (oz) 0	Folic acid (mcg) 54
Protein (g) 3.8	Nuts (oz) 0	Vitamin B_{12} (mcg) 0.1

Glistening Gazpacho

Preparation time: 25 minutes	*4 servings (about 1 cup each)* *111 calories per serving, 80% from fat*

RealAge effect if eaten 12 times a year:	RealAge-effect ingredients:
5.2 days younger	Onion, bell peppers, tomatoes, olive oil, cucumber (potassium, flavonoids, carotenoids, lycopene, folate, healthy fats)

ingredients

1 cup each diced (¼-inch) peeled cucumber, red or orange bell pepper, and seeded ripe tomato

¼ cup finely minced red onion

1 cup tomato juice

3 tablespoons red wine vinegar

3 tablespoons extra-virgin olive oil

2 dashes (or to taste) hot pepper sauce

Salt and freshly ground black pepper, to taste

Optional: chopped fresh parsley or cilantro, diced avocado

preparation

Place all ingredients except garnishes in large bowl and combine. Allow to sit for about 5 minutes. Coarsely purée about half the mixture in a blender or food processor and return it to the bowl. Stir well to combine thoroughly and refrigerate for at least 2 hours and up to 8 hours before serving. Garnish sparingly with parsley, cilantro, or avocado, if desired.

substitutions: Try V8 juice instead of tomato juice.

tips: This soup is very refreshing on a hot summer day. Serve it with a glass of chilled red wine, bowls of olives and nuts, and a side of salad for a quick, nutritious, delicious lunch.

nutritional analysis

Total fat (g) 9.8	Sodium (mg) 220	Vitamin A (RE) 73
Fat calories (kc) 89	Calcium (mg) 16	Beta-carotene (RE) 256
Cholesterol (mg) 0	Magnesium (mg) 20	Vitamin C (mg) 45
Saturated fat (g) 1.4	Zinc (mg) 0.3	Vitamin E (mg) 2.05
Polyunsaturated fat (g) 0.9	Selenium (mcg) 13	Thiamin B1 (mg) 0.08
Monounsaturated fat (g) 7.2	Potassium (mg) 324	Riboflavin B2 (mg) 0.05
Fiber (g) 2.0	Flavonoids (oz) 9.8	Niacin B3 (mg) 0.8
Carbohydrates (g) 8.5	Lycopene (oz) 6.4	Vitamin B6 (mg) 0.19
Sugar (g) 4.0	Fish (oz) 0	Folic acid (mcg) 29
Protein (g) 1.2	Nuts (oz) 0	Vitamin B12 (mcg) 0

FOR DINNER

Grilled Tuna Niçoise with Tarragon Mesclun

■ ■ ■ ■

Preparation time: 8 minutes	*4 servings*
Cooking time: 10 minutes	*291 calories per serving, 24% from fat*

RealAge effect if eaten 12 times a year:	**RealAge-effect ingredients:**
A good source of protective polyunsaturated omega-3 fatty acids, and a treasure trove of monounsaturated fats, too, this recipe will make you 5.5 days younger.	Tuna, olive oil, green beans, salad greens, tomatoes (healthy protein, healthy fat, antioxidants, potassium, B vitamins, including folic acid and B_{12}, lycopene)

ingredients

2 tablespoons olive oil

1 tablespoon coarse-grained mustard, such as Pommery or Country Dijon

3 tablespoons tarragon white wine vinegar

1 teaspoon dried tarragon

¾ teaspoon salt

½ teaspoon freshly ground black pepper

4 (4-ounce) fresh tuna steaks, cut about ½ inch thick

1 pound small red boiling waxy potatoes

8 ounces whole fresh green beans

8 cups (10 ounces) mesclun (assorted young salad greens) or torn salad greens, loosely packed

16 grape, teardrop, or cherry tomatoes (optional)

preparation

In a small bowl, combine oil, mustard, vinegar, tarragon, salt, and pepper; mix well. Brush 1½ tablespoons of the mixture over tuna; set tuna and remaining dressing aside.

Rinse potatoes and green beans but do not dry. Place potatoes in an 8-inch square baking dish or microwave-safe casserole. Cover; cook at high power for 3 minutes. Add green beans; cover and continue to cook at high power 4 minutes or until vegetables are tender. Transfer to a colander and rinse with cold water to stop the cooking and cool the vegetables.

Meanwhile, heat a ridged grill pan over medium-high heat. Add tuna; cook 2 minutes per side or until seared and still very pink in center. (If a ridged grill pan is not available, tuna may be broiled 3 to 4 inches from heat for 3 minutes per side, or grilled outside over a bed of medium-hot coals.)

Arrange greens on four serving plates. Quarter the potatoes and cut green beans in half if large; arrange over greens. Top with tuna and drizzle with reserved dressing. Garnish with tomatoes, if desired.

substitutions: Salmon or Pacific halibut may replace tuna; cook to desired doneness. White wine or champagne vinegar may replace tarragon vinegar. The result will be just a little less complex and herbal.

tips: An outdoor grill will add smokiness to the tuna. For a beautiful presentation, arrange the potatoes around the edges of the salad; arrange the green beans around the outside, too, like spokes in a bicycle wheel.

nutritional analysis

Total fat (g) 8.1	Sodium (mg) 556	Vitamin A (RE) 950
Fat calories (kc) 76	Calcium (mg) 94	Beta-carotene (RE) 428
Cholesterol (mg) 41.7	Magnesium (mg) 109	Vitamin C (mg) 43
Saturated fat (g) 1.3	Zinc (mg) 1.8	Vitamin E (mg) 2.67
Polyunsaturated fat (g) 2.0	Selenium (mcg) 90	Thiamin B_1 (mg) 0.5
Monounsaturated fat (g) 4.5	Potassium (mg) 1268	Riboflavin B_2 (mg) 0.5
Fiber (g) 5.3	Flavonoids (mg) 2.0	Niacin B_3 (mg) 11.6
Carbohydrates (g) 32.5	Lycopene (mg) 1.0	Vitamin B_6 (mg) 0.9
Sugar (g) 4.9	Fish (oz) 1.0	Folic acid (mcg) 184
Protein (g) 30.6	Nuts (oz) 0	Vitamin B_{12} (mcg) 9.3

Milanese Gnocchi (Dumplings) and Vegetable Stew

■ ■ ■ ■

Preparation time: 10 minutes	*4 servings*
Cooking time: 10 minutes	*363 calories per serving, 26% from fat*

RealAge effect if eaten 12 times a year:	RealAge-effect ingredients:
Bursting with age-reducing phytochemicals, one bowlful makes your RealAge 4.7 days younger.	Olive oil, garlic, tomatoes, escarole (monounsaturated fat, lycopene, flavonoids, calcium, potassium, selenium, antioxidants)

ingredients

2 teaspoons olive oil (taken from the container of sun-dried tomatoes packed in oil, see below)

3 garlic cloves, minced

3 cups low-salt chicken broth

1 package (16 ounces) shelf-stable (nonrefrigerated, vacuum-packed) spinach or potato gnocchi (dumplings), such as Bellino brand

¼ cup sliced well-drained sun-dried tomatoes packed in oil, such as Sonoma brand

2 cups packed torn escarole

1 cup diced plum tomatoes

½ cup (2 ounces) crumbled Gorgonzola cheese

1 tablespoon chopped fresh sage or 1 teaspoon dried sage

Crushed red pepper flakes or sun-dried tomato bits or flakes (optional)

preparation

Heat a large, deep skillet over medium-high heat. Add oil, then garlic; cook 30 seconds, stirring frequently. Add broth; bring to a boil over high heat.

Add gnocchi and sun-dried tomatoes; simmer 3 to 4 minutes or until gnocchi begin to float. Stir in escarole; simmer 1 minute. Stir in plum tomatoes; ladle into shallow bowls. Top with cheese, sage, and pepper flakes or sun-dried tomato flakes, if desired.

substitutions: Frisée (curly endive) may replace escarole, and vegetable broth may replace chicken broth.

tips: This big, warm stew has a soft and chewy texture. For a pleasant textural contrast, sprinkle sun-dried tomato flakes on top just before serving, and don't forget to top with Gorgonzola cheese. The dish becomes brightly lit, with little streaks of white, salty, melted flavor.

nutritional analysis

Total fat (g) 10.8	Sodium (mg) 862	Vitamin A (RE) 236
Fat calories (kc) 97	Calcium (mg) 328	Beta-carotene (RE) 269
Cholesterol (mg) 30	Magnesium (mg) 33	Vitamin C (mg) 12
Saturated fat (g) 2.2	Zinc (mg) 1.9	Vitamin E (mg) 3
Polyunsaturated fat (g) 1.3	Selenium (mcg) 8	Thiamin B_1 (mg) 0.2
Monounsaturated fat (g) 7.3	Potassium (mg) 400	Riboflavin B_2 (mg) 0.3
Fiber (g) 2.2	Flavonoids (mg) 1.8	Niacin B_3 (mg) 3.8
Carbohydrates (g) 68	Lycopene (mg) 2.4	Vitamin B_6 (mg) 0.1
Sugar (g) 1.8	Fish (oz) 0	Folic acid (mcg) 54
Protein (g) 20.4	Nuts (oz) 0	Vitamin B_{12} (mcg) 0.7

Cajun Couscous-Crusted Monkfish

Preparation time: 12 minutes	*4 servings*
Cooking time: 8 minutes	*282 calories per serving, 16% from fat*

RealAge effect if eaten 12 times a year:	**RealAge-effect ingredients:**
3.5 days younger	Whole wheat couscous, egg white, monkfish, tofu (fiber, potassium, magnesium, selenium, healthy protein, healthy fat)

ingredients

⅔ cup uncooked whole wheat couscous

2 to 3 teaspoons Cajun seasonings, as desired

1 egg white

1 tablespoon skim milk or nonfat soy milk

1 pound skinless monkfish fillet

Cooking oil spray

4 ounces (½ cup) extra-firm light silken tofu, such as Mori-Nu brand

1 tablespoon light mayonnaise

2 tablespoons sweet pickle relish

1 teaspoon each seasoned rice vinegar and Dijon mustard

½ teaspoon chopped fresh dill

¼ teaspoon salt

Optional garnishes: lemon wedges, dill sprigs

preparation

Combine couscous and seasonings in a pie plate or shallow dish. In another pie plate, beat egg white until frothy; stir in milk. Cut monkfish crosswise into ¾-inch medallions. Dip in egg white mixture, turning to coat. Roll in couscous mixture, patting to coat.

Heat a large nonstick skillet over medium heat until hot. Coat heavily with cooking oil spray. Add fish and coat with additional cooking oil spray. Do not crowd pan. Cook fish in batches or use two skillets, if necessary. Cook 3 to 4 minutes per side or until fish is opaque and firm to the touch.

Meanwhile, blend tofu and mayonnaise in a food processor or blender until fairly smooth. Stir in pickle relish, vinegar, mustard, dill, and salt. Serve fish with sauce and garnish as desired.

substitutions: Diced sweet or dill pickles may replace pickle relish, and Creole or blackening seasoning mix may replace Cajun seasonings. The tail of the anglerfish, monkfish (also referred to as lotte) is a low-fat fish with a firm texture and mild, sweet flavor. If not available, substitute with Pacific halibut fillets that have been cut crosswise into ¾-inch-thick slices.

nutritional analysis

Total fat (g) 5.0
Fat calories (kc) 44.6
Cholesterol (mg) 36.3
Saturated fat (g) 1.2
Polyunsaturated fat (g) 2.5
Monounsaturated fat (g) 2.1
Fiber (g) 5.2
Carbohydrates (g) 27.5
Sugar (g) 0.3
Protein (g) 29.9

Sodium (mg) 163
Calcium (mg) 103
Magnesium (mg) 134
Zinc (mg) 1.0
Selenium (mcg) 53
Potassium (mg) 589
Flavonoids (mg) 0
Lycopene (mg) 0
Fish (oz) 4
Nuts (oz) 0

Vitamin A (RE) 49
Beta-carotene (RE) 6
Vitamin C (mg) 0.5
Vitamin E (mg) 1.0
Thiamin B_1 (mg) 0.1
Riboflavin B_2 (mg) 0.2
Niacin B_3 (mg) 7.2
Vitamin B_6 (mg) 0.4
Folic acid (mcg) 24
Vitamin B_{12} (mcg) 1.2

Ratatouille Pasta

■ ■ ■ ■

Preparation time: 10 minutes
Cooking time: 20 minutes

4 servings
394 calories per serving, 9% from fat

RealAge effect if eaten 12 times a year:

Age-reducing fiber, generous amounts of garlic, and lycopene-packed tomatoes make your RealAge 7.8 days younger.

RealAge-effect ingredients:

Whole-grain pasta, eggplant, olive oil, onion, bell pepper, tomatoes, garlic, salad greens (lycopene, flavonoids, calcium, magnesium, potassium, fiber, folic acid, vitamin C, vitamin B_3)

ingredients

12 ounces whole wheat spaghetti

1 dried ancho or pasilla chile

3 cups diced (½-inch cubes) unpeeled eggplant (8 ounces)

2 teaspoons olive oil

1 medium red onion, coarsely chopped

1 yellow or red bell pepper, coarsely chopped

6 garlic cloves, sliced

2 cans (14½ ounces each) stewed tomatoes, undrained, coarsely chopped

1 cup packed mesclun (mixed baby salad greens)

1 tablespoon chopped fresh thyme or lemon thyme

preparation

Cook pasta according to package directions. Meanwhile, heat a large, deep skillet over medium-high heat until hot. Add the chile; cook, turning until fragrant and toasted, about 1 minute. When the chile is cool enough to handle, discard its stem and set the seeds aside for a garnish. Chop the chile.

Add eggplant to hot skillet; cook until browned, about 4 minutes, stirring frequently. Add oil, then chopped onion, bell pepper, and garlic; cook 3 minutes, stirring occasionally. Add tomatoes and chile. Reduce heat; simmer uncovered 10 minutes or until vegetables are tender and sauce thickens. Remove from heat; stir in salad greens. Salt to taste. Drain pasta; transfer to four serving plates. Top with sauce. Garnish with reserved chile seeds and thyme.

substitutions: One-fourth teaspoon crushed red pepper flakes or 1 teaspoon ancho chile powder may substitute for the chile. Omit the toasting step and add the flakes or powder along with the tomatoes. Arugula or mizuna may replace mesclun salad greens.

tips: This pasta dish is loosely based on ratatouille, a traditional French side dish from the region of Provence. Dried pasilla chile provides a slightly sweet-hot flavor. Look for the chiles in Mexican grocery stores or in the ethnic section of your supermarket. Toasting the chile in a dry skillet before chopping brings out the aroma and flavor.

nutritional analysis

Total fat (g) 4.0	Sodium (mg) 466	Vitamin A (RE) 163
Fat calories (kc) 36	Calcium (mg) 106	Beta-carotene (RE) 816
Cholesterol (mg) 0	Magnesium (mg) 58	Vitamin C (mg) 78
Saturated fat (g) 0.5	Zinc (mg) 1.1	Vitamin E (mg) 1.1
Polyunsaturated fat (g) 0.6	Selenium (mcg) 2	Thiamin B_1 (mg) 0.3
Monounsaturated fat (g) 1.8	Potassium (mg) 823	Riboflavin B_2 (mg) 0.1
Fiber (g) 5.6	Flavonoids (mg) 5.1	Niacin B_3 (mg) 2.5
Carbohydrates (g) 37.6	Lycopene (mg) 7.3	Vitamin B_6 (mg) 0.3
Sugar (g) 8.6	Fish (oz) 0	Folic acid (mcg) 41
Protein (g) 6.4	Nuts (oz) 0	Vitamin B_{12} (mcg) 0

Smoky BBQ Soy Kabobs

■ ■ ■ ■

Preparation time: 25 minutes	*4 servings*
Cooking time: 10 minutes	*204 calories per serving, 14% from fat*

RealAge effect if eaten 12 times a year:	RealAge-effect ingredients:
Amazingly loaded with fiber and vitamin C, just one serving makes your RealAge 11.8 days younger.	Tofu, zucchini, bell peppers, squash, mushrooms, onion, chiles, olive oil (healthy protein, calcium, folic acid, antioxidants, healthy fat, fiber, magnesium, zinc, selenium, potassium, beta-carotene, vitamin B_3)

ingredients

24 ounces extra-firm low-fat tofu, such as Mori-Nu brand

3 each medium zucchini and yellow crookneck squash, cut into thick slices

1 red bell pepper, cut into 1-inch squares

16 small to medium button mushrooms

1 small red onion, cut through the core into thin wedges

1¼ cups bottled barbecue sauce, such as K. C. Masterpiece or Trader Joe's brands

2 teaspoons puréed chipotle chiles in adobo sauce

Olive oil cooking spray

½ teaspoon each salt and freshly ground black pepper

preparation

Heat broiler. Press tofu between paper towels to absorb excess moisture. Cut into 1½-inch squares. Alternately thread tofu and vegetables onto metal skewers (or bamboo skewers that have been soaked in cold water for 10 minutes).

In a small bowl, combine barbecue sauce and chipotle chiles. Coat a jelly-roll pan or cookie sheet with cooking oil spray. Arrange skewers on pan; brush liberally on both sides with barbecue sauce mixture, reserving some in bottom of bowl. Broil 4 to 5 inches from heat source 5 minutes per side or until deeply browned. Brush with reserved barbecue sauce mixture from bowl; sprinkle with salt and pepper.

substitutions: For a smokier flavor, use hickory-flavored barbecue sauce.

tips: Coating the kabobs with extra sauce again right after they are broiled brightens the vegetable flavor and is worth the extra effort.

nutritional analysis

Total fat (g) 3.2
Fat calories (kc) 29
Cholesterol (mg) 0
Saturated fat (g) 0.2
Polyunsaturated fat (g) 2.3
Monounsaturated fat (g) 0.9
Fiber (g) 13.1
Carbohydrates (g) 39.3
Sugar (g) 18.2
Protein (g) 36.6

Sodium (mg) 1116
Calcium (mg) 460
Magnesium (mg) 313
Zinc (mg) 4.5
Selenium (mcg) 29
Potassium (mg) 2264
Flavonoids (mg) 0.6
Lycopene (mg) 0.7
Fish (oz) 0
Nuts (oz) 0

Vitamin A (RE) 306
Beta-carotene (RE) 1777
Vitamin C (mg) 78
Vitamin E (mg) 1.91
Thiamin B_1 (mg) 0.78
Riboflavin B_2 (mg) 0.63
Niacin B_3 (mg) 6.1
Vitamin B_6 (mg) 0.86
Folic acid (mcg) 202
Vitamin B_{12} (mcg) 0

Stir-Fried Sea Scallops and Summer Squash over Minted Couscous

Preparation time: 15 minutes
Cooking time: 12 minutes

4 servings
435 calories per serving, 4% from fat

RealAge effect if eaten 12 times a year:
Very low in fat and high in potassium, this dish will make your RealAge 5.1 days younger.

RealAge-effect ingredients:
Bell pepper, whole wheat couscous, prunes, squash, mint (healthy protein, calcium, magnesium, zinc, selenium, potassium, vitamin B_3, folic acid, vitamin B_{12}, antioxidants, fiber)

ingredients

¼ cup each light soy sauce and orange marmalade

2 tablespoons rice vinegar or seasoned rice vinegar

16 sea scallops (about 1 pound)

1 cup whole wheat couscous, uncooked

8 pitted dried prunes, coarsely chopped

Cooking oil spray

1 red or yellow bell pepper, seeded, cut into 1-inch chunks

8 ounces baby pattypan squash, sliced

¼ cup chopped mint leaves

preparation

In a medium bowl, combine soy sauce, marmalade, and vinegar. Transfer ¼ cup of the mixture to a medium saucepan; set aside. Toss scallops with remaining soy sauce mixture in bowl; let marinate at room temperature 10 minutes while preparing vegetables.

Meanwhile, add 1¾ cups water to the soy sauce mixture in saucepan; bring to a simmer. Stir in couscous and prunes. Cover; remove from heat and let stand 5 minutes or until liquid is absorbed.

Heat a large nonstick skillet over medium-high heat until hot. Coat with cooking oil spray. Transfer scallops from marinade to hot skillet; reserve marinade. Cook scallops on one side (don't turn them over) for only 2 minutes or until glazed; transfer scallops and juices from skillet to a bowl or plate; set aside. Recoat skillet with cooking oil spray. Add bell pepper and squash; stir-fry 3 minutes. Add reserved marinade from bowl; cook 1 minute. Add reserved scallops with juices; stir-fry 1 to 2 minutes or until scallops are opaque and vegetables are crisp-tender.

Stir mint into couscous; transfer to four serving plates. Top with scallop mixture and serve with additional soy sauce, if desired.

substitutions: Zucchini or yellow summer squash may replace baby pattypan squash, and dried apricots may replace prunes.

tips: Rinse sea scallops in cold water and pat dry with paper towels before marinating: They will take the marinade more readily and will caramelize in the pan to a beautiful golden brown.

nutritional analysis

Total fat (g) 1.9	Sodium (mg) 803	Vitamin A (RE) 274
Fat calories (kc) 16.8	Calcium (mg) 113	Beta carotene (RE) 1478
Cholesterol (mg) 37	Magnesium (mg) 159	Vitamin C (mg) 30
Saturated fat (g) 0.2	Zinc (mg) 2.3	Vitamin E (mg) 0.2
Polyunsaturated fat (g) 0.6	Selenium (mcg) 94	Thiamin B_1 (mg) 0.3
Monounsaturated fat (g) 0.5	Potassium (mg) 1517	Riboflavin B_2 (mg) 0.4
Fiber (g) 16.2	Flavonoids (mg) 0	Niacin B_3 (mg) 6.2
Carbohydrates (g) 71	Lycopene (mg) 0.7	Vitamin B_5 (mg) 0.7
Sugar (g) 51.1	Fish (oz) 0	Folic acid (mcg) 54
Protein (g) 30.5	Nuts (oz) 0	Vitamin B_{12} (mcg) 1.7

Teriyaki Tofu with Red Bell Pepper and Shiitakes over Jasmine Rice

■ ■ ■ ■

Preparation time: 20 minutes
Cooking time: 12 minutes

4 servings
514 calories per serving, 26% from fat

RealAge effect if eaten 12 times a year:	**RealAge-effect ingredients:**
High in potassium and unexpectedly rich in folate, this recipe makes your RealAge 8.9 days younger.	Garlic, tofu, broccoli, asparagus, mushrooms, bell peppers (healthy protein, healthy fat, potassium, antioxidants, folic acid)

ingredients

3 tablespoons dark sesame oil

2 tablespoons light teriyaki sauce, such as Kikkoman brand

4 garlic cloves, minced

½ teaspoon five-spice powder

12 ounces baked teriyaki-flavored tofu, such as Soy Deli brand, cut into 1-inch squares

4 cups each broccoli florets and sliced asparagus spears (2-inch pieces)

2 cups each sliced shiitake mushrooms and diced red bell pepper

1 cup vegetable broth or stock, such as Pacific brand

2 teaspoons Chinese hot chili sauce (optional)

3 cups hot cooked jasmine rice (an aromatic white rice)

preparation

In a large bowl, combine 2 tablespoons of the oil, the teriyaki sauce, garlic, and five-spice powder; mix well. Add tofu, tossing to coat.

Heat a Dutch oven over medium-high heat. Add remaining 1 tablespoon oil, then tofu mixture. Stir-fry 1 minute. Add broccoli and asparagus; stir-fry 2 minutes. Add mushrooms and bell pepper; stir-fry 2 minutes. Add broth; stir-fry 2 minutes. Stir in hot chili sauce, if desired. Transfer to four shallow bowls; serve with rice.

substitutions: Sliced bok choy may replace the broccoli, and regular long-grain white rice may replace the jasmine rice (aromatic as it is). Chunks of chicken breast could be substituted for the baked tofu, although the chicken will need to marinate 10 minutes to absorb the teriyaki flavor.

tips: Using a large, heavy-bottomed pot makes it easy to move the vegetables around so they cook evenly. A large, heavy-bottomed wok would work well here, too.

nutritional analysis

Total fat (g) 14.9	Sodium (mg) 1087	Vitamin A (RE) 183
Fat calories (kc) 134	Calcium (mg) 272	Beta-carotene (RE) 927
Cholesterol (mg) 0.3	Magnesium (mg) 152	Vitamin C (mg) 126
Saturated fat (g) 1.7	Zinc (mg) 3.6	Vitamin E (mg) 1.1
Polyunsaturated fat (g) 9.0	Selenium (mcg) 37	Thiamin B_1 (mg) 1.1
Monounsaturated fat (g) 6.2	Potassium (mg) 952	Riboflavin B_2 (mg) 0.5
Fiber (g) 6.1	Flavonoids (mg) 4.4	Niacin B_3 (mg) 9.4
Carbohydrates (g) 127	Lycopene (mg) 0	Vitamin B_6 (mg) 0.7
Sugar (g) 3.4	Fish (oz) 0	Folic acid (mcg) 120
Protein (g) 29.1	Nuts (oz) 0	Vitamin B_{12} (mcg) 0.1

Wasabi Mashed Potatoes with Caramelized Sweet Onions

■　■　■　■

Preparation time: 10 minutes	*4 servings*
Cooking time: 20 minutes	*305 calories per serving, 19% from fat*

RealAge effect if eaten 12 times a year:	**RealAge-effect ingredients:**
3.1 days younger. This recipe can be hot.	Onions, buttermilk, olive oil (potassium, calcium, healthy fats)

ingredients

2 pounds red potatoes or red steamers, scrubbed

1¼ tablespoons extra-virgin olive oil

2 cups chopped sweet or yellow onions

1¼ teaspoons salt

1¼ cups 1% low-fat buttermilk

1 tablespoon wasabi powder (see Substitutions)

preparation

Bring a large pot of water to a simmer. Cut potatoes into 1-inch chunks. Add to water; return to a simmer. Simmer uncovered until potatoes are tender when pierced with tip of a knife, about 14 minutes.

Meanwhile, heat a medium saucepan over medium-high heat. Add oil, then onions. Cook 8 to 10 minutes or until onions begin to brown, stirring occasionally. Remove from heat.

Drain potatoes; return to same pot. Sprinkle salt over potatoes; cook over medium heat 30 seconds to dry potatoes. Add buttermilk and wasabi powder; turn off heat. Mash with a potato masher until desired consistency. Stir in onion mixture; transfer to serving plates.

substitutions: Red potatoes kept at room temperature for a few days make fluffy mashed potatoes, but Yukon Gold or russets may replace them, with some extra effort: add a little more buttermilk, as the russets and Yukon Golds have a drier texture.

Wasabi is a root found in Japan. The pungent green Wasabi paste may replace the powder for an even hotter, cleaner heat in the dish.

tips: Caramelizing the onions adds sweetness, bringing out their natural sugars and replacing the roundness your palate may expect from butter or cream. Another way to accomplish this goal is to add a head of peeled, mashed roasted garlic to the pot just before mashing. Roast garlic by cutting off the top of the head, wrapping it in aluminum foil with a teaspoon of olive oil, and placing it in a 500-degree toaster oven for 12 to 15 minutes. Cool, peel, and mash the garlic.

nutritional analysis

Total fat (g) 6.4	Sodium (mg) 822	Vitamin A (RE) 7
Fat calories (kc) 57.6	Calcium (mg) 113	Beta-carotene (RE) 0
Cholesterol (mg) 2.7	Magnesium (mg) 66	Vitamin C (mg) 35
Saturated fat (g) 1.2	Zinc (mg) 1.1	Vitamin E (mg) 1.3
Polyunsaturated fat (g) 0.6	Selenium (mcg) 4	Thiamin B_1 (mg) 0.3
Monounsaturated fat (g) 4.2	Potassium (mg) 1095	Riboflavin B_2 (mg) 0.2
Fiber (g) 4.7	Flavonoids (mg) 2.8	Niacin B_3 (mg) 3.4
Carbohydrates (g) 56.1	Lycopene (mg) 0	Vitamin B_6 (mg) 0.8
Sugar (g) 9.5	Fish (oz) 0	Folic acid (mcg) 42
Protein (g) 7.6	Nuts (oz) 0	Vitamin B_{12} (mcg) 0.2

FOR DESSERT

Succulent Ripe Berry Parfait

■ ■ ■ ■

Preparation time: 15 minutes	*4 servings* *245 calories per serving, 9% from fat*

RealAge effect if eaten 12 times a year:	RealAge-effect ingredients:
Blueberries, raspberries, and strawberries have incredibly high antioxidant capacities— and they're delicious, to boot. This parfait will make your RealAge 8.4 days younger.	Berries, nuts, yogurt, melon, whole-grain cereal, soy yogurt (antioxidants, calcium, healthy protein, magnesium, selenium, potassium, vitamin B$_3$, folic acid, flavonoids, fiber)

ingredients

24 ounces low-fat soy vanilla yogurt, such as White Wave brand

4 teaspoons honey

½ teaspoon pure vanilla extract

1 cup hulled, quartered strawberries

1 cup raspberries

1 cup blueberries

1 cup diced honeydew melon

½ cup Grape-Nuts (or similar) cereal

preparation

In a medium bowl, combine yogurt, honey, and vanilla; mix well. In four large goblets or clear dessert dishes, arrange fruit and yogurt mixture in four layers. Top with cereal.

substitutions: Low-fat vanilla yogurt may replace soy yogurt, blackberries may replace blueberries, and cantaloupe may replace honeydew melon.

tips: Look for especially juicy melon—its ripeness will help sweeten the dish. The crunch of the cereal is a chef's way to keep you interested: the rough texture contrasts with the smoothness of the yogurt and the firm flesh of the fruit to make your mouth go "Wow!" Keep the melon diced medium: it's easier to eat small chunks rather than big ones, and the melon will go farther.

nutritional analysis

Total fat (g) 4.0
Fat calories (kc) 36
Cholesterol (mg) 0
Saturated fat (g) 0.4
Polyunsaturated fat (g) 1.7
Monounsaturated fat (g) 0.7
Fiber (g) 6.6
Carbohydrates (g) 36
Sugar (g) 16.7
Protein (g) 7.6

Sodium (mg) 128
Calcium (mg) 30
Magnesium (mg) 58
Zinc (mg) 1.0
Selenium (mcg) 6
Potassium (mg) 561
Flavonoids (mg) 1.1
Lycopene (mg) 0
Fish (oz) 0
Nuts (oz) 0

Vitamin A (RE) 203
Beta-carotene (RE) 95
Vitamin C (mg) 44
Vitamin E (mg) 0.3
Thiamin B_1 (mg) 0.5
Riboflavin B_2 (mg) 0.4
Niacin B_3 (mg) 3.6
Vitamin B_6 (mg) 0.4
Folic acid (mcg) 70
Vitamin B_{12} (mcg) 0.8

Caramelized Ripe Tropical Fruit

■ ■ ■ ■

Preparation time: 10 minutes
Cooking time: 6 minutes

4 servings
228 calories per serving, 19.7% from fat

RealAge effect if eaten 12 times a year:	**RealAge-effect ingredients:**
Can dessert be this good for you? You bet. The alcohol (just a little), plus the flavonoids in chocolate (just a little more), oh, and the banana combine to make you 0.8 days younger.	Bananas, pineapple, alcohol, chocolate (potassium, fiber, calcium, magnesium, potassium, folic acid, fiber, antioxidants)

ingredients

Cooking oil spray

2 ripe but firm bananas, peeled, halved lengthwise

4 wedges (1½ inches thick) cored fresh ripe pineapple

½ cup dark rum

¼ teaspoon ground allspice

1 tablespoon dark brown sugar

8 small (¼ cup) scoops low-fat chocolate ice cream

preparation

Heat a large nonstick skillet over medium-high heat until hot. Coat with cooking oil spray. Add bananas in one layer; cook 30 to 40 seconds per side or until well browned. Transfer to four serving plates; set aside. Add pineapple to same skillet; cook 1 minute per side or until golden brown and hot. Transfer to serving plates.

Reduce heat under the skillet to low and add rum and allspice. Cook until mixture reduces by half, about 30 seconds, stirring constantly. Drizzle mixture over fruit; top with brown sugar. Serve with ice cream.

substitutions: Rather than wedges, you may cut cored fresh pineapple into four 1½-inch-thick rings. Sweet ground cinnamon substitutes well for allspice—use twice as much cinnamon as allspice.

tips: Leave the fruit in the pan long enough for the fruit to darken; you want the natural sugar inside to come out. You'll scoop it all back up again by deglazing the pan with the rum.

nutritional analysis

Total fat (g) 5.0	Sodium (mg) 32	Vitamin A (RE) 40
Fat calories (kc) 45	Calcium (mg) 56	Beta-carotene (RE) 39
Cholesterol (mg) 15	Magnesium (mg) 33	Vitamin C (mg) 18
Saturated fat (g) 2.5	Zinc (mg) 0.5	Vitamin E (mg) 0.3
Polyunsaturated fat (g) 0.7	Selenium (mcg) 0	Thiamin B_1 (mg) 0.1
Monounsaturated fat (g) 1.2	Potassium (mg) 397	Riboflavin B_2 (mg) 0.2
Fiber (g) 1.9	Flavonoids (mg) 0.4	Niacin B_3 (mg) 0.7
Carbohydrates (g) 35	Lycopene (mg) 0	Vitamin B_6 (mg) 0.4
Sugar (g) 21.6	Fish (oz) 0	Folic acid (mcg) 21
Protein (g) 1.2	Nuts (oz) 0	Vitamin B_{12} (mcg) 0.2

Chocolate Soy Sundae Smoothie

■ ■ ■ ■

Preparation time: 5 minutes

4 (8-ounce) servings
145 calories per serving, 24.7% from fat

RealAge effect if eaten 12 times a year:

Loaded with isoflavones from two soy foods, and with a surprisingly hefty fiber count, this quickie will make your RealAge 5.5 days younger.

RealAge-effect ingredients:

Soy milk, bananas, berries (healthy protein, antioxidants, flavonoids, potassium)

ingredients

2 cups low-fat (1%) chocolate soy milk, such as Silk brand

1 cup frozen chocolate nondairy soy dessert, such as Soy Delicious brand

24 frozen medium strawberries

1 medium banana, broken into chunks

¼ cup chocolate syrup such as Drucker's (optional)

Multicolored sprinkles (optional)

preparation

Combine all ingredients except sprinkles in blender container. Cover and blend at high speed until thick and smooth. Pour into frosted mugs; garnish with sprinkles, if desired.

substitutions: Low-fat Tofutti (a nondairy soy-based ice cream substitute) may replace the chocolate nondairy soy dessert. Fresh strawberries will work instead of the frozen ones, but the drink will not be as cold or as thick.

tips: For a thicker, colder shake, slice and freeze the banana the night before.

nutritional analysis

Total fat (g) 4.0	Sodium (mg) 32	Vitamin A (RE) 9
Fat calories (kc) 36	Calcium (mg) 21	Beta-carotene (RE) 57
Cholesterol (mg) 0	Magnesium (mg) 59	Vitamin C (mg) 39
Saturated fat (g) 0.5	Zinc (mg) 0.7	Vitamin E (mg) 0.2
Polyunsaturated fat (g) 1.6	Selenium (mcg) 1	Thiamin B_1 (mg) 0.3
Monounsaturated fat (g) 0.7	Potassium (mg) 523	Riboflavin B_2 (mg) 0.2
Fiber (g) 4.5	Flavonoids (mg) 2.2	Niacin B_3 (mg) 0.7
Carbohydrates (g) 25	Lycopene (mg) 0	Vitamin B_6 (mg) 0.3
Sugar (g) 18	Fish (oz) 0	Folic acid (mcg) 20
Protein (g) 6.0	Nuts (oz) 0	Vitamin B_{12} (mcg) 0

Sliced Peaches with Raspberries, Blueberries, and Chocolate Chips

THIS RECIPE IS A REALAGE SPECIAL
CREATED BY GALE GAND.

■ ■ ■ ■

| Preparation time: 10 minutes | 4 servings |
| | 75 calories per serving, 25% from fat |

| **RealAge effect if eaten 12 times a year:** | **RealAge-effect ingredients:** |
| 3.7 days younger | Peaches, berries (flavonoids, potassium, antioxidants, fiber) |

ingredients

2 large or 4 small ripe peaches, sliced

1 teaspoon cinnamon

Pinch of nutmeg

½ cup (2 ounces) fresh raspberries

½ cup (2 ounces) fresh blueberries

3 tablespoons (1 ounce) mini-chocolate chips (real cocoa, not milk chocolate)

preparation

Combine sliced peaches with cinnamon and nutmeg; transfer to four serving plates. Top peaches with raspberries, blueberries, and chocolate chips.

substitutions: Unpeeled sliced nectarines may replace the peaches, and blackberries may replace the raspberries. White peaches are especially succulent and sweet; look for them in the summer.

tips: Keeping the well-washed skin on the peaches increases the amount of dietary fiber in this simple, easy dish. A drizzle of liqueur—perhaps Chambord, a raspberry liqueur—would make this simple dessert elegant.

nutritional analysis

Total fat (g) 2.1	Sodium (mg) 1.9	Vitamin A (RE) 33
Fat calories (kc) 19	Calcium (mg) 22	Beta-carotene (RE) 159
Cholesterol (mg) 0	Magnesium (mg) 10	Vitamin C (mg) 8
Saturated fat (g) 1.4	Zinc (mg) 0.1	Vitamin E (mg) 0.1
Polyunsaturated fat (g) 0.2	Selenium (mcg) 1	Thiamin B_1 (mg) 0.02
Monounsaturated fat (g) 0.8	Potassium (mg) 147	Riboflavin B_2 (mg) 0.1
Fiber (g) 2.7	Flavonoids (mg) 0.5	Niacin B_3 (mg) 0.6
Carbohydrates (g) 12.5	Lycopene (mg) 0	Vitamin B_6 (mg) 0.02
Sugar (g) 9.4	Fish (oz) 0	Folic acid (mcg) 7
Protein (g) 1.0	Nuts (oz) 0	Vitamin B_{12} (mcg) 0

Autumn Produce

Many fruits and vegetables are at their peak at the beginning of autumn. Juicy apples, sweet peppers, winter squash, and cranberries are some of our favorites.

Autumn Produce Chart

Vegetable/Fruit	Buying and Using
Apples	➤ **When:** Most apples are best in August and September. There are hundreds of varieties, some ripe as early as March and some as late as November. (Most apples available in winter have more crunchy texture than flavor.) The smells of freshly pressed apple cider and apple pies in the oven are sure signs of autumn. The assortments of colors and flavors make apples a very versatile fruit. ➤ **What to Look For:** Apples have the best, juiciest flavor right after they're harvested. You'll find a nice variety at the farmers' market, probably ones you've never seen before; ask for samples. A ready-to-eat apple feels a little heavy for its size, is aromatic and firm, and has no soft spots or cracks. Avoid apples with wormholes. ➤ **Why:** Apples are a great RealAge snack. There are plenty of age-reducing flavonoids and fiber in their skin. Because of the high flavonoid content, eating apples decreases the risk of asthma, in addition to other age-reducing benefits. So, the saying "An apple a day keeps the doctor away" really is based on science. ➤ **How to Use:** Different varieties are best for cooking, baking, eating raw, and pressing. I like Fuji, Mutsu, and Pink Lady for eating. For a great, filling snack, dip three apple slices into a little melted chocolate. Just microwave chocolate chips (made from true-dark, cocoa-based chocolate, not milk chocolate) in a microwave-proof tumbler until very fluid, approximately 45 seconds. Dip slices into the chocolate, scrape the excess onto one side, place the slices on a plate lined with waxed paper, and refrigerate for approximately 10 minutes, until set. The right amount of cocoa fat is

Cooking the RealAge Way

approximately 7 grams, or 16 chips, per person using regular-size chocolate chips. (Mike uses Wegmans, Food Club, or Ghirardelli chocolate chips.) Try this snack trick with strawberries, too. Kids love it when we make these for a late afternoon snack.

Although apples can be used in salads and meat dishes, they're usually associated with desserts, such as apple pie and cobbler. (Try chocolate-dipped as a desert, too). Apples can be stemmed, cored, diced, and cooked with a little juice or water and a big cinnamon stick to make a delicious homemade applesauce.

Beans, shelling

➤ **When:** Beans are plentiful in the fall. They stimulate thoughts of warm, hearty soups and satisfying, filling stews.

➤ **What to Look For:** Beans are available already shelled and in the pod. The farmer harvests the pods but usually sells beans shelled. Actually, they're protected by their pod, which holds the flavorful bean. Try cranberry beans—they look just like crimson speckled jewels. The pod should be leathery, and you should be able to feel the bean inside the pod. The pod should be moist but not wet; the beans themselves are moist. Pods that are wet are susceptible to mold and injury.

➤ **Why:** Beans are rich in the RealAge-smart nutrients fiber and potassium.

➤ **How to Use:** Beans can also be dried for later use, used in soups and stews, mixed with stewed tomatoes and chiles, or blended into a party dip with roasted garlic, yogurt, and fresh herbs. Shelled beans cook more quickly than dried beans. We have received many thank-you e-mails regarding the Portuguese Bean Soup recipe in *The RealAge Diet* book. We hope you'll also enjoy the Rich and Spicy Black Bean Soup on page 291 of this chapter.

Broccoli

➤ **When:** Broccoli is available all year, with a peak season from August through October and even earlier in the South and West. Fresh broccoli has a sweet and mild flavor that makes it perfect for a large variety of dishes.

➤ **What to Look For:** Look for slender, firm stalks. The florets should be tight. Avoid stalks with yellow or limp florets and leaves. Size doesn't count with broccoli: small florets are just as likely to be flavorful as large ones.

➤ **Why:** Broccoli is rich in flavonoids, so it makes you younger every time you enjoy it. And it is a great source of vitamin C, calcium, potassium, and lutein, so your immune system, arteries, bones, and eyes are all younger because you ate broccoli.

➤ **How to Use:** Broccoli can be eaten raw as a snack, with dips, or in salads. It can also be boiled, steamed, sautéed, and added to a teriyaki stir-fry. Toss broccoli florets with garlic oil and sesame seeds and roast them at high temperature just until they begin to darken. Eat the leaves and stem, too: cut off the toughest part of the stem and peel away the remaining rough skin. Then slice the stem into broccoli stars!

Brussels sprouts

➤ **When:** Brussels sprouts are available from late August through March but are best in October and November (except in the West, where they're best in winter). Buy Brussels sprouts on their stalk whenever you can, as it's often a good indication they've just been harvested.

➤ **What to Look For:** Find Brussels sprouts on the stalk and cook them soon after purchasing. Loose sprouts should not have any yellow leaves or brown butts. The sprouts themselves should be tight and firm. At a farmers' market, ask when they were harvested.

➤ **Why:** Thanks to their vitamin C, potassium, selenium, and fiber, Brussels sprouts are a *great*—not just a good—choice that can make you younger.

➤ **How to Use:** Brussels sprouts can be steamed or boiled and are usually not eaten raw unless sliced very fine. They usually need seasoning and cooking to bring out their sweetness and flavor. Try minced leek, fresh dill, and caraway seeds as seasonings.

Cooking by the Seasons

A favorite way to prepare Brussels sprouts is with freshly grated pecorino or Parmesan cheese: separate the leaves of each sprout (it's easier than it sounds), sauté garlic and onion in olive oil, wilt the leaves in a hot pan, simmer them in chicken stock, and shake on the cheese.

Cauliflower

➤ **When:** Cauliflower is another vegetable you can find all year. Its peak season is at the end of summer and the beginning of autumn (except in the South and West, where cauliflower is better in winter and spring, respectively).

➤ **What to Look For:** The florets should be close together and smooth. If they've started to separate, the flavor will be stronger, like cabbage. Avoid cauliflower that is turning dark in spots. Pick a cauliflower still slightly covered by its green veil.

➤ **Why:** Cauliflower is RealAge-wise. It's packed with vitamin C, folate, and flavonoids, and decreases aging of the immune system. As is true for all cruciferous vegetables, consumption of cauliflower is associated with a decreased incidence of several cancers, including breast and colon cancer, and a decreased risk of aging of the eyes.

➤ **How to Use:** Serve raw or steam just until firm; add to soups, stews, salads, and pastas and other grain dishes. Roasted cauliflower—separated into large florets and roasted at a high temperature (start with 450 degrees for 15 minutes, and adjust to taste)—is a wonderful treat. Roasted cauliflower soup is even better; combine roasted cauliflower with roasted chestnuts or chestnut purée.

Chestnuts

➤ **When:** The aroma of roasting chestnuts is a sure sign that fall is here and winter isn't far ahead. Fresh chestnuts, most of which are imported, are available from September through February. Those grown in the United States (largely in California) are at their peak in October and November.

➤ **What to Look For:** Choose firm, plump chestnuts that have no blemishes on their shells.

Vegetable/Fruit	Buying and Using

➤ **Why:** Chestnuts contain healthy (age-reducing) fat and protein.

➤ **How to Use:** Chestnuts can be boiled, roasted, candied, puréed, and preserved. They're commonly used in desserts, stuffing, and soup. Dried chestnuts and chestnut flour are also available.

Cranberries

➤ **When:** The peak market period for cranberries is October through December.

➤ **What to Look For:** Look for plump red berries that are not discolored, shriveled, or mashed. It's very easy to freeze cranberries (just put them in the freezer), and they freeze very well.

➤ **Why:** These berries are loaded with age-reducing nutrients, such as flavonoids.

➤ **How to Use:** The tart flavor of cranberries makes them a nice accompaniment to mildly flavored foods. Raw cranberries, however, are too tart for most people, so the berries are usually dried or cooked. Use cranberries in scones, muffins, breads, and desserts. Cooked cranberries can also be used in salads, or as an accompaniment to poultry. Cranberries are synonymous with Thanksgiving and, in many households, appear on the table as a sauce. Cranberry-ginger chutney, a good alternative to cranberry sauce, can be made by simmering cranberries with fresh and candied ginger and adding orange juice and raisins.

Fennel

➤ **When:** Fennel is especially available in the fall, particularly September.

➤ **What to Look For:** Heads of fennel should feel firm, solid, and moist. The greens should still be attached. Buy bulbs that have a healthy root and a smooth outer layer, and that feel heavy for their size.

➤ **Why:** Fennel contains vitamins B_1, B_2, B_3, and C.

➤ **How to Use:** Fennel has a distinctive licorice flavor; if an aroma is present, it will likely be faint. The whole plant (bulb and stalks) can

Vegetable/Fruit	Buying and Using

be used instead of, or in addition to, celery. The stalks can be thinly sliced 4 to 5 inches up from the bulb; save the rest of the stalk for stock. The outer layer and the root portion are tough; peel away one or two stalks, divide in half, and cut out the remaining root. Fennel can be eaten raw, baked, braised, grilled, sautéed, steamed, and used in salads, sauces, and stuffing. I like to caramelize fennel with olive oil, sweet onions, and fennel seeds, and sprinkle it with Maytag Blue or fresh goat cheese for a quick and easy pizza. Also, the leaves can be used as a garnish or in a salad, and the seeds can be used to flavor sausage and beans.

Mushrooms

➤ **When:** Mushrooms are edible fungi. They are sought for their woodsy flavor, their meatiness, and their earthy character, all of which complement many fall recipes. Mushrooms come in many varieties, the peak months being September and October. Some special varieties—morels, in particular—pop up in April and May.

➤ **What to Look For:** Mushrooms should be firm. The stem should not be separating from the cap, a condition that indicates age. Open gills are desirable in portobello mushrooms and acceptable in others, if the mushroom is not soft or discolored.

➤ **Why:** Mushrooms contain age-reducing potassium and selenium.

➤ **How to Use:** Mushrooms can be dried for later use, sautéed, grilled, and used in sauces or in combination with other dishes. Mushrooms are like onions: there aren't many main dishes they don't improve. They are versatile, and add body and flavor to many dishes. I love their texture. To store, keep mushrooms refrigerated in an open paper bag.

Pears

➤ **When:** Pears are at their best from August through October. They're better soft than firm. As they age, their sweet flavor develops, and their flesh becomes gently soft. Buy pears slightly firm; they'll ripen in just a few days, at home. Look for Seckel pears in fall—tiny, beautiful, intensely flavored, perfect.

➤ **What to Look For:** Pears should have a good aroma and be slightly firm. A ripe pear will feel heavy for its size. It will soften and become more fragrant as it ripens.

➤ **Why:** Pears are rich in flavonoids and fiber, and both make your RealAge younger.

➤ **How to Use:** Pears can be eaten plain, poached, or sautéed, or used in desserts and sauces. Like apples, some pears are best for cooking purposes (not many varieties, however, as their delicate flavor disappears). A delicious way to prepare pears is to poach them whole in red wine and cloves and then drizzle them with chocolate. (See APPLES for how to prepare the chocolate drizzle.)

Pecans

➤ **When:** Unshelled pecans are available throughout the year; their peak season is during the autumn. Pecans are a wonderful, underappreciated age-reducing food choice.

➤ **What to Look For:** Choose unshelled pecans by their clean, unblemished, uncracked shells: they look like footballs with blunt ends. The kernel should not rattle in the shell when shaken, as it may have dried up and become inedible.

➤ **Why:** Pecans contain great RealAge-healthy fats and proteins.

➤ **How to Use:** Pecans are famous for their use in pies, stuffings, pasta, and many desserts. Toasted pecans are a great snack, but remember, a few is optimal to make you younger. Put them on a sheet pan at 350 degrees for 8 to 10 minutes or until they begin to darken. Add a little salt, let them cool, and store them in a clear container.

Persimmons

➤ **When:** Persimmons are available from October to February. Although they're gaining in popularity, you still might not be familiar with these fruits.

➤ **What to Look For:** There are many kinds of persimmons, and this is one fruit you should sample first. Seek assistance in selecting ripe ones. For Hachiya persimmons—the ones that look like a heart—

Vegetable/Fruit	Buying and Using

the softer and more fragrant, the better. Also, Hachiya persimmons should have a uniform, all-over orange color. Fuyu persimmons, which are flat like a squat tomato, should be firm and have a deep orange-red color.

➤ **Why:** Persimmons are rich in the RealAge nutrients fiber, vitamin C, and potassium.

➤ **How to Use:** Use persimmons in ice creams, custards, or sherbet, or as fresh fruit and in salads. For a sweet-hot exotic dip, puree persimmons in a blender with roasted garlic, a little habanero chile, and raspberry vinegar.

Pomegranates

➤ **When:** In the United States, pomegranates are available in October and November. Underappreciated as a fruit, they often simply adorn mantelpieces at Christmas.

➤ **What to Look For:** Pomegranates should feel heavy for their size, which means they're full of juice. An occasional crack on the surface can be a sign of ripeness, but avoid those with penetrating cracks or sunken pockets of skin. Pomegranates are not usually fragrant.

➤ **Why:** Pomegranates are loaded with age-reducing fiber and potassium.

➤ **How to Use:** Pomegranate seeds are eaten raw and are used in salads and as a garnish. They can be cooked and added to compotes or sauces. To obtain the seeds, slice a thin piece off the crown. Then slit the skin with a knife from top to bottom, in four sections, to reveal the seeds. If you don't want the seeds, roll the pomegranate around with slight pressure and cut open a small slit to drain the juice. Look for pomegranate molasses in specialty shops; it's simply reduced juice, and it's heavenly—sweet and tart at the same time.

Potatoes, mature

➤ **When:** In the cooler climates, mature potatoes are in peak season in September and October. They have a thicker skin and a grainier texture than new (baby) potatoes. Look for special varieties just for fun: Purple Peruvians, fingerlings, Yukon Golds, Yellow Finns. All have lovely color and firm texture and are fun to eat.

➤ **What to Look For:** Small potatoes tend to have a more delicate flavor than larger ones. Avoid potatoes with sprouts and any hint of green skin, which can be toxic. Flesh that is soft or discolored is also undesirable.

➤ **How to Use:** Although they're delicious on their own, potatoes are a good accompaniment to other foods as well. Remember to decrease the blood sugar-raising effect of potatoes by enjoying a little healthy fat, such as a small amount of guacamole or olive oil on a small slice of whole-grain bread 8 or 10 minutes beforehand.

Potatoes should be washed thoroughly, but peeling is usually not necessary. Potatoes are boiled, grilled, roasted, or sliced to make a gratin. Russets make very flaky baked potatoes. To store, keep potatoes in a cool, dark, dry place in an open paper bag.

Radicchio (Italian chicory)

➤ **When:** This leafy vegetable is popular in Italy and is now gaining recognition here. A small, cabbage-like vegetable with beautiful magenta-ivory streaks, radicchio is a member of the chicory family. In cooler climates, it's ready for harvest by mid-fall. You'll probably find leaves and small heads of radicchio at your farmers' market.

➤ **What to Look For:** If it is the cabbage-type radicchio, the head should be closed and tight. If it is not, still avoid leaves that are brown or decaying. Leaves should be firm and crisp, but not so heavy that they break away from the core, indicating age.

➤ **Why:** The folate, flavonoids, and potassium in radicchio make your RealAge younger.

➤ **How to Use:** Radicchio can be used raw in mixed green salads and as a sandwich ingredient. It can also be sautéed and added to a warm salad or risotto. Grilled smoky radicchio—caramelized and sweet-sour—is truly delicious.

247

Vegetable/Fruit	Buying and Using
Sweet peppers, bell peppers	➤ **When:** A green pepper is a pepper that was picked before it was mature. Left on the vine, it develops into a sweet pepper. In late August and September, sweet peppers come alive with a multitude of colors (purples, yellows, oranges, reds, chocolate brown) and variations of sweetness. Bell peppers are the most common sweet peppers eaten in the United States. ➤ **What to Look For:** Sweet peppers are mature. Their skin should be glossy and smooth without wrinkling or punctures. Look for moist green stems that indicate they are freshly picked. Sweet peppers should feel heavy for their size, indicating ripeness. ➤ **Why:** Sweet peppers are rich in vitamin C, flavonoids, and fiber. ➤ **How to Use:** Enjoy raw sweet peppers as crudités or chopped in salads. They can also be grilled, sautéed, and stuffed, or used in soups, spreads, sauces, and stews. The purple peppers hold their color when sliced fresh but turn dark green when cooked.
Winter squash (acorn squash, butternut squash, Delicata, Hubbard squash, turbans, Red Kuri, Kabochas, pumpkins)	➤ **When:** The harvest of winter squash is from September to the first serious frost in winter. Winter squash develop tough skins, which give them protection against predators and a long shelf life. Although squash appear in a variety of enchanting shapes and sizes, they almost always have sweet yellow or orange flesh. ➤ **What to Look For:** Look for hard, unblemished skin with a firm and smooth texture, and heaviness for its size. A truly bright sheen on the skin indicates the squash isn't ripe. If stored at room temperature, winter squash tend to improve in flavor after a few weeks; if stored in a cool dry place, they can last up to 6 months. ➤ **Why:** The potassium, folate, essential amino acids, and fiber in winter squash contribute to their large RealAge benefit. ➤ **How to Use:** You can bake, roast, or steam winter squash. They can be used in soups (puréed or chunky), breads, and desserts (especially pumpkin). Cut the squash into small pieces and add to

stews. Roast cubes of butternut squash with chunks of potato. Roast slices of winter squash at high heat and cover them with an orange-cranberry sauce. For a special RealAge fall dinner, fill scooped-out, baked Kabochas with wild rice and berries, drizzle with balsamic vinegar, and sprinkle with toasted pistachios.

Sweet potatoes

➤ **When:** Fresh sweet potatoes are available sporadically throughout the year, although not as readily during the summer. Their peak season lasts from October to December. You might think potatoes store well, but not sweet potatoes. Try to use them within a week.

➤ **What to Look For:** Sweet potatoes should have a smooth surface and no pits. Avoid potatoes that are shriveled, have black patches, or are sprouting.

➤ **Why:** Like squash, sweet potatoes have the RealAge-healthy nutrients folate and essential amino acids. In fact, a sweet potato has more than twice as much folate (50 mcg) as an ordinary potato.

➤ **How to Use:** Sweet potatoes have so much flavor, they're good just baked or steamed. They make a wonderful soup and can be added to stews. Sweet potatoes are also good grilled and roasted on an open fire. They're famously adaptable for custards and pie.

Recipes Using Autumn Produce

FOR BREAKFAST

Double Apple Cinnamon Smoothie

Preparation time: 5 minutes	*4 (8-ounce) servings* *204 calories per serving, 15% from fat*

RealAge effect if eaten 12 times a year:	RealAge-effect ingredients:
Rich in potassium, which lowers blood pressure and makes your RealAge younger, twelve of these 8-ounce cups of this smoothie lowers your RealAge by 1.9 days.	Apple juice, applesauce, soy milk (potassium, calcium, flavonoids, antioxidants, healthy protein)

ingredients

½ cup frozen apple juice concentrate, not thawed

1 cup cinnamon applesauce, such as Mott's brand

1¼ cups vanilla or plain fat-free or light soy milk

1½ cups low-fat vanilla frozen yogurt

¼ teaspoon apple pie spice

preparation

Combine all ingredients in blender container. Cover; blend at high speed for 1 minute. Pour into frosty mugs, if desired.

substitutions: Allspice may replace the apple pie spice. If you can't find cinnamon applesauce, add ¼ teaspoon cinnamon to a cup of applesauce.

tips: Blending for a full minute dissolves the tiny bit of graininess from the applesauce. Blend the smoothie at your blender's highest setting to get extra lift and lightness in each mouthful. If you like it a little less sweet, use half of the apple juice concentrate.

nutritional analysis

Total fat (g) 3.4
Fat calories (kc) 30.5
Cholesterol (mg) 5.6
Saturated fat (g) 1.3
Polyunsaturated fat (g) 1.0
Monounsaturated fat (g) 1.1
Fiber (g) 2.7
Carbohydrates (g) 34.9
Sugar (g) 8.9
Protein (g) 9.1

Sodium (mg) 266
Calcium (mg) 220
Magnesium (mg) 39
Zinc (mg) 1.2
Selenium (mcg) 12
Potassium (mg) 565
Flavonoids (mg) 3.7
Lycopene (mg) 0
Fish (oz) 0
Nuts (oz) 0

Vitamin A (RE) 22
Beta-carotene (RE) 24
Vitamin C (mg) 3
Vitamin E (mg) 0.5
Thiamin B_1 (mg) 0.3
Riboflavin B_2 (mg) 0.4
Niacin B_3 (mg) 1.4
Vitamin B_6 (mg) 0.1
Folic acid (mcg) 22
Vitamin B_{12} (mcg) 0.5

Apricot Breakfast Polenta

■ ■ ■ ■

Preparation time: 5 minutes	*4 servings*
Cooking time: 10 minutes	*289 calories per serving, 14% from fat*

RealAge effect if eaten 12 times a year:	**RealAge-effect ingredients:**
Bursting with potassium and omega-3 fatty acids, our breakfast polenta makes your RealAge 8.4 days younger.	Apricot nectar, apricots, walnuts, cornmeal (fiber, magnesium, potassium, folic acid, antioxidants, lycopene, healthy fats)

ingredients

1 can (11.5 ounces) apricot nectar, such as Libby's-Kern's brand

1 cup coarsely chopped dried apricots

1 tube (16 ounces) plain prepared polenta (cornmeal), cut crosswise into 12 slices

Butter-flavored cooking oil spray

¼ to ½ cup coarsely chopped walnuts, toasted

1 tablespoon honey (optional)

preparation

In a small saucepan, combine nectar and apricots; bring to a simmer over high heat. Reduce heat; simmer uncovered 6 to 7 minutes or until sauce thickens.

Meanwhile, heat broiler. Arrange cornmeal slices on a baking sheet or jelly-roll pan; coat with cooking oil spray. Broil 3 to 4 inches from heat 4 to 5 minutes per side or until browned. Transfer to four serving plates; top with apricot sauce and walnuts. Drizzle with honey, if desired.

substitutions: Dried fruit bits, such as Sunsweet brand, may replace apricots, and corn nuts or toasted soy nuts may replace walnuts.

tips: A few snips of mint leaves will add color, flavor, and no calories to the dish.

nutritional analysis

Total fat (g) 4.6
Fat calories (kc) 117
Cholesterol (mg) 0
Saturated fat (g) 0.8
Polyunsaturated fat (g) 1.8
Monounsaturated fat (g) 1.0
Fiber (g) 7.6
Carbohydrates (g) 48.4
Sugar (g) 15.6
Protein (g) 7.2

Sodium (mg) 385
Calcium (mg) 74
Magnesium (mg) 55
Zinc (mg) 1
Selenium (mcg) 8
Potassium (mg) 535
Flavonoids (mg) 0
Lycopene (mg) 2
Fish (oz) 0
Nuts (oz) 0.4

Vitamin A (RE) 278
Beta-carotene (RE) 1605
Vitamin C (mg) 2
Vitamin E (mg) 0.8
Thiamin B_1 (mg) 0.1
Riboflavin B_2 (mg) 0.1
Niacin B_3 (mg) 1.6
Vitamin B_6 (mg) 0.2
Folic acid (mcg) 16
Vitamin B_{12} (mcg) 0.1

Fabulous French Toast with Spiced Fruit and Powdered Sugar

■ ■ ■ ■

Preparation time: 8 minutes
Cooking time: 12 minutes

4 servings
335 calories per serving, 6% from fat

RealAge effect if eaten 12 times a year:

The natural goodness of soy protein reduces aging of the coronary arteries (now an FDA-approved claim). This powerful breakfast carries a RealAge benefit of 8.9 days younger.

RealAge-effect ingredients:

Apple juice, fruit, egg whites, soy milk, whole grains (fiber, flavonoids, antioxidants, folic acid, potassium, healthy protein)

ingredients

2 cups unfiltered apple juice or apple cider

1 cinnamon stick or ¼ teaspoon cinnamon

1 cup mixed dried fruit bits, such as Sunsweet brand

2 egg whites, beaten until frothy

½ cup nonfat vanilla soy milk

⅛ teaspoon nutmeg

Butter-flavored cooking oil spray

8 slices whole wheat or multigrain bread, such as Natural Ovens brand

2 teaspoons confectioners' sugar

preparation

Combine juice and cinnamon stick or cinnamon in a small saucepan. Bring to a boil over high heat; boil gently 3 minutes to reduce slightly. Add fruit bits; simmer uncovered 8 minutes or until fruit is tender and sauce thickens. Discard cinnamon stick.

Meanwhile, combine egg whites, soy milk, and nutmeg in a pie plate or shallow dish. Heat a large nonstick griddle or skillet over medium heat. Coat skillet with cooking oil spray. Dip each slice of bread into milk mixture, turning to coat both sides lightly. Cook on hot griddle 2 to 3 minutes per side or until golden brown. Transfer to four serving plates; top with fruit mixture. Place confectioners' sugar in strainer; shake over French toast to dust lightly with sugar.

substitutions: Diced dried apples or apricots may be substituted for fruit bits. One-half cup liquid egg substitute may replace egg whites.

tips: Reducing the apple cider is an easy way to add extra flavor to this topping. During the simmering time, the water evaporates, leaving a more concentrated flavor behind. Do not soak the bread in the milk mixture too long or the French toast will become soggy. A quick turn of the bread in the milk mixture will suffice.

nutritional analysis

Total fat (g) 2.3	Sodium (mg) 384	Vitamin A (RE) 75
Fat calories (kc) 21	Calcium (mg) 65	Beta-carotene (RE) 450
Cholesterol (mg) 0	Magnesium (mg) 75	Vitamin C (mg) 2
Saturated fat (g) 0.1	Zinc (mg) 1.2	Vitamin E (mg) 0.20
Polyunsaturated fat (g) 0.3	Selenium (mcg) 29	Thiamin B_1 (mg) 0.30
Monounsaturated fat (g) 0.1	Potassium (mg) 597	Riboflavin B_2 (mg) 0.3
Fiber (g) 10.1	Flavonoids (mg) 2	Niacin B_3 (mg) 0.8
Carbohydrates (g) 49.6	Lycopene (mg) 0	Vitamin B_6 (mg) 0.2
Sugar (g) 20.5	Fish (oz) 0	Folic acid (mcg) 32
Protein (g) 9.0	Nuts (oz) 0	Vitamin B_{12} (mcg) 0.04

FOR BRUNCH

Sweet Potato Pancakes with Apple and Cinnamon

■ ■ ■ ■

Preparation time: 10 minutes	*4 servings*
Cooking time: 8 minutes (griddle),	*191 calories per serving, 18.7% from fat*
16 minutes (2 skillets)	

RealAge effect if eaten 12 times a year:	**RealAge-effect ingredients:**
This recipe makes your RealAge 5.7 days younger.	Sweet potatoes, apple, applesauce, egg whites (flavonoids, potassium, fiber, vitamin C, vitamin B$_6$, healthy protein)

ingredients

1 large sweet potato (about 12 ounces), scrubbed

1 small Granny Smith apple

¼ cup all-purpose flour

1 egg white

1 whole egg

½ teaspoon salt

½ teaspoon cinnamon

Butter-flavored cooking oil spray

½ cup chunky applesauce or cinnamon applesauce

¼ cup fat-free or low-fat sour cream (optional)

preparation

Shred sweet potato and apple (by hand or in a food processor fitted with the shredding blade); transfer to a medium bowl. Add flour, egg white, egg, salt, and cinnamon; mix well.

Heat a large nonstick griddle or two skillets over medium heat until hot. Coat with cooking oil spray. Drop sweet potato batter by ¼ cupfuls; press down with back of spatula to form 3-inch patties. Cook 4 minutes per side or until golden brown and cooked through.

Transfer to warmed serving plates; top with applesauce and, if desired, sour cream.

substitutions: One-half cup liquid egg may replace the 1 egg white and 1 whole egg. Ground cloves may replace the cinnamon; use just ¼ teaspoon, because a little goes a long way.

tips: Use a nested metal ¼-cup measure to drop the sweet potato into neat rounds. Flattening with the spatula ensures that the pancakes cook through. The cooked pancakes may be kept warm on serving plates in a 200-degree oven as they are made.

nutritional analysis

Total fat (g) 4.0	Sodium (mg) 367	Vitamin A (RE) 1881
Fat calories (kc) 35.8	Calcium (mg) 75	Beta-carotene (RE) 11,137
Cholesterol (mg) 53.3	Magnesium (mg) 22	Vitamin C (mg) 23
Saturated fat (g) 2.4	Zinc (mg) 0.5	Vitamin E (mg) 4
Polyunsaturated fat (g) 0.4	Selenium (mcg) 7	Thiamin B_1 (mg) 0.1
Monounsaturated fat (g) 0.8	Potassium (mg) 404	Riboflavin B_2 (mg) 0.2
Fiber (g) 3.8	Flavonoids (mg) 2.6	Niacin B_3 (mg) 1.1
Carbohydrates (g) 35.5	Lycopene (mg) 0	Vitamin B_6 (mg) 0.3
Sugar (g) 13.8	Fish (oz) 0	Folic acid (mcg) 29
Protein (g) 4.4	Nuts (oz) 0	Vitamin B_{12} (mcg) 0.1

Tunisian Egg Scramble with Golden Raisins and Paprika

Preparation time: 10 minutes	*4 servings*
Cooking time: 5 minutes	*246 calories per serving, 30.0% from fat*

RealAge effect if eaten 12 times a year:	**RealAge-effect ingredients:**
This scramble has every B vitamin we track— B_1, B_2, B_3, B_6, B_{12}—plus folate. Its RA effect is terrific: 3.2 days younger.	Onion, egg whites, olives, raisins, parsley, whole wheat (B vitamins, including folic acid)

ingredients

2 medium poblano chiles

2 teaspoons olive oil

½ cup chopped onion

5 large egg whites plus 2 large eggs

½ teaspoon each salt and ground cumin

¼ teaspoon paprika, preferably hot Hungarian, such as Szeged brand

¼ cup each chopped pitted Kalamata olives, golden raisins, and flat-leaf parsley

4 whole wheat pitas (pocket breads), such as Sahara brand, toasted or warmed

preparation

Heat broiler. Split chiles lengthwise in half; discard stems and seeds. Place cut side down on foil-lined baking sheet. Broil 3 to 4 inches from heat source until skin blackens, about 8 minutes. Wrap chiles in foil; let cool 5 minutes. Unwrap chiles; discard blackened skin and cut chiles into strips.

Meanwhile, heat a large nonstick skillet over medium-high heat. Add oil, then onion; cook 4 minutes, stirring occasionally. Beat together egg whites, eggs, salt, cumin, and paprika; add to skillet and cook 1 minute, stirring constantly. Stir sliced chiles, olives, raisins, and parsley into egg mixture; continue cooking until eggs are desired doneness. Serve over pita bread.

substitutions: 1¾ cups egg substitute may replace the egg whites and eggs without any loss of flavor.

tips: Good, rich, plain yogurt, especially soy yogurt, and pickled capers (which are, actually, flower buds!) are other flavorful toppings that can make this intriguing dish even better.

nutritional analysis

Total fat (g) 8.1	Sodium (mg) 752	Vitamin A (RE) 76
Fat calories (kc) 73	Calcium (mg) 73	Beta-carotene (RE) 177
Cholesterol (mg) 106	Magnesium (mg) 27	Vitamin C (mg) 17
Saturated fat (g) 1.4	Zinc (mg) 0.8	Vitamin E (mg) 1.1
Polyunsaturated fat (g) 0.8	Selenium (mcg) 19	Thiamin B_1 (mg) 0.2
Monounsaturated fat (g) 4.3	Potassium (mg) 286	Riboflavin B_2 (mg) 0.5
Fiber (g) 2.1	Flavonoids (mg) 0.7	Niacin B_3 (mg) 1.7
Carbohydrates (g) 32	Lycopene (mg) 0	Vitamin B_6 (mg) 0.1
Sugar (g) 6.6	Fish (oz) 0	Folic acid (mcg) 48
Protein (g) 13.5	Nuts (oz) 0	Vitamin B_{12} (mcg) 0.4

FOR LUNCH

Multi-Mushroom Risotto

■ ■ ■ ■

Preparation time: 10 minutes	*4 servings*
Cooking time: 25 minutes	*502 calories per serving, 14% from fat*

RealAge effect if eaten 12 times a year:	**RealAge-effect ingredients:**
Low in fat and very low in sodium, our risotto is bursting with B vitamins, especially niacin. It makes your RealAge 5.3 days younger.	Mushrooms, olive oil, shallots, spinach, walnuts (B vitamins, potassium, flavonoids, healthy fats, calcium)

ingredients

3½ cups fat-free beef or mushroom broth

½ ounce dried porcini mushrooms

1 tablespoon olive oil

1 cup sliced shallots (about 3 large)

2 (4-ounce) packages sliced exotic mushrooms, such as Pennsylvania Farms brand

1½ cups Arborio rice (see Tips)

Salt and freshly ground black pepper to taste

4 cups packed baby spinach leaves

2 ounces Parmigiano-Reggiano cheese

2 tablespoons chopped fresh thyme or toasted walnuts (optional)

preparation

Place broth in a medium saucepan. Use scissors or kitchen shears to cut porcini mushrooms into ½-inch pieces; add to broth. Bring to a simmer over high heat. Reduce heat; keep broth at a constant gentle simmer while preparing risotto.

Heat a large, deep skillet over medium-high heat. Add oil and shallots; cook 2 minutes, stirring occasionally. Add mushrooms; cook 4 minutes, stirring occasionally. Add rice; cook and stir 1 minute. Add 1 cup simmering porcini-broth mixture to skillet. Cook, stirring frequently until broth is absorbed. Continue adding broth ½ cup at a time, keeping rice mixture at a constant simmer and stirring until broth is absorbed. Repeat process until rice is cooked just through, about 18 minutes total. When all broth mixture is used, stir in salt and pepper to taste and check rice for doneness. If rice is too firm, add ½ cup hot water and continue to cook and stir. Mixture should have a creamy texture.

Arrange 1 cup spinach on each of four large plates. Spoon risotto over spinach to wilt. Using a swivel-bladed vegetable peeler or cheese plane, shave cheese over risotto. Sprinkle with thyme or walnuts, or both, if desired.

substitutions: Crimini mushrooms may replace all or part of the exotic mushrooms, and low-salt chicken broth may replace the beef or mushroom broth. Button mushrooms will give you more mushrooms, but not more mushroom flavor.

tips: Arborio rice is an Italian medium-grain rice. To add a subtle wine flavor to the risotto, add ½ cup dry vermouth or dry white wine to the sautéed rice and let the rice absorb the wine before adding the broth. The alcohol evaporates quickly, and the whole dish is transformed—just a tinge of lemon-like pucker behind every rich and creamy bite.

nutritional analysis

Total fat (g) 7.4	Sodium (mg) 430	Vitamin A (RE) 154
Fat calories (kc) 67	Calcium (mg) 193	Beta-carotene (RE) 42
Cholesterol (mg) 14.5	Magnesium (mg) 62	Vitamin C (mg) 36
Saturated fat (g) 1.4	Zinc (mg) 2.2	Vitamin E (mg) 3.1
Polyunsaturated fat (g) 1.3	Selenium (mcg) 30	Thiamin B_1 (mg) 0.5
Monounsaturated fat (g) 3.4	Potassium (mg) 683	Riboflavin B_2 (mg) 0.5
Fiber (g) 6.2	Flavonoids (mg) 1.7	Niacin B_3 (mg) 8.2
Carbohydrates (g) 71.2	Lycopene (mg) 0	Vitamin B_6 (mg) 0.3
Sugar (g) 5.2	Fish (oz) 0	Folic acid (mcg) 73
Protein (g) 15.7	Nuts (oz) 0	Vitamin B_{12} (mcg) 0.3

Broccoli Toasters

■ ■ ■ ■

Preparation time: 15 minutes	*4 servings*
Cooking time: 10 minutes	*224 calories per serving, 21% from fat*

RealAge effect if eaten 12 times a year:	**RealAge-effect ingredients:**
10.4 days younger	Olive oil, onions, broccoli, whole grains, tofu, parsley, lemon juice (calcium, magnesium, potassium, selenium, vitamin C, folic acid, fiber, flavonoids, healthy fats)

ingredients

¾ cup (6 ounces) extra-firm light silken tofu, such as Mori-Nu brand

2 tablespoons chopped flat-leaf parsley

1½ tablespoons lemon juice

1 tablespoon water

½ teaspoon salt

1 tablespoon olive oil

1 cup thinly sliced red onion

3 cups chopped broccoli florets

¼ teaspoon freshly ground black pepper

¼ cup barbecue sauce

4 whole wheat or whole-grain English muffins, split, toasted

preparation

Combine tofu, parsley, lemon juice, water, and ¼ teaspoon of the salt in a blender container or food processor. Blend until smooth; set aside.

Heat a large nonstick skillet over medium-high heat. Add oil, then onion; cook 4 minutes, stirring occasionally. Add broccoli, remaining ¼ teaspoon salt, and pepper; cook 4 minutes, stirring occasionally. Add barbecue sauce; continue cooking 2 minutes or until thickened. Spoon broccoli mixture evenly over bottom halves of muffins. Top with tofu dressing and muffin tops.

substitutions: Any sweet onion will work. Try Walla Wallas and Vidalias; both are specialty onions, and both are occasionally eaten out of hand! Seasoned rice wine vinegar can substitute for the lemon juice; it's a little milder and smoother than lemon juice, and good by itself as a dressing.

tips: Although this sandwich can be made with a little grated melted cheese on top (try smoked Gouda), it's tangy with lemony smooth tofu and sweet with the barbecue sauce. Double this recipe—everyone will want two of these sandwiches, at least.

nutritional analysis

Total fat (g) 5.6	Sodium (mg) 902	Vitamin A (RE) 126
Fat calories (kc) 51	Calcium (mg) 116	Beta-carotene (RE) 754
Cholesterol (mg) 0	Magnesium (mg) 82	Vitamin C (mg) 70
Saturated fat (g) 0.9	Zinc (mg) 1.5	Vitamin E (mg) 1.1
Polyunsaturated fat (g) 1.4	Selenium (mcg) 24	Thiamin B_1 (mg) 0.3
Monounsaturated fat (g) 3.2	Potassium (mg) 500	Riboflavin B_2 (mg) 0.2
Fiber (g) 10.1	Flavonoids (mg) 4.7	Niacin B_3 (mg) 2.6
Carbohydrates (g) 37	Lycopene (mg) 0	Vitamin B_6 (mg) 0.3
Sugar (g) 6.0	Fish (ounce) 0	Folic acid (mcg) 98
Protein (g) 9.0	Nuts (oz) 0	Vitamin B_{12} (mcg) 0

Two-Bean Chili with Avocado and Salsa

■ ■ ■ ■

Preparation time: 5 minutes
Cooking time: 30 minutes

4 servings (approximately 7 cups total)
332 calories per serving, 31% from fat

RealAge effect if eaten 12 times a year:	RealAge-effect ingredients:
What a difference a bean makes! Full of protein and energy, plus the monounsaturated fat of avocado, this dish makes your RealAge 8.3 days younger.	Onion, canola or olive oil, salsa, beans, tomatoes, avocado (fiber, potassium, magnesium, healthy protein, healthy fat, lycopene, flavonoids, beta-carotene, folic acid)

ingredients

2 teaspoons canola or olive oil

1 large white onion, chopped

2 teaspoons dried oregano leaves, preferably Mexican

½ cup salsa, preferably guajillo chile salsa, such as Frontera Foods brand

1 can (15 to 16 ounces) black or kidney beans, rinsed and drained

1 can (15 to 16 ounces) pinto beans, rinsed and drained

2 cans (14½ ounces each) diced tomatoes or diced tomatoes with green chiles, undrained

1 ripe medium avocado, peeled, seeded, and diced

¼ cup chopped cilantro

preparation

Heat a large saucepan over medium-high heat. Add oil, then onion and oregano. Cook 3 minutes, stirring occasionally. Add salsa, beans, and tomatoes. Cover; bring to a boil over high heat. Reduce heat; simmer 25 minutes. Ladle into bowls; top with avocado and cilantro.

substitutions: Fresh Italian flat-leaf parsley can be used instead of cilantro for those who prefer the bright, clean mineral flavors of parsley to the perfume and pungency of cilantro. This seasonal recipe uses Fuerte avocados, which seem to peak in fall and winter. If you use Haas avocados, the recipe becomes a spring and summer treat, as Haas peak in spring and summer.

tips: Leftover chili may be covered and refrigerated up to 3 days or frozen up to 3 months. The chili may be drained or cooked uncovered to thicken and used as a burrito filling.

nutritional analysis

Total fat (g) 11	Sodium (mg) 757	Vitamin A (RE) 108
Fat calories (kc) 99	Calcium (mg) 61	Beta-carotene (RE) 227
Cholesterol (mg) 0	Magnesium (mg) 92	Vitamin C (mg) 22
Saturated fat (g) 1.6	Zinc (mg) 1.3	Vitamin E (mg) 1.5
Polyunsaturated fat (g) 1.3	Selenium (mcg) 2	Thiamin B_1 (mg) 0.3
Monounsaturated fat (g) 6.6	Potassium (mg) 834	Riboflavin B_2 (mg) 0.1
Fiber (g) 6.0	Flavonoids (mg) 5.8	Niacin B_3 (mg) 2.3
Carbohydrates (g) 32	Lycopene (mg) 15	Vitamin B_6 (mg) 0.3
Sugar (g) 4.1	Fish (oz) 0	Folic acid (mcg) 170
Protein (g) 9.9	Nuts (oz) 0	Vitamin B_{12} (mcg) 0

Cooking the RealAge Way

Veggie-Salsa Soup

Preparation time: 15 minutes	*4 servings*
Cooking time: 20 minutes	*73 calories per serving, 3% from fat*

RealAge effect if eaten 12 times a year:	RealAge-effect ingredients:
7.4 days younger	Onion, carrots, cauliflower, soy milk, salsa, garlic (potassium, flavonoids, lycopene, calcium)

ingredients

Cooking oil spray

1 cup each small cauliflower florets, chopped onion, and chopped carrot

2 garlic cloves, minced

3 cups low-salt vegetable broth

½ teaspoon salt

¼ teaspoon freshly ground black pepper

½ cup canned evaporated skim milk

½ cup chipotle chile salsa

¼ cup chopped cilantro or parsley

preparation

Heat a large saucepan over medium heat. Coat with cooking oil spray. Add cauliflower, onion, carrot, and garlic; cook 5 minutes, stirring occasionally. Add broth, salt and pepper; bring to a boil over high heat. Reduce heat; cover and simmer 15 minutes or until vegetables are very tender. Using a slotted spoon, transfer vegetables to a blender or food processor, leaving sauce in saucepan. Add evaporated skim milk and blend until smooth. Return soup to saucepan; add salsa, stir, and heat through. Stir in cilantro; ladle into shallow bowls.

substitutions: Chicken broth will work just as well as vegetable broth, and will provide a little additional lean protein. Fat-free half-and-half (skim milk with natural thickeners) would work very well in place of evaporated skim milk and would be a little sweeter and creamier.

tips: For a slightly more exotic, brighter flavor, add half a teaspoon of ground cumin to the broth at the beginning of cooking. The slight spiciness of the cumin (especially if the salsa also contains a touch of cumin) will tingle your tongue with every spoonful of soup.

nutritional analysis

Total fat (g) 0.25	Sodium (mg) 554	Vitamin A (RE) 997
Fat calories (kc) 2	Calcium (mg) 135	Beta-carotene (RE) 5520
Cholesterol (mg) 2.0	Magnesium (mg) 25	Vitamin C (mg) 37
Saturated fat (g) 0.1	Zinc (mg) 0.7	Vitamin E (mg) 0.3
Polyunsaturated fat (g) 0.1	Selenium (mcg) 8	Thiamin B_1 (mg) 0.1
Monounsaturated fat (g) 0.1	Potassium (mg) 632	Riboflavin B_2 (mg) 0.2
Fiber (g) 2.5	Flavonoids (mg) 1.9	Niacin B_3 (mg) 3.4
Carbohydrates (g) 15.0	Lycopene (mg) 8.4	Vitamin B_6 (mg) 0.2
Sugar (g) 3.7	Fish (oz) 0	Folic acid (mcg) 42
Protein (g) 8.0	Nuts (oz) 0	Vitamin B_{12} (mcg) 0.3

FOR DINNER

Double Sesame Salmon with Mango-Avocado Salsa

Preparation time: 15 minutes	*4 servings*
Cooking time: 6 minutes	*319 calories per serving, 38% from fat*

RealAge effect if eaten 12 times a year:	RealAge-effect ingredients:
With much more omega-3 fatty acid than omega-6, this is the tastiest way we know to get your essential fatty acids and make your RealAge 4.2 days younger.	Salmon, sesame seeds, mango, avocado (healthy fat, healthy protein, potassium, B_{12}, folate)

ingredients

¼ cup plus 2 tablespoons hot mango chutney, such as Crosse & Blackwell brand,
  large pieces of mango chopped

4 (5- to 6-ounce) salmon fillets with skin

¾ teaspoon salt

1 tablespoon mixed white and black sesame seeds (see Substitutions)

1 tablespoon seasoned rice wine vinegar

1 cup diced ripe fresh mango

½ ripe medium avocado, diced

2 tablespoons chopped cilantro

preparation

Heat broiler. Spread 2 tablespoons chutney over skinless side of fish. Sprinkle
½ teaspoon salt and the sesame seeds over fish, patting to coat. Place salmon on rack
of broiler pan, skin side down. Broil 4 to 5 inches from heat for 5 to 6 minutes, or
until fish is opaque in the center.

Meanwhile, combine remaining ¼ cup chutney with vinegar and remaining
¼ teaspoon salt. Stir in mango, avocado, and cilantro. Serve salsa over fish.

substitutions: Black sesame seeds can be found at Asian grocery stores or the ethnic
section of select supermarkets. If not available, use 1 tablespoon of regular white
sesame seeds. A tablespoon of Eden Shake may also be used. This bottled table
condiment consists of white and black sesame seeds, seaweed flakes, and seasonings,
and can be found at health food stores and some supermarkets. This recipe also works
with striped bass fillets.

tips: Chutney and other thick, sweet toppings are great glazes for fish. The fish doesn't
need to marinate because the flavor is baked right on. Try orange marmalade or
whole raspberry preserves. Experimenting in the kitchen is a very good thing.

nutritional analysis

Total fat (g) 13.6
Fat calories (kc) 123
Cholesterol (mg) 100
Saturated fat (g) 1.1
Polyunsaturated fat (g) 3.7
Monounsaturated fat (g) 5.4
Fiber (g) 4.0
Carbohydrates (g) 44.4
Sugar (g) 6.2
Protein (g) 25.7

Sodium (mg) 580
Calcium (mg) 157
Magnesium (mg) 76
Zinc (mg) 1.6
Selenium (mcg) 0
Potassium (mg) 386
Flavonoids (mg) 0
Lycopene (mg) 0
Fish (oz) 5.5
Nuts (oz) 0

Vitamin A (RE) 209
Beta-carotene (RE) 272
Vitamin C (mg) 22
Vitamin E (mg) 4.4
Thiamin B$_1$ (mg) 0.3
Riboflavin B$_2$ (mg) 0.4
Niacin B$_3$ (mg) 7.2
Vitamin B$_6$ (mg) 0.3
Folic acid (mcg) 49
Vitamin B$_{12}$ (mcg) 5

Pistachio Pilaf with Butternut Squash and Gingered Cranberry Sauce

Preparation time: 8 minutes
Cooking time: 20 minutes

4 servings
363 calories per serving, 22% from fat

RealAge effect if eaten 12 times a year:

High in potassium, flavonoids, and fiber, this beautifully colored fork-tender dish makes your RealAge 8.7 days younger.

RealAge-effect ingredients:

Wheat pilaf, olive oil, squash, cranberry juice, pistachios (healthy protein, calcium, magnesium, zinc, selenium, potassium, vitamin B$_3$, folic acid, fiber, healthy fats, flavonoids, antioxidants)

ingredients

1 box (6 ounces) wheat pilaf mix, such as Near East brand

1 tablespoon olive oil

1 large butternut squash, about 2½ pounds

½ cup plus 3 tablespoons cranberry chutney, such as Crosse & Blackwell brand

¼ cup cranberry juice cocktail

2 tablespoons chopped crystallized ginger

⅓ cup coarsely chopped pistachios, toasted

preparation

Prepare pilaf according to package directions using 1 tablespoon olive oil rather than butter. Meanwhile, cut squash in half lengthwise; discard seeds and membrane. Cut squash halves crosswise into quarters, then cut each quarter lengthwise into four wedges, forming 16 pieces of squash. Place squash skin side down in a microwave-safe dish. Brush 3 tablespoons of the chutney over squash flesh. Cover with waxed paper; microwave at high power until squash is fork-tender, 12 to 16 minutes, rotating dish twice if microwave oven does not have a turntable.

Meanwhile, in a small saucepan, combine remaining ½ cup chutney, cranberry juice, and ginger. Bring to a simmer over medium heat. Simmer 2 to 3 minutes or until slightly thickened.

Transfer pilaf to serving plates; top with squash. Spoon sauce over all; top with pistachios.

substitutions: This is a very flexible recipe. Acorn squash may replace butternut squash (both are "winter" varieties), white grape juice may replace cranberry juice cocktail, mango or peach chutney may replace cranberry chutney, and soy nuts may replace pistachios.

tips: Leave the skin on the squash: it's not as slippery and is easier to cut up when unpeeled. The olive oil in the pilaf adds a little roundness to the grains. Try new varieties, too—wild rice, roasted garlic, and more.

nutritional analysis

Total fat (g) 9.0	Sodium (mg) 520	Vitamin A (RE) 797
Fat calories (kc) 81.3	Calcium (mg) 87	Beta-carotene (RE) 4766
Cholesterol (mg) 0	Magnesium (mg) 123	Vitamin C (mg) 28
Saturated fat (g) 1.2	Zinc (mg) 1.2	Vitamin E (mg) 1.2
Polyunsaturated fat (g) 1.3	Selenium (mcg) 2	Thiamin B_1 (mg) 0.3
Monounsaturated fat (g) 5.9	Potassium (mg) 671	Riboflavin B_2 (mg) 0.1
Fiber (g) 13.4	Flavonoids (mg) 10.5	Niacin B_3 (mg) 3.5
Carbohydrates (g) 67.3	Lycopene (mg) 0	Vitamin B_6 (mg) 0.3
Sugar (g) 7.0	Fish (oz) 0	Folic acid (mcg) 48
Protein (g) 8.4	Nuts (oz) 0.4	Vitamin B_{12} (mcg) 0

Caribbean Chicken with Black Beans, Sweet Potato, and Lime

■ ■ ■ ■

Preparation time: 10 minutes	*4 servings*
Cooking time: 20 minutes	*289 calories per serving, 13% from fat*

RealAge effect if eaten 12 times a year:	**RealAge-effect ingredients:**
Substituting protein for aging fat and cholesterol helps you become 4.2 days younger.	Olive oil, onion, sweet potato, chicken, beans, (healthy fat, protein, carotenoids, fiber, potassium, folate, niacin)

ingredients

2 teaspoons canola or olive oil

1 medium white onion, chopped

1 medium sweet potato (8 ounces), unpeeled, diced (½-inch chunks)

4 teaspoons Caribbean jerk seasonings, such as McCormick brand

1 cup low-salt chicken broth

2 bay leaves (optional)

4 (4-ounce) skinless, boneless chicken breast halves

Cooking oil spray

1 can (15 to 16 ounces) black beans, rinsed and drained

¼ teaspoon salt

1 lime

Optional condiments: Pickapeppa Sauce (see Tips), mango chutney, plain yogurt, chopped cilantro

preparation

Heat a large, deep skillet over medium-high heat. Add oil, then onion. Cook 5 minutes, stirring frequently. Stir in sweet potato. Sprinkle 2 teaspoons of the seasonings over vegetables; cook 1 minute. Add broth and, if desired, bay leaves; simmer uncovered 10 minutes.

Meanwhile, sprinkle remaining 2 teaspoons seasonings over chicken; coat chicken with cooking oil spray. Grill over medium coals, broil 4 to 5 inches from heat, or cook in a ridged grill pan over medium heat until chicken is just cooked through, 4 to 5 minutes per side.

Stir black beans and salt into the sweet potato mixture. Finely shred or zest enough lime peel to measure ½ teaspoon; stir into bean mixture. Cut lime into four quarters; set aside. Continue cooking bean mixture 4 to 5 minutes or until sweet potato is tender. If bay leaves have been used, discard them. Transfer bean mixture to four serving plates; top with chicken and serve with lime wedges. Top chicken with condiments as desired.

substitutions: Blackened seasoning mix may replace the Caribbean jerk seasoning mix; ½ teaspoon Old Bay seasoning may replace bay leaves.

tips: Pickapeppa Sauce, a mild, sweet brown sauce from Jamaica, may be found in the condiment section of your supermarket.

Adding the black beans at the end of cooking keeps the onion from darkening. Also, the beans pick up just enough seasoning from the stock and the lime to become more flavorful.

nutritional analysis

Total fat (g) 4.3	Sodium (mg) 836	Vitamin A (RE) 1269
Fat calories (kc) 39	Calcium (mg) 75	Beta-carotene (RE) 7424
Cholesterol (mg) 96	Magnesium (mg) 124	Vitamin C (mg) 21
Saturated fat (g) 0.4	Zinc (mg) 2.7	Vitamin E (mg) 3.4
Polyunsaturated fat (g) 1.3	Selenium (mcg) 34	Thiamin B_1 (mg) 0.4
Monounsaturated fat (g) 2.6	Potassium (mg) 978	Riboflavin B_2 (mg) 0.3
Fiber (g) 6.8	Flavonoids (mg) 1.0	Niacin B_3 (mg) 16
Carbohydrates (g) 44	Lycopene (mg) 0	Vitamin B_6 (mg) 0.88
Sugar (g) 7.2	Fish (oz) 0	Folic acid (mcg) 188
Protein (g) 46	Nuts (oz) 0	Vitamin B_{12} (mcg) 0.4

Coriander-Crusted Sea Bass and Asparagus over Sweet Potato Purée

■ ■ ■ ■

Preparation time: 12 minutes	*4 servings*
Cooking time: 18 minutes	*540 calories per serving, 20% from fat*

RealAge effect if eaten 12 times a year:	**RealAge-effect ingredients:**
The carotenoids in sweet potatoes and the omega-3s in fish combine to make you 14.2 days younger.	Sea bass, olive oil, asparagus, pistachios, sweet potatoes (carotenoids, healthy protein, healthy fat, potassium, fiber, selenium, folate, vitamin C)

ingredients

2 large sweet potatoes (about 1¼ pounds)

1 bunch (about 14 ounces) asparagus spears

2½ teaspoons olive oil

4 (4-ounce) sea bass fillets, cut 1 to 1¼ inches thick

2 teaspoons ground coriander

1¼ teaspoons salt

¼ teaspoon cayenne pepper

2 teaspoons coriander seeds

¼ cup low-salt chicken broth or reserved sweet potato cooking water

¼ cup chopped toasted pistachios

preparation

Heat oven to 425 degrees. Bring a large saucepan of salted water to a simmer. Cut sweet potatoes into 1-inch chunks. Cook in simmering water, uncovered, about 15 minutes or until tender.

Meanwhile, arrange asparagus in a shallow baking dish. Add ½ teaspoon oil, turning asparagus to coat with oil. Bake 8 to 10 minutes or until crisp-tender, depending on thickness of asparagus.

Rinse and pat fish dry with paper towel. Rub 1 teaspoon of the oil over meaty side of fish; sprinkle ground coriander, ½ teaspoon salt, and cayenne pepper over fish. Press coriander seeds into fish. Heat a large nonstick ovenproof skillet over medium-high heat until hot. Add fish, seasoned side down. Cook 3 minutes or until fish is browned and seared. Turn fish over; transfer skillet to oven. Bake 8 to 10 minutes or until fish is opaque and slightly firm to touch.

Drain sweet potatoes; return to saucepan. Add remaining 1 teaspoon oil, remaining ¾ teaspoon salt, and chicken broth. Mash with a potato masher. Transfer to four serving plates. Top with fish and asparagus. Garnish with nuts.

substitutions: Striped bass may replace the sea bass, and boniato (commonly referred to as "Cuban sweet potato") may replace the sweet potato. The boniato, which has white flesh, should be peeled. It needs a few more minutes of simmering to become tender, and more chicken broth, than the yellow- or orange-fleshed sweet potato does, but is deliciously filling.

tips: Coriander is the seed that gives rise to cilantro, but you might never guess that relationship as their flavors are so different.

nutritional analysis

Total fat (g) 12.0	Sodium (mg) 178	Vitamin A (RE) 6345
Fat calories (kc) 108.1	Calcium (mg) 135	Beta-carotene (RE) 37,203
Cholesterol (mg) 60.1	Magnesium (mg) 156	Vitamin C (mg) 99
Saturated fat (g) 2.7	Zinc (mg) 2.3	Vitamin E (mg) 17
Polyunsaturated fat (g) 3.6	Selenium (mcg) 143	Thiamin B_1 (mg) 0.5
Monounsaturated fat (g) 4.7	Potassium (mg) 1752	Riboflavin B_2 (mg) 0.7
Fiber (g) 10.4	Flavonoids (mg) 0	Niacin B_3 (mg) 5.3
Carbohydrates (g) 75	Lycopene (mg) 0	Vitamin B_6 (mg) 1.4
Sugar (g) 34	Fish (oz) 4	Folic acid (mcg) 176
Protein (g) 36	Nuts (oz) 0.3	Vitamin B_{12} (mcg) 0.4

Grilled Portobello Mushroom Barley Pilaf with Pine Nuts and Arugula

Preparation time: 5 minutes	*4 servings*
Cooking time: 15 minutes	*251 calories per serving, 21.5% from fat*

RealAge effect if eaten 12 times a year:	**RealAge-effect ingredients:**
High in fiber and low in fat, this choice makes a terrific dinner: It makes your RealAge 4.2 days younger.	Mushrooms, barley, arugula, nuts (fiber, healthy fat, potassium, vitamin B_3, folic acid)

ingredients

$\frac{1}{2}$ cup balsamic vinegar

4 large portobello mushrooms (about 1 pound)

Garlic-flavored cooking oil spray

$\frac{1}{2}$ teaspoon freshly ground black pepper

$\frac{3}{4}$ teaspoon salt

1 cup quick-cooking barley, such as Mother's brand

2 cups low-salt chicken or mushroom broth

3 cups packed arugula leaves

$\frac{1}{4}$ cup pine nuts, toasted

preparation

Place vinegar in a small nonreactive saucepan; bring to a boil over high heat. Boil gently uncovered until reduced to ¼ cup, 3 to 4 minutes.

Meanwhile, remove stems from mushrooms; chop stems and set aside. Coat mushroom caps with cooking oil spray; sprinkle with the pepper and ½ teaspoon of the salt. Grill over medium coals or broil 4 to 5 inches from heat source for 4 to 5 minutes per side or until tender.

Heat a medium saucepan over medium-high heat. Coat with cooking oil spray; add chopped mushroom stems and stir-fry 1 minute. Add barley; stir-fry 1 minute. Add broth and remaining ¼ teaspoon salt; bring to a boil. Reduce heat; cover and simmer 10 to 12 minutes or until liquid is absorbed. Stir in 2 cups of the arugula until wilted (about 30 seconds). Transfer mixture to serving plates.

Arrange grilled mushrooms over barley mixture; top with remaining 1 cup arugula and the pine nuts. Drizzle reduced vinegar over all.

substitutions: Toasted chopped Brazil nuts may replace pine nuts, and baby spinach leaves may replace arugula.

tips: Chopping and then cooking the mushroom stems adds flavor to the grain. Make sure you include the stems, except for the very tough end, which you can save for stock or compost.

nutritional analysis

Total fat (g) 6	Sodium (mg) 405	Vitamin A (RE) 80
Fat calories (kc) 54	Calcium (mg) 50	Beta-carotene (RE) 120
Cholesterol (mg) 0.5	Magnesium (mg) 55	Vitamin C (mg) 7
Saturated fat (g) 0.9	Zinc (mg) 2.3	Vitamin E (mg) 0.9
Polyunsaturated fat (g) 1.3	Selenium (mcg) 106	Thiamin B_1 (mg) 0.3
Monounsaturated fat (g) 3.2	Potassium (mg) 833	Riboflavin B_2 (mg) 0.7
Fiber (g) 9.9	Flavonoids (mg) 0.2	Niacin B_3 (mg) 9.0
Carbohydrates (g) 43.9	Lycopene (mg) 0	Vitamin B_6 (mg) 0.3
Sugar (g) 2.7	Fish (oz) 0	Folic acid (mcg) 104
Protein (g) 9.2	Nuts (oz) 0.5	Vitamin B_{12} (mcg) 0.1

Golden Polenta with Exotic Mushroom Ragout

■ ■ ■ ■

Preparation time: 10 minutes	*4 servings*
Cooking time: 20 minutes	*274 calories per serving, 29% from fat*

RealAge effect if eaten 12 times a year:	**RealAge-effect ingredients:**
With its powerhouse of B vitamins, carotenoids from the carrots, and a little healthy fat, this soothing fall dish makes your RealAge 4.6 days younger.	Olive oil, cornmeal, onions, carrots, mushrooms (B vitamins, carotenoids, potassium, healthy fats)

ingredients

3½ cups low-salt chicken or vegetable broth

1 cup (6 ounces) cornmeal, preferably stone-ground

2 teaspoons olive oil

½ cup sliced shallots or chopped yellow onion

1½ cups thickly sliced carrots

2 packages (4 ounces each) mixed sliced exotic mushrooms, such as Pennsylvania Farms
   brand

1½ cups (4 ounces) sliced button or crimini mushrooms

2 tablespoons dry sherry

1 tablespoon chopped fresh thyme or 1 teaspoon dried

¾ teaspoon salt

½ teaspoon freshly ground black pepper

½ cup (2 ounces) crumbled herbed feta or herbed goat cheese

preparation

Combine 3 cups broth and cornmeal in a large saucepan. Mix well with a wire whisk. Bring to a simmer over medium heat, whisking occasionally. Simmer uncovered over low heat 15 to 18 minutes or until very thick, whisking frequently. Remove from heat; cover and keep warm.

Place a large, deep skillet over medium heat until hot. Add oil, then shallots and carrots; sauté 5 minutes. Add mushrooms; sauté 5 minutes. Add remaining ½ cup broth, sherry, thyme, salt, and pepper. Simmer uncovered 5 minutes or until carrots are tender, stirring occasionally.

Spread polenta over four warmed serving plates. Top with mushroom ragout and cheese. Garnish with additional chopped fresh thyme and freshly ground black pepper, if desired.

substitutions: If sliced exotic mushrooms (a combination of crimini, oyster, and shiitake mushrooms) are not available, substitute 8 ounces fresh shiitake mushrooms. Save the tough stems for stock, and slice the caps for the dish. Cubed unpeeled sweet potatoes—Garnets are some of the sweetest—can substitute for carrots.

tips: Look for exotic mushrooms in the produce section of your supermarket. Mushroom stock—homemade or purchased—adds depth of flavor. For even more intensity, find mushroom soy sauce—I love Pearl River brand's deep, dark layers of flavor.

nutritional analysis

Total fat (g) 8.9	Sodium (mg) 782	Vitamin A (RE) 36
Fat calories (kc) 80	Calcium (mg) 89	Beta-carotene (RE) 0.4
Cholesterol (mg) 13.3	Magnesium (mg) 32	Vitamin C (mg) 6
Saturated fat (g) 2.9	Zinc (mg) 1.6	Vitamin E (mg) 0.55
Polyunsaturated fat (g) 1.0	Selenium (mcg) 0	Thiamin B_1 (mg) 0.2
Monounsaturated fat (g) 3.0	Potassium (mg) 611	Riboflavin B_2 (mg) 0.6
Fiber (g) 3.6	Flavonoids (mg) 0.7	Niacin B_3 (mg) 7.0
Carbohydrates (g) 40.6	Lycopene (mg) 0	Vitamin B_6 (mg) 0.3
Sugar (g) 2.2	Fish (oz) 0	Folic acid (mcg) 51
Protein (g) 11.9	Nuts (oz) 0	Vitamin B_{12} (mcg) 0.5

Rainbow Shrimp Moo Shu Roll-Ups

Preparation time: 20 minutes	*4 servings (2 roll-ups per serving)*
Cooking time: 5 minutes	*270 calories per serving, 6% from fat*

RealAge effect if eaten 12 times a year:	**RealAge-effect ingredients:**
Full of complex carbohydrates, but virtually no sugar, eating this makes your RealAge 11.8 days younger.	Chile purée, bell peppers, coleslaw, onions, whole wheat (fiber, antioxidants, potassium)

ingredients

12 ounces uncooked peeled and deveined small, medium, or halved large shrimp, thawed if frozen

2 tablespoons chile purée, such as Lee Kum Kee or China Bowl brands

Garlic-flavored cooking oil spray

1 each red and yellow bell pepper, cut into short, thin strips

4 cups coleslaw mix (shredded cabbage and carrots)

8 green onions, cut into 1/2-inch slices

1/4 cup oyster sauce, such as Dynasty or Kame brands

1 tablespoon cornstarch

8 (10-inch) whole wheat or honey whole wheat flour tortillas, such as Tumaro's brand, warmed

2 teaspoons coriander seeds, coarsely crushed (optional)

preparation

In a medium bowl, combine shrimp and chile purée, tossing to coat. Heat a Dutch oven or large saucepan over medium heat; coat with cooking oil spray. Add shrimp; stir-fry 1 minute. Add bell peppers, coleslaw mix, and green onions; stir-fry 1 minute. Add oyster sauce; stir-fry 2 minutes or until shrimp are opaque and vegetables are crisp-tender.

Combine cornstarch with 1 tablespoon cold water; mix well. Stir into shrimp mixture; cook 1 minute or until thickened, stirring constantly. Spoon mixture down center of tortillas; sprinkle coriander seeds over mixture, if desired. Fold one end of tortilla over filling; roll up burrito fashion.

substitutions: Shredded napa cabbage may replace the coleslaw mix, and hoisin sauce may replace the oyster sauce.

tips: Adding the cornstarch slurry at the end of cooking helps to keep the juices inside the vegetables. The touch of crushed coriander seed is worth the extra effort. Just a little gives a bit of spiciness to the dish.

nutritional analysis

Total fat (g) 1.9
Fat calories (kc) 17
Cholesterol (mg) 183.0
Saturated fat (g) 0.1
Polyunsaturated fat (g) 0.8
Monounsaturated fat (g) 0.8
Fiber (g) 7.2
Carbohydrates (g) 57.4
Sugar (g) 2.1
Protein (g) 25.3

Sodium (mg) 968
Calcium (mg) 195
Magnesium (mg) 62
Zinc (mg) 2.8
Selenium (mcg) 65
Potassium (mg) 569
Flavonoids (mg) 1.6
Lycopene (mg) 0.7
Fish (oz) 0
Nuts (oz) 0

Vitamin A (RE) 246
Beta-carotene (RE) 601
Vitamin C (mg) 83
Vitamin E (mg) 10.1
Thiamin B_1 (mg) 0.17
Riboflavin B_2 (mg) 0.30
Niacin B_3 (mg) 4.9
Vitamin B_6 (mg) 0.4
Folic acid (mcg) 55
Vitamin B_{12} (mcg) 1.4

Warm Chinese Greens with Shiitake Mushrooms and Five-Spice Pancakes

Preparation time: 10 minutes
Cooking time: 15 minutes

4 servings
201 calories per serving, 30% from fat

RealAge effect if eaten 12 times a year:	RealAge-effect ingredients:
Rich with potassium, high in fiber, and filled with phytonutrients, these greens make your RealAge 12.0 days younger.	Egg whites, kale, onions, mushrooms, sesame oil (fiber, phytonutrients, flavonoids, healthy protein, calcium, magnesium, potassium, selenium, beta-carotene, folic acid, and vitamins E and B_6)

ingredients

2 large eggs plus 2 large egg whites

1/2 teaspoon Chinese five-spice powder

1 teaspoon salt

2 teaspoons dark sesame oil

1 pound kale

1 1/2 cups chopped white onion

8 ounces shiitake mushrooms, stems discarded and caps halved or quartered, if large

2 tablespoons hoisin sauce, such as Kame brand

preparation

Beat together eggs, egg whites, five-spice powder, and ¼ teaspoon of the salt. Heat a 9- or 10-inch nonstick skillet over medium-high heat. Add 1 teaspoon of the oil, swirling to coat pan. Add egg mixture; spread into a thin layer and cook 2 minutes or until bottom of pancake is set. With a large spatula, carefully turn pancake; continue to cook 1 minute or until eggs are set. Set aside to cool.

Rinse kale but do not dry. Cut crosswise into ½-inch slices, discarding tough stems; set aside. Heat a Dutch oven over medium-high heat. Add remaining 1 teaspoon oil and onion; cook 3 minutes, stirring occasionally. Add mushrooms; cook 2 minutes, stirring occasionally. Add kale and hoisin sauce. Toss well, then cover and let steam for 1½ minutes. Meanwhile, cut the egg pancake into ½-inch strips; cut strips into 2-inch pieces.

Uncover and shake the wilted greens mixture. Add pancake strips and remaining ¾ teaspoon salt; toss well. Transfer to serving plates.

substitutions: Small, fresh mustard greens may replace kale; the dish will be a little more zingy and slightly hot. Be sure to cut away the large stems. Look for kale with firm green leaves that stay upright and bounce back when bent. Specialty markets may carry Lacinato or "dinosaur" kale, which is forest green, has thinner stems, cooks more quickly, and is lance-straight instead of quilted. If you find it, buy it: it will give you a completely new flavor and texture for kale—softer, sweeter.

tips: Steaming cooking greens enables thorough cooking—their water comes out as they steam and coats the mushrooms and onions. You'll end up with just one-fourth of what you started with. Greens can reduce by three-fourths after just 90 seconds in the pot.

nutritional analysis

Total fat (g) 6.6	Sodium (mg) 832	Vitamin A (RE) 887
Fat calories (kc) 59.8	Calcium (mg) 128	Beta-carotene (RE) 834
Cholesterol (mg) 106	Magnesium (mg) 60	Vitamin C (mg) 52
Saturated fat (g) 1.3	Zinc (mg) 1.5	Vitamin E (mg) 9.5
Polyunsaturated fat (g) 1.9	Selenium (mcg) 34	Thiamin B_1 (mg) 0.3
Monounsaturated fat (g) 2.1	Potassium (mg) 660	Riboflavin B_2 (mg) 0.6
Fiber (g) 8.3	Flavonoids (mg) 3.3	Niacin B_3 (mg) 4
Carbohydrates (g) 26.0	Lycopene (mg) 0	Vitamin B_6 (mg) 0.4
Sugar (g) 5.9	Fish (oz) 0	Folic acid (mcg) 64
Protein (g) 11.3	Nuts (oz) 0	Vitamin B_{12} (mcg) 0.3

FOR DESSERT

Sweet Baked Apples with Cherries and Citrus

■ ■ ■ ■

Preparation time: 2 minutes	*4 servings*
Cooking time: 18 minutes	*105 calories per serving, 5% from fat*

RealAge effect if eaten 12 times a year:	**RealAge-effect ingredients:**
A great natural source of vitamin A, citrus fruits add freshness, sprightliness, and extra minerals, too, making your RealAge 1.1 days younger.	Apples, cherries, tangerines, apple juice (fiber, antioxidants, flavonoids, potassium)

ingredients

2 large baking apples, such as Rome Beauty

1¼ cups apple juice, preferably unfiltered organic juice

½ cup (2 ounces) dried pitted cherries

¼ teaspoon ground cloves

2 seedless clementines or tangerines, peeled, separated into segments

Mint sprigs (optional)

preparation

Heat oven to 400 degrees. Cut apples in half; cut out and discard core, seeds, and stems. Place ¼ cup of the apple juice in an 8-inch baking dish or casserole. Place apples cut sides down over juice. Bake 15 to 18 minutes or until apples are tender.

Meanwhile, simmer remaining 1 cup apple juice in a small saucepan over medium-high heat 5 minutes. Add cherries and cloves; reduce heat and simmer uncovered 10 minutes, or until cherries are plumped, stirring occasionally. Remove from heat; stir in citrus sections.

Arrange apple halves cut sides up on serving dishes. Pour any remaining liquid from dish into cherry mixture and spoon the mixture over apples. Garnish with mint sprigs, if desired.

substitutions: Dried cranberries may replace cherries. Baking apples cook more quickly and develop a softer texture when baked than eating apples. McIntosh apples are another good choice for this recipe.

tips: A little ground clove goes a long way; its zippiness is a perfect complement to this fall/winter dessert. Try studding each apple with two whole cloves, so that they are submerged in the apple juice as the apples bake. Remove the cloves before eating the apple, which will now be scented with zingy spice.

nutritional analysis

Total fat (g) 0.5	Sodium (mg) 6	Vitamin A (RE) 45
Fat calories (kc) 4.8	Calcium (mg) 18	Beta-carotene (RE) 273
Cholesterol (mg) 0	Magnesium (mg) 13	Vitamin C (mg) 18
Saturated fat (g) 0.1	Zinc (mg) 0.2	Vitamin E (mg) 0.4
Polyunsaturated fat (g) 0.2	Selenium (mcg) 2	Thiamin B_1 (mg) 0.1
Monounsaturated fat (g) 0.1	Potassium (mg) 272	Riboflavin B_2 (mg) 0.04
Fiber (g) 2.8	Flavonoids (mg) 3.9	Niacin B_3 (mg) 0.2
Carbohydrates (g) 26.4	Lycopene (mg) 0	Vitamin B_6 (mg) 0.1
Sugar (g) 22.8	Fish (oz) 0	Folic acid (mcg) 11
Protein (g) 0.7	Nuts (oz) 0	Vitamin B_{12} (mcg) 0

Triple Apple Sauté

■ ■ ■ ■

Preparation time: 12 minutes	4 servings
Cooking time: 12 minutes	199 calories per serving, 10% from fat

RealAge effect if eaten 12 times a year:	**RealAge-effect ingredients:**
With blood pressure–reducing potassium and hefty amounts of fiber and isoflavones, all underlined by monounsaturated oil, this RealAge-reducer weighs in at 2.9 days younger.	Apples, nuts, apple juice (potassium, fiber, isoflavones, flavonoids, healthy fat)

ingredients

3 large or 4 small cooking apples, such as Ambrosia or Jonagold (1½ pounds)

¼ cup apple butter

¼ cup unsweetened apple juice or cider

½ teaspoon five-spice powder (see Tips)

¼ cup chopped Brazil nuts or walnuts, toasted

½ cup nonfat or low-fat vanilla frozen yogurt, such as Häagen Dazs

preparation

Cut apples into quarters; discard stems, core, and seeds. Cut apple quarters into thin slices. Heat a large nonstick skillet over medium-high heat until hot. Add apples; cook until apples begin to brown, about 4 minutes, tossing occasionally. Stir in apple butter, apple juice, and five-spice powder; continue to cook 5 to 8 minutes or until apples are tender and sauce thickens, tossing frequently. Transfer to serving plates; top with nuts. Serve with frozen yogurt.

substitutions: One-half teaspoon cinnamon may be substituted for the five-spice powder; the flavor will be softer and sweeter.

tips: Five-spice powder is a combination of Chinese spices that usually includes cinnamon, cloves, fennel seed, star anise, and Szechwan peppercorns. Look for the spice mix in the Asian section of your supermarket or by the other spices.

As the apples brown and caramelize in the pan, their own natural sugars add to the rich sauce.

nutritional analysis

Total fat (g) 2.3
Fat calories (kc) 20
Cholesterol (mg) 1.1
Saturated fat (g) 0.3
Polyunsaturated fat (g) 0.9
Monounsaturated fat (g) 0.4
Fiber (g) 7.3
Carbohydrates (g) 62
Sugar (g) 34.8
Protein (g) 4.1

Sodium (mg) 21
Calcium (mg) 62
Magnesium (mg) 27
Zinc (mg) 0.4
Selenium (mcg) 4
Potassium (mg) 403
Flavonoids (mg) 5.1
Lycopene (mg) 0
Fish (oz) 0
Nuts (oz) 0.3

Vitamin A (RE) 29
Beta-carotene (RE) 16
Vitamin C (mg) 6
Vitamin E (mg) 0.51
Thiamin B_1 (mg) 0.1
Riboflavin B_2 (mg) 0.1
Niacin B_3 (mg) 0.5
Vitamin B_6 (mg) 0.2
Folic acid (mcg) 7
Vitamin B_{12} (mcg) 0

Roasted Pears with Raspberry Coulis, Chocolate, and Pistachios

■ ■ ■ ■

Preparation time: 3 minutes	*4 servings*
Cooking time: 27 minutes	*172 calories per serving, 27.3% from fat*

RealAge effect if eaten 12 times a year:	RealAge-effect ingredients:
Can chocolate make you younger? You bet— as long as it is real (cocoa-based) chocolate and you eat it first! The RA factor for this delicious bit of paradise: at least 2.6 days younger.	Pears, grape juice, berries, pistachios, chocolate (antioxidants, healthy fats, potassium, fiber)

ingredients

2 large Bartlett, Comice, or Anjou pears, preferably red

1 cup white grape juice, such as Welch's brand

1 package (12 ounces) frozen unsweetened raspberries, thawed, or 2 cups fresh raspberries

2 tablespoons mini-chocolate chips (from cocoa—real chocolate, not milk chocolate)

3 tablespoons coarsely chopped pistachios, toasted

Mint sprigs (optional)

preparation

Heat oven to 400 degrees. Cut each pear in half; remove core with a melon baller or metal measuring teaspoon. Arrange pears, cut sides down, in a shallow baking dish. Pour grape juice over pears. Bake 18 to 20 minutes or until pears are tender when pierced with the tip of a paring knife.

Meanwhile, purée raspberries in food processor; strain and discard seeds. Transfer roasted pears to serving plates, cut sides up; sprinkle chocolate chips over the pears (the heat of the pears will melt the chips). Combine puréed raspberries and liquid remaining in baking dish in a small saucepan. Cook over high heat until sauce has reduced to ¾ cup, 6 to 8 minutes. Spoon sauce over and around pears; sprinkle with pistachios and garnish with mint sprigs, if desired.

substitutions: If you have champagne or white wine and not white grape juice, then use it without fear, and with a teaspoon of sugar. Sliced toasted almonds or chopped hazelnuts may replace pistachios, and blackberries or strawberries may replace raspberries.

tips: Toast the pistachios by baking them at 350 degrees for approximately 6 minutes. Using mini-chocolate chips makes the chocolate flavor go further by packing in the most chips per tablespoon.

nutritional analysis

Total fat (g) 5.2	Sodium (mg) 7	Vitamin A (RE) 14
Fat calories (kc) 47	Calcium (mg) 45	Beta-carotene (RE) 50
Cholesterol (mg) 0	Magnesium (mg) 32	Vitamin C (mg) 15
Saturated fat (g) 1.4	Zinc (mg) 0.4	Vitamin E (mg) 0.9
Polyunsaturated fat (g) 0.7	Selenium (mcg) 2	Thiamin B_1 (mg) 0.1
Monounsaturated fat (g) 2.6	Potassium (mg) 344	Riboflavin B_2 (mg) 0.1
Fiber (g) 4.9	Flavonoids (mg) 0	Niacin B_3 (mg) 0.7
Carbohydrates (g) 31.8	Lycopene (mg) 0	Vitamin B_6 (mg) 0.15
Sugar (g) 24.0	Fish (oz) 0	Folic acid (mcg) 24
Protein (g) 2.7	Nuts (oz) 0.2	Vitamin B_{12} (mcg) 0

Maple Cranberry-Topped Frozen Yogurt

Preparation time: 5 minutes	*4 servings*
Cooking time: 8 minutes	*193 calories per serving, 5% from fat*

RealAge effect if eaten 12 times a year:	**RealAge-effect ingredients:**
Low in saturated fat, this dish still tastes like a million bucks *and* takes 2.6 days off your RealAge.	Cranberries, orange juice, orange peel (flavonoids, antioxidants, folic acid, calcium, potassium)

ingredients

1 cup fresh or frozen cranberries

1 cup orange juice

½ cup dried cranberries

3 tablespoons pure maple syrup

1⅓ cups low-fat vanilla frozen yogurt

1 teaspoon finely shredded orange peel

preparation

Combine fresh or frozen cranberries, orange juice, and dried cranberries in a medium saucepan. Bring to a boil over high heat. Reduce heat; simmer uncovered 7 to 8 minutes or until cranberries are popped and sauce thickens slightly. Remove from heat; stir in syrup. Serve warm, at room temperature, or chilled over frozen yogurt. Garnish with orange peel.

substitutions: Coffee frozen yogurt may replace the vanilla, and dried cherries may replace the cranberries. If you use coffee frozen yogurt and can find a great-tasting brand, you can use its fat-free version; if you use vanilla, however, choose the 1%-fat variety instead of the fat-free version.

tips: Splashing 2 teaspoons of Cointreau, Grand Marnier, or Triple Sec over the top adds an elegant touch of orange-flavored liqueur. Try any or all. Combining fresh and dried fruit is an easy way to double flavor: Fresh fruit always has more juiciness, and dried fruit always has more sweetness. Together, they pack a flavor wallop.

nutritional analysis

Total fat (g) 1.1	Sodium (mg) 77	Vitamin A (RE) 31
Fat calories (kc) 10	Calcium (mg) 141	Beta-carotene (RE) 107
Cholesterol (mg) 4.2	Magnesium (mg) 22	Vitamin C (mg) 39
Saturated fat (g) 0.7	Zinc (mg) 0.7	Vitamin E (mg) 0.03
Polyunsaturated fat (g) 0.2	Selenium (mcg) 3	Thiamin B_1 (mg) 0.1
Monounsaturated fat (g) 0.4	Potassium (mg) 332	Riboflavin B_2 (mg) 0.2
Fiber (g) 1.7	Flavonoids (mg) 10.7	Niacin B_3 (mg) 0.5
Carbohydrates (g) 30.1	Lycopene (mg) 0	Vitamin B_6 (mg) 0.1
Sugar (g) 22.2	Fish (oz) 0	Folic acid (mcg) 45
Protein (g) 4.4	Nuts (oz) 0	Vitamin B_{12} (mcg) 0.4

⁂ Winter Produce ⁂

You might think that nothing can grow in the winter, but some fruits and vegetables reach maturity and their peak of flavor at this time. In fact, some that stay in the ground develop extra sweetness during colder months. Winter's vegetables are appropriate for heartier dishes such as soups, stews, casseroles, and "skillets" (one-dish meals cooked in a skillet).

Winter Produce Chart

Vegetable/Fruit	Buying and Using
Broccoli rabe (rapini)	➤ **When:** Broccoli rabe is a leafy green vegetable related to both the cabbage and turnip. It's at its peak in the winter. This vegetable is another made popular by Italian cuisine. Unlike broccoli, it's the leaves that people want from broccoli rabe, not just the florets. ➤ **What to Look For:** Look for a deep green color, tender stems, and few (if any) yellow flowers. Choose smaller bunches without thick stems; they will be tender, a little spicy, and delicious. ➤ **Why:** The great amount of flavonoids and the potassium in broccoli rabe make your RealAge younger. ➤ **How to Use:** Try broccoli rabe sautéed, cut up in soups and salads, or served with pasta. If briefly cooked, it has a nutty, slightly bitter taste and crunchy texture that are well complemented by garlic and oil. Try broccoli rabe served with a mild grain, such as couscous or bulgur.
Cabbage	➤ **When:** Cabbage is related to many other brassicas (members of the mustard family)—broccoli, kale, Brussels sprouts, and cauliflower. Cabbage is often used in late fall and winter (January through May for the South and West). Cabbage keeps for months, is inexpensive, and is a wonderful staple. It comes in red (purple) and green. ➤ **What to Look For:** Cabbage should be firm, have a bright color, and feel heavy for its size. Avoid wilted leaves. Beware of (and avoid)

Cooking the RealAge Way

worm holes and dry, cracked leaves—an indication the cabbage was harvested some time ago. In general, the darker the color, the more intense the flavor.

➤ **Why:** A flavonoid-rich vegetable, cabbage makes your immune system younger. Its consumption has a documented association with a decreased risk of breast, prostate, and colon cancers.

➤ **How to Use:** Shred cabbage for salads or spicy coleslaw—perhaps with chiles and cumin seeds. Sauté cabbage with a little of your favorite flavored olive oil and onions. Use cabbage as a topping for hearty stews, such as posole (a Latin American chili-hominy stew) and crockpot chili. Steam whole quarters and serve with a tangy whole-grain mustard or horseradish cream. Grate with apples and beets for a crunchy winter salad.

Celery

➤ **When:** Celery is available year-round. Summer through late fall are peak seasons for the Midwest, East, and Northwest. Winter is peak season in the West and South, although celery pops up in the spring in the Midwest. Celery is available in the colder months because it can withstand freezing weather.

➤ **What to Look For:** Celery stalks should be bunched together closely. The stalks and the leaves should be green and crisp, not yellow or soft. Reject celery that bends at all when you pick it up.

➤ **Why:** Just crunching celery decreases my stress and makes me younger (hope it does that for you, too).

➤ **How to Use:** Celery can be eaten raw or cut up and added to soups, stews, and stir-fries. Some cooks use celery to reduce the amount of salt that needs to be added to their dishes, as the sodium content of celery is higher (but not high overall) than that of most vegetables. Use finely minced celery leaves as a garnish, as a substitute for an herb in a salad, or over the top of a stew or casserole. Also see CELERY ROOT.

Celery root (celeriac)

➤ **When:** Celery root is also available year-round but is usually best harvested in late fall and winter. Its slightly sweet, meaty flavor—like a potato with a touch of celery—actually improves with the cold. Sometimes celery roots stay in the ground until the following spring.

➤ **What to Look For:** Celery root is a storage root crop, so shelf life is more important than freshness. However, when pulled out of the ground, the celery leaves and stalks should be upright, firm, tall, and deep green. The root itself is huge and hairy; it can weigh 2 pounds or more, and lots of small roots spring off the main root.

➤ **How to Use:** Don't eat the leaves and stalks of celery root; they're much tougher and stringier than ordinary celery. Peel the root with a sharp knife, cutting off the outer skin. Then cut the pure white flesh into cubes or batons (pieces the shape of french fries) and steam, roast, boil, mash, or purée. You can combine these with large cubes of sweet potato, rutabaga, and potato, plus olive oil, garlic, and rosemary. Then roast this mixture at 450 degrees until slightly crispy and darkened, about 20 minutes.

Citrus fruits

➤ **When:** Citrus fruits are grown in warmer climates and are available all year. The freshest fruit is available in the winter. Look for firm, fragrant, in-season citrus at the farmers' market.

➤ **What to Look For:** Citrus fruits should feel heavy for their size. This heavy feeling indicates a juicy fruit. Avoid shriveled fruits, which have lost moisture, and blotchy fruits, which have been damaged. To determine sweetness, ask for a sample.

➤ **Why:** Most citrus fruits have a great deal of age-reducing potassium and vitamin C.

➤ **How to Use:** Citrus fruits should be peeled and eaten whole, although they can be juiced. They can be added to fruit and grain salads, used to brighten the flavor of almost any main dish (especially fish), or just eaten plain.

Cooking by the Seasons

Vegetable/Fruit	Buying and Using
Greens (beet greens, Swiss chard, collards, dandelion greens, kale, mustard greens, purslane, turnip greens)	➤ **When:** These greens can withstand a chill, which accounts for their peak in the winter season. Look for specialty cooking greens, too: Lacinato kale is buttery and cooks quickly; and rainbow chard is streaked gorgeously with red, orange, and yellow. ➤ **What to Look For:** In general, greens should look fresh and have no yellowing. Smaller leaves usually have a milder flavor. ➤ **Why:** Loaded with lutein, these greens keep your eyes young. ➤ **How to Use:** Baby turnips and baby beets sometimes have greens that are delicate enough to be used in a mesclun (an assortment of edible raw baby greens). Young chard, kale, and dandelion greens can be used raw in salads, but the other greens should be cooked. Braise, sauté, or steam them with seasonings or use them in soups.
Parsnips	➤ **When:** Fresh parsnips peak during fall and winter. Parsnips are planted in the spring but take up to 6 months to mature, making them a winter vegetable. They are very, very sweet when cooked. Like celery root, parsnips develop some of their sweetness as they stay in the ground. ➤ **What to Look For:** Parsnips should feel rigid; those that are soft are older and less sweet. Although larger parsnips tend to have a sweeter flavor and more color, huge parsnips—10 inches long or more—tend to be fibrous and woody; avoid them. Parsnips should have smooth skin, with no dents or other injuries. ➤ **Why:** Parsnips are a good source of fiber and are high in potassium, magnesium, and vitamins B_1, B_2 and C. ➤ **How to Use:** Parsnip greens should be discarded, and parsnips should not be eaten raw. They can be whipped, glazed, roasted, or cut into cubes for soups and stews.
Rutabagas	➤ **When:** This root vegetable is available year-round, with a peak season of July through April. However, because they store so well, rutabagas are considered a winter vegetable.

➤ **What to Look For:** Rutabagas should have a smooth skin. Larger ones tend to have stronger flavor. Do not buy rutabagas if they've been waxed, or if their greens are reappearing after their tops have been cut off.

➤ **Why:** Rutabagas are high in vitamin C, and are a good source of calcium, potassium, and magnesium.

➤ **How to Use:** Use a paring knife or a chef's knife to cut off the peel and the tough outer layer of flesh. Simmer rutabagas and mash and purée them with potatoes and sweet potatoes. Simmer them in soups and stews. Roast cubes of rutabaga with cubes of other root vegetables at a high temperature, after a quick toss with olive oil, salt, and pepper.

Turnips

➤ **When:** Although fresh turnips are available year-round, their peak season is late fall to early spring. Turnips are good to have on hand, as they don't deteriorate rapidly and can make a tasty treat.

➤ **What to Look For:** The greens should look fresh and the skin smooth. Don't buy turnips if their tops have been removed (the turnips may have been stored) or if their greens are trying to reappear after the top has been removed (the turnips will be starchy and not a bit juicy). In general, the smaller the turnip, the milder the flavor.

➤ **Why:** Turnips have large amounts of vitamin C, folate, and potassium that make you younger.

➤ **How to Use:** Turnips are actually sweet if you know how to find them and cook them. For tennis ball-size turnips, cut off the top and peel the turnip; use baby turnips whole. Roast turnips and beets together to bring out their sweetness, and to create an attractive pairing. Simmer turnips in soups and stews, and with other vegetables that are naturally sweet, such as carrots and sweet potatoes.

Cooking by the Seasons

Cooking the RealAge Way

Recipes Using Winter Produce

FOR BREAKFAST

Toasted Oatmeal with Double Mango and Toasted Walnuts

Preparation time: 5 minutes	*4 servings*
Cooking time: 15 minutes	*475 calories per serving, 33% from fat*

RealAge effect if eaten 12 times a year:	**RealAge-effect ingredients:**
Potassium and fiber, plus the linolenic acid in walnuts (an omega-3 fatty acid), make your RealAge 11.8 days younger.	Oats, walnuts, soy milk, mango, nuts (fiber, healthy fats, potassium, calcium, magnesium, folic acid)

ingredients

3 cups old-fashioned oats, uncooked

½ cup coarsely chopped walnuts

4 cups skim milk or fat-free soy milk

½ cup diced dried mango

¼ teaspoon salt

⅛ teaspoon ground nutmeg

1 large ripe fresh mango, diced (2 cups)

preparation

Heat oven to 400 degrees. Spread oats in a single layer on a jelly-roll pan. Place nuts on a small baking sheet. Bake oats and nuts 6 to 7 minutes or until lightly toasted. Set nuts and oats aside separately.

Combine milk, dried mango, salt, and nutmeg in a medium saucepan; bring just to a simmer over high heat. Reduce heat to low; add toasted oats. Simmer 5 to 8 minutes or until thickened, stirring only once or twice. Transfer to four serving bowls; top with fresh mango and toasted nuts. Serve with additional milk, if desired.

substitutions: Dried strawberries or golden raisins may replace dried mango; 2 cups sliced strawberries may replace fresh mango. Brazil nuts may replace walnuts. One-half teaspoon cinnamon may replace nutmeg. For a lighter, less aggressive flavor, use true cinnamon, sometimes called Ceylonese cinnamon, if you can find it.

tips: Toasting rolled oats is one way to boost flavor without adding calories or unhealthy fats. Over-stirring the oatmeal changes the texture from smooth to too smooth and a little pasty. Just let the simmering milk do its job.

nutritional analysis

Total fat (g) 17.5
Fat calories (kc) 158
Cholesterol (mg) 0
Saturated fat (g) 1.8
Polyunsaturated fat (g) 9.3
Monounsaturated fat (g) 4.1
Fiber (g) 9.3
Carbohydrates (g) 64.6
Sugar (g) 16.2
Protein (g) 20.7

Sodium (mg) 33
Calcium (mg) 61
Magnesium (mg) 176
Zinc (mg) 3.0
Selenium (mcg) 36
Potassium (mg) 793
Flavonoids (mg) 0
Lycopene (mg) 0
Fish (oz) 0
Nuts (oz) 0.6

Vitamin A (RE) 428
Beta-carotene (RE) 447
Vitamin C (mg) 29
Vitamin E (mg) 2.2
Thiamin B_1 (mg) 0.9
Riboflavin B_2 (mg) 0.3
Niacin B_3 (mg) 1.5
Vitamin B_6 (mg) 0.40
Folic acid (mcg) 48
Vitamin B_{12} (mcg) 0

Toasted Quinoa with Prunes and Lemon

Preparation time: 5 minutes
Cooking time: 15 minutes

4 servings
479 calories per serving, 8% from fat

RealAge effect if eaten 12 times a year:

Brimming with protein, potassium, and fiber, and each bowlful makes your RealAge 11.4 days younger.

RealAge-effect ingredients:

Quinoa, prunes, grape juice (fiber, potassium, magnesium, calcium, vitamin C, niacin, folic acid, healthy protein)

ingredients

1½ cups quinoa, uncooked (see Tips)

3 cups water

¼ teaspoon salt

1 package (12 ounces) lemon-essence prunes, such as Sunsweet brand

¾ cup white grape juice

1 (3-inch) cinnamon stick, canela or Mexican preferred (optional)

½ cup plain low-fat yogurt

preparation

Heat a medium saucepan over medium heat. Add quinoa; cook 4 minutes or until fragrant and lightly toasted, stirring frequently. Add water and salt; bring to a simmer. Simmer uncovered 15 minutes or until thickened, stirring occasionally.

Meanwhile, cut prunes into bite-sized pieces. In a small saucepan, combine prunes, grape juice, and, if desired, cinnamon stick. Bring to a simmer over high heat. Reduce heat; simmer uncovered 4 to 5 minutes or until prunes are soft and sauce has thickened, stirring occasionally. Remove cinnamon stick if using. Transfer quinoa to shallow serving bowls; top with warm prune mixture and yogurt.

substitutions: Wheatena cereal may replace quinoa. Prepare the cereal according to package directions. Try to get the quinoa, just once—it makes a big difference.

tips: Quinoa (pronounced KEEN-*wa*) is a weed of the high Andes that is high in protein and minerals. For all practical purposes, it is treated as a grain. Toasting quinoa adds nuttiness and crunch. Expect the husks to pop up like a dust storm when you pour the grain in the pan—they'll just float away.

Mexican cinnamon also makes a difference here. Canela cinnamon is softer, richer, rounder, and fruitier in flavor than the cinnamon sticks you find in spice bottles. To grind your own, save the stick from this recipe, dry it out, and add it to a coffee grinder with three or four others—you'll never go back to store-bought cinnamon powder again.

nutritional analysis

Total fat (g) 5.3	Sodium (mg) 186	Vitamin A (RE) 212
Fat calories (kc) 47.5	Calcium (mg) 164	Beta-carotene (RE) 1240
Cholesterol (mg) 1.8	Magnesium (mg) 212	Vitamin C (mg) 135
Saturated fat (g) 0.8	Zinc (mg) 3.1	Vitamin E (mg) 0.1
Polyunsaturated fat (g) 1.8	Selenium (mcg) 3	Thiamin B_1 (mg) 0.4
Monounsaturated fat (g) 1.5	Potassium (mg) 1602	Riboflavin B_2 (mg) 0.6
Fiber (g) 10.8	Flavonoids (mg) 0	Niacin B_3 (mg) 4.5
Carbohydrates (g) 137.3	Lycopene (mg) 0	Vitamin B_6 (mg) 0.5
Sugar (g) 73.5	Fish (oz) 0	Folic acid (mcg) 142
Protein (g) 14.1	Nuts (oz) 0	Vitamin B_{12} (mcg) 0.1

FOR LUNCH/STARTERS

Rich and Spicy Black Bean Soup

■ ■ ■ ■

Preparation time: 10 minutes
Cooking time: 21 minutes

4 servings
186 calories per serving, 9% from fat

RealAge effect if eaten 12 times a year:	**RealAge-effect ingredients:**
Loaded with the antioxidant lycopene, and not weighed down at all with fat, this deep, dark bowl of rustic goodness makes you 8.1 days younger.	Onion, garlic, tomatoes, salsa, beans, cilantro (fiber, healthy protein, calcium, magnesium, zinc, selenium, potassium, vitamin B_3, folic acid, lycopene, antioxidants, healthy fats, flavonoids)

ingredients

1 teaspoon canola oil

1 small red or yellow onion, chopped

3 garlic cloves, minced

1 teaspoon each ground coriander and ground cumin

1¾ cups low-salt chicken broth

1 can (14½ ounces) diced tomatoes, undrained

2 cans (15 or 16 ounces each) black beans, rinsed and drained

⅓ cup chipotle chile salsa or cooking sauce, preferably Frontera Foods brand

¼ cup chopped cilantro

Optional garnishes: low-fat sour cream, crushed baked tortilla chips

preparation

Heat a large saucepan over medium heat. Add oil, then onion. Cook 5 minutes, stirring occasionally. Add garlic, coriander, and cumin; cook 1 minute.

Add broth and tomatoes; bring to a boil over high heat. Stir in beans and salsa. Reduce heat; simmer uncovered 15 minutes, stirring occasionally. Remove from heat; stir in cilantro. Ladle into bowls; garnish as desired.

substitutions: Canned diced tomatoes with green chiles such as Muir Glen brand may be substituted for diced tomatoes, and vegetable broth may replace chicken broth. Crunchy banana chips, if they're dried and not deep-fried, can easily replace tortilla chips.

tips: This treat can be enjoyed year-round. To quickly separate a head of garlic into cloves, press it firmly with the heel of your hand or smash it with the bottom of a heavy pot. Each head contains approximately 12 cloves of garlic. To loosen the papery skin and quickly peel the garlic, smash the clove with the side of a chef's knife.

nutritional analysis

Total fat (g) 3.0	Sodium (mg) 699	Vitamin A (RE) 69
Fat calories (kc) 27	Calcium (mg) 116	Beta-carotene (RE) 411
Cholesterol (mg) 0.4	Magnesium (mg) 167	Vitamin C (mg) 19
Saturated fat (g) 0.45	Zinc (mg) 2.7	Vitamin E (mg) 0.5
Polyunsaturated fat (g) 1.0	Selenium (mcg) 5	Thiamin B_1 (mg) 0.6
Monounsaturated fat (g) 1.6	Potassium (mg) 1158	Riboflavin B_2 (mg) 0.2
Fiber (g) 10.2	Flavonoids (mg) 2.9	Niacin B_3 (mg) 3.4
Carbohydrates (g) 59.5	Lycopene (mg) 8.9	Vitamin B_6 (mg) 0.3
Sugar (g) 3.4	Fish (oz) 0	Folic acid (mcg) 331
Protein (g) 22.9	Nuts (oz) 0	Vitamin B_{12} (mcg) 0.1

Classic Split Pea Soup

■ ■ ■ ■

Preparation time: 5 minutes	*4 servings*
Cooking time: 45 minutes to 2 hours	*310 calories per serving, 3% from fat*

RealAge effect if eaten 12 times a year:	**RealAge-effect ingredients:**
This makes your RealAge 7.3 days younger.	Onion, carrot, split peas (flavonoids, potassium, calcium, folic acid)

ingredients

1 medium onion

1 large carrot

2 cups green or yellow split peas

6½ cups water

1 tablespoon chile-garlic paste or purée

Sea salt and freshly ground black pepper to taste

preparation

Finely chop onion and carrot. Combine all ingredients and simmer covered on low heat for 1 hour, or until peas are tender and soup thickens.

substitutions: Yellow curry paste may substitute for the chile-garlic paste or purée.

tips: Simple is sometimes better—if the vegetables are of the highest quality, you'll taste it in this recipe. To add richness (and protein), use chicken stock instead of water, and top with crumbled feta and/or toasted pistachios.

nutritional analysis

Total fat (g) 1.0	Sodium (mg) 20	Vitamin A (RE) 516
Fat calories (kc) 9	Calcium (mg) 49	Beta-carotene (RE) 3083
Cholesterol (mg) 0	Magnesium (mg) 26	Vitamin C (mg) 47
Saturated fat (g) 0	Zinc (mg) 0.4	Vitamin E (mg) 0.3
Polyunsaturated fat (g) 0.1	Selenium (mcg) 2	Thiamin B_1 (mg) 0.1
Monounsaturated fat (g) 0	Potassium (mg) 248	Riboflavin B_2 (mg) 0.1
Fiber (g) 2.9	Flavonoids (mg) 1.7	Niacin B_3 (mg) 0.6
Carbohydrates (g) 9.7	Lycopene (mg) 0	Vitamin B_6 (mg) 0.2
Sugar (g) 3.4	Fish (oz) 0	Folic acid (mcg) 38
Protein (g) 2.5	Nuts (oz) 0	Vitamin B_{12} (mcg) 0

Curried Lentil Soup

■ ■ ■ ■

Preparation time: 5 minutes
Cooking time: 25 minutes

4 servings (approximately 6 cups total)
285 calories per serving, 14% from fat

RealAge effect if eaten 12 times a year:

A blockbuster for beta-carotene, this winner of a main dish makes your RealAge 4.6 days younger.

RealAge-effect ingredients:

Carrots, lentils, onion, red wine, yogurt, cilantro (magnesium, calcium, selenium, potassium, vitamin B$_3$, folic acid, antioxidants, fiber, flavonoids, healthy protein)

ingredients

1 carton (8 ounces) plain fat-free or low-fat yogurt

2 teaspoons canola oil

1 large white onion, chopped

2 large carrots, thinly sliced

¾ cup red lentils

2 teaspoons curry powder, preferably Madras curry powder (see Tips)

4¼ cups low-salt chicken or vegetable broth

1 cup fruity red wine such as merlot

¾ teaspoon salt

¼ cup chopped cilantro

preparation

Place a strainer over a bowl; line with a double thickness of paper towels. Place yogurt in strainer to drain and thicken while you prepare the soup.

Heat a large saucepan over medium-high heat. Add oil, then onion; cook 5 minutes, stirring occasionally. Stir in carrots, lentils, and curry powder; cook 1 minute. Stir in broth, wine, and salt; cover and bring to a boil over high heat. Reduce heat and simmer uncovered 18 to 20 minutes or until lentils and vegetables are tender. Ladle into soup bowls; top with thickened yogurt and cilantro.

substitutions: Garam masala may replace curry powder for a richer, rounder flavor. Garam masala is an Indian blend of dry-roasted and ground Indian spices such as curry powder, cloves, coriander, cumin, cinnamon, fennel, mace, nutmeg, black pepper, and dried chiles. Look for it in Middle Eastern or Indian markets and in the gourmet section of some supermarkets. Additional chicken or vegetable broth may replace red wine; it will give a cleaner, more beany taste to the soup. For a spicier soup, add ¼ teaspoon cayenne pepper along with the salt.

tips: Madras curry powder, representative of curries from southern India, is highly seasoned, pungent, and hot.

Strain the yogurt in the refrigerator the day before to make a tart "cream cheese" you can flavor with minced garlic and Tabasco sauce for a beautiful garnish.

nutritional analysis

Total fat (g) 4.4	Sodium (mg) 633	Vitamin A (RE) 1024
Fat calories (kc) 40	Calcium (mg) 154	Beta-carotene (RE) 6076
Cholesterol (mg) 4.6	Magnesium (mg) 68.6	Vitamin C (mg) 7
Saturated fat (g) 1.4	Zinc (mg) 2.4	Vitamin E (mg) 0.6
Polyunsaturated fat (g) 0.7	Selenium (mcg) 24	Thiamin B_1 (mg) 0.3
Monounsaturated fat (g) 2.3	Potassium (mg) 1011	Riboflavin B_2 (mg) 0.3
Fiber (g) 7.1	Flavonoids (mg) 2.1	Niacin B_3 (mg) 5.2
Carbohydrates (g) 34.7	Lycopene (mg) 0	Vitamin B_6 (mg) 0.4
Sugar (g) 8.1	Fish (oz) 0	Folic acid (mcg) 225
Protein (g) 19.2	Nuts (oz) 0	Vitamin B_{12} (mcg) 0.6

Pasta e Fagioli (Pasta and Bean) Soup

■ ■ ■ ■

Preparation time: 8 minutes	*4 (1½-cup) servings*
Cooking time: 20 minutes	*268 calories per serving, 12% from fat*

RealAge effect if eaten 12 times a year:	RealAge-effect ingredients:
10.0 days younger	Carrots, tomatoes, peas, beans, olive oil, garlic, whole wheat pasta (fiber, lycopene, calcium, potassium, folic acid, healthy fats)

ingredients

1 teaspoon olive oil

2 carrots, thinly sliced

4 garlic cloves, minced

¼ teaspoon crushed red pepper flakes

3 cups low-salt vegetable or chicken broth

½ cup (2 ounces) uncooked whole wheat gemelli (small twisted pasta), such as Eden brand, or ditalini (small tube pasta) or small shell pasta

1 can (14½ ounces) seasoned diced tomatoes, undrained (such as Muir Glen brand)

1 can (15 to 16 ounces) kidney beans or red beans, rinsed and drained

½ cup frozen baby peas, thawed

¼ cup chopped fresh basil or flat-leaf parsley

¼ cup grated Romano or Asiago cheese

preparation

Heat a large saucepan over medium heat. Add olive oil and carrots; cook 2 minutes. Stir in garlic and red pepper flakes; cook 1 minute. Add broth and pasta; bring to a boil over high heat. Reduce heat; simmer 10 minutes. Stir in tomatoes and beans; return to a simmer and cook 5 minutes or until pasta is tender. Stir in peas; heat through. Ladle into shallow bowls; top with basil and cheese.

substitutions: Freshly shelled peas may be substituted for frozen peas; stir them into the soup with the tomatoes and beans. Great Northern or cannellini beans may replace the kidney or red beans.

tips: Leftover soup will keep up to 3 days in the refrigerator or up to 3 months in the freezer. For extra flavor, drizzle a small amount of rosemary-infused olive oil (Boyajian makes a delicious one) over the soup just before serving.

nutritional analysis

Total fat (g) 3.5	Sodium (mg) 684	Vitamin A (RE) 11
Fat calories (kc) 32	Calcium (mg) 245	Beta-carotene (RE) 6583
Cholesterol (mg) 27.1	Magnesium (mg) 44	Vitamin C (mg) 29
Saturated fat (g) 0.7	Zinc (mg) 2.1	Vitamin E (mg) 0.8
Polyunsaturated fat (g) 1.0	Selenium (mcg) 12	Thiamin B_1 (mg) 0.3
Monounsaturated fat (g) 2.0	Potassium (mg) 888	Riboflavin B_2 (mg) 0.3
Fiber (g) 8.9	Flavonoids (mg) 2.2	Niacin B_3 (mg) 5
Carbohydrates (g) 40.9	Lycopene (mg) 3.3	Vitamin B_6 (mg) 0.8
Sugar (g) 8.6	Fish (oz) 0	Folic acid (mcg) 55
Protein (g) 19.3	Nuts (oz) 0	Vitamin B_{12} (mcg) 0.4

FOR DINNER

Barbecued Red Snapper with Spicy Red Beans and Rice

■   ■   ■   ■

Preparation time: 8 minutes	*4 servings*
Cooking time: 12 minutes	*642 calories per serving, 9% from fat*

RealAge effect if eaten 12 times a year:	**RealAge-effect ingredients:**
With more RealAge-reducing omega-3s than omega-6s, serving this makes your RealAge 11.4 days younger.	Vegetable juice, red snapper, kale, beans (healthy protein, healthy fat, fiber, potassium, antioxidants, B vitamins)

ingredients

⅓ cup hickory barbecue sauce, such as KC Masterpiece brand

2 teaspoons Caribbean jerk seasoning mix, such as McCormick brand

1½ cups spicy vegetable juice, such as Spicy V8 brand

2 cups quick-cooking brown rice, such as Uncle Ben's brand

4 (4- to 5-ounce) skinless red snapper fish fillets

3 cups packed sliced kale or collard greens

1 can (15 or 16 ounces) red beans, rinsed and drained

2 tablespoons light sour cream

preparation

Prepare charcoal or gas grill. Combine barbecue sauce and jerk seasoning; mix well. Brush 3 tablespoons of the mixture over fish; set aside.

In a small bowl, set aside 1 tablespoon of vegetable juice. In a large deep skillet, combine remaining barbecue sauce mixture, remaining vegetable juice, and 1 cup water; bring to a simmer. Stir in rice; cover and simmer 8 minutes.

Grill fish over medium-hot coals (or over medium-high heat in a ridged grill pan) 3 to 4 minutes per side or until fish is opaque and firm to the touch. Meanwhile, stir kale and beans into rice mixture. Cover and continue to simmer 3 to 4 minutes or until kale is wilted and liquid is absorbed.

Transfer rice mixture to four serving plates; top with fish. Add sour cream to reserved 1 tablespoon vegetable juice; mix well. Drizzle over fish and rice.

substitutions: Halibut or scrod may replace red snapper; Cajun or blackened seasonings may replace jerk seasoning; other cooking greens, such as mustard, may replace kale, although the taste will be sharper and not as sweet.

tips: Cooking kale brings out its sweetness. The heat of the rice and beans continues to soften its flavor as the dish cooks. The same is true for other cooking greens—collards, mustard, turnip, dandelion. Try Red Russian kale; it's especially flavorful and easy to cook. Also, when selecting snapper, choose firm, clear, and clean fillets that are not a bit mushy or fishy smelling.

nutritional analysis

Total fat (g) 6.5	Sodium (mg) 921	Vitamin A (RE) 908
Fat calories (kc) 58.4	Calcium (mg) 186	Beta-carotene (RE) 922
Cholesterol (mg) 49.5	Magnesium (mg) 209	Vitamin C (mg) 64.0
Saturated fat (g) 1.3	Zinc (mg) 3.6	Vitamin E (mg) 9
Polyunsaturated fat (g) 2.6	Selenium (mcg) 5	Thiamin B_1 (mg) 0.6
Monounsaturated fat (g) 2.8	Potassium (mg) 1475	Riboflavin B_2 (mg) 0.2
Fiber (g) 15.0	Flavonoids (mg) 3.2	Niacin B_3 (mg) 7.0
Carbohydrates (g) 101	Lycopene (mg) 1.6	Vitamin B_6 (mg) 1.7
Sugar (g) 9.5	Fish (oz) 4.5	Folic acid (mcg) 72
Protein (g) 42.4	Nuts (oz) 0	Vitamin B_{12} (mcg) 3.9

Cioppino (Seafood Stew)

■ ■ ■ ■

Preparation time: 8 minutes	*4 servings*
Cooking time: 15 minutes	*281 calories per serving, 26% from fat*

RealAge effect if eaten 12 times a year:	**RealAge-effect ingredients:**
1.2 days younger. Low-fat, low-calorie, and high in lycopene, this one's an easy winner.	Tomatoes, olive oil, garlic, alcohol, onion, halibut (healthy fats, healthy protein, lycopene, potassium, flavonoids)

ingredients

1 tablespoon olive oil

1 cup chopped white onion

4 garlic cloves, minced

¼ cup dry white wine or vermouth (optional)

1 bottle (8 ounces) clam juice

1 can (14¼ ounces) "pasta-ready" or Italian seasoned diced tomatoes, undrained, such as Contadina Del Monte brand

1 teaspoon each dried basil and Mexican oregano

¼ teaspoon crushed red pepper flakes (optional)

8 ounces skinless halibut fish fillets, cut into 1-inch chunks

½ pound uncooked peeled and deveined medium shrimp

preparation

Heat a large, deep skillet over medium-high heat. Add oil and onion; cook 3 minutes, stirring occasionally. Add garlic; cook 1 minute, stirring once. If desired, add wine or vermouth; cook 30 seconds. Add clam juice, tomatoes, basil, oregano, and, if desired, red pepper flakes; bring to a simmer. Reduce heat; simmer uncovered 8 minutes.

Stir in fish and shrimp. Cook until fish and shrimp are opaque, about 5 minutes. Ladle into shallow bowls.

substitutions: Red snapper or 8 ounces halved sea scallops may replace the fish fillets.

tips: Although the wine or vermouth (we like vermouth) is optional, it does add a dimension of flavor—a little puckery, a little like the sea. Almost all the alcohol disappears with cooking. When time is short, use cans of "pasta-ready" or "recipe-ready" tomatoes that are already peeled, seasoned, and diced. They're a perfect shortcut.

nutritional analysis

Total fat (g) 8.1	Sodium (mg) 719	Vitamin A (RE) 121
Fat calories (kc) 73	Calcium (mg) 111	Beta-carotene (RE) 367
Cholesterol (mg) 40.4	Magnesium (mg) 123	Vitamin C (mg) 24
Saturated fat (g) 1.2	Zinc (mg) 2.0	Vitamin E (mg) 1.2
Polyunsaturated fat (g) 1.7	Selenium (mcg) 82	Thiamin B_1 (mg) 0.30
Monounsaturated fat (g) 3.7	Potassium (mg) 923	Riboflavin B_2 (mg) 0.3
Fiber (g) 4.4	Flavonoids (mg) 3.4	Niacin B_3 (mg) 7.6
Carbohydrates (g) 22.7	Lycopene (mg) 3.2	Vitamin B_6 (mg) 0.5
Sugar (g) 7.7	Fish (oz) 2	Folic acid (mcg) 64
Protein (g) 27.5	Nuts (oz) 0	Vitamin B_{12} (mcg) 8.0

Grilled Sea Bass with Asian Red Lentils and Kale

■ ■ ■ ■

Preparation time: 10 minutes	*4 servings*
Cooking time: 20 minutes	*294 calories per serving, 12% from fat*

RealAge effect if eaten 12 times a year:	**RealAge-effect ingredients:**
The antioxidants in this incredibly delicious dish are too numerous to mention—but let it be said that this dish makes your RealAge 10.4 days younger.	Sea bass, garlic, lentils, kale, sesame seeds (antioxidants, healthy protein, healthy fat, fiber, potassium, magnesium, calcium, folate, vitamin E)

ingredients

1 pound fresh sea bass fillet, cut into four portions about ½ inch thick

2 tablespoons soy sauce

1 tablespoon mirin (rice wine)

2 garlic cloves, minced

1 teaspoon finely grated fresh ginger

1 teaspoon dark sesame oil

1 cup red lentils

2 cups low-salt chicken broth

4 cups packed sliced kale (4 ounces)

2 teaspoons sesame seeds, toasted (optional)

preparation

Prepare a charcoal or gas grill. Place fish on a shallow plate. Combine soy sauce, mirin, garlic, ginger, and sesame oil; mix well. Pour over fish, turning to coat. Let stand 10 minutes.

Meanwhile, combine lentils and broth in a large, deep skillet. Bring to a boil over high heat. Reduce heat; simmer uncovered 10 minutes; stirring occasionally. Add kale; cover and simmer 5 minutes or until lentils and kale are tender, stirring once.

Drain fish, reserving marinade. Grill over medium-high heat 3 to 4 minutes per side or until fish is opaque in center. Transfer marinade to a small saucepan; add 1 tablespoon water. Bring to a boil; boil gently 30 seconds.

Spoon lentil mixture onto four warmed serving plates; top with fish. Sprinkle with sesame seeds, if desired. Drizzle boiled marinade over fish and lentil mixture.

substitutions: This versatile recipe swings all ways. Halibut, red snapper, or striped bass may replace the sea bass; tamari may replace soy sauce; dry sherry may replace mirin; vegetable broth may replace chicken broth; and Swiss chard or beet greens may replace kale. French green lentils may substitute for red lentils; cook them until tender.

tips: Red lentils cook more quickly than green or brown lentils; they are done when they are just past al dente. They should be soft but not mushy. Sea bass fillets are easy to cook; cook them only until they are opaque in the center or firm to the touch. If they are thicker than ½ inch, add a minute or two to the grilling time. The fish may also be cooked in a preheated ridged grill pan over medium-high heat.

nutritional analysis

Total fat (g) 4.0	Sodium (mg) 657	Vitamin A (RE) 1035
Fat calories (kc) 36	Calcium (mg) 155	Beta-carotene (RE) 966
Cholesterol (mg) 60.5	Magnesium (mg) 124	Vitamin C (mg) 57
Saturated fat (g) 0.6	Zinc (mg) 1.9	Vitamin E (mg) 12
Polyunsaturated fat (g) 1.8	Selenium (mcg) 18	Thiamin B_1 (mg) 0.4
Monounsaturated fat (g) 1.6	Potassium (mg) 908	Riboflavin B_2 (mg) 0.4
Fiber (g) 8.9	Flavonoids (mg) 0.3	Niacin B_3 (mg) 6.0
Carbohydrates (g) 25	Lycopene (mg) 0	Vitamin B_6 (mg) 0.8
Sugar (g) 4.9	Fish (oz) 4	Folic acid (mcg) 62
Protein (g) 36.7	Nuts (oz) 0	Vitamin B_{12} (mcg) 0.5

Poached Salmon with Sautéed Kale and Cherry Tomatoes

■ ■ ■ ■

Preparation time: 10 minutes	*4 servings*
Cooking time: 20 minutes	*255 calories per serving, 35% from fat*

RealAge effect if eaten 12 times a year:	**RealAge-effect ingredients:**
8.2 days younger	Salmon, lemon juice, kale, olive oil, shallots, tomatoes, wine (healthy protein, healthy fats, alcohol, potassium, flavonoids, lycopene)

ingredients

1 cup each dry white wine and water

2 tablespoons lemon juice

1½ teaspoons each crushed dried rosemary and dried dill

4 (4- to 5-ounce) skinless salmon fillets

2 teaspoons olive oil

6 small shallots, sliced (½ cup)

½ bunch kale (8 ounces), coarse stalks discarded, leaves coarsely chopped

4 small plum tomatoes, quartered

¾ teaspoon salt

¼ teaspoon freshly ground black pepper

2 tablespoons chopped fresh dill (optional)

Lemon wedges (optional)

preparation

In a large deep skillet, combine wine, water, lemon juice, rosemary, and dill. Bring to a boil over high heat. Reduce heat; simmer uncovered 10 minutes. Add salmon; poach gently until salmon is opaque and firm to the touch, 3 to 5 minutes.

Meanwhile, heat a Dutch oven over medium-high heat. Add oil, then shallots. Cook 1 minute, stirring frequently. Reduce heat to medium. Add kale. Cover and cook until kale is wilted, about 3 minutes. Uncover; continue cooking kale, turning with tongs until tender, about 3 minutes. Add tomatoes, salt, and pepper; heat through. Transfer vegetables to serving plates. Using a slotted spatula, drain salmon; place over vegetables. Garnish with fresh dill and lemon wedges, if desired.

substitutions: Salmon steaks, cut through the bone, work well here, too. You can leave the skin on, from start to finish. If you can find it, try Lacinato kale (or dinosaur kale). Stemmed and washed, it has more delicate flavor and texture than most kale. Otherwise, whole-leaf spinach can substitute for kale. Broth can substitute for wine, and your favorite skinned fish can substitute for salmon.

tips: A drizzle of olive oil or horseradish sour cream will add extra moisture to this dish, as will more chopped fresh dill. However, poaching the salmon gently and not excessively is the best way to preserve moisture.

nutritional analysis

Total fat (g) 10	Sodium (mg) 522	Vitamin A (RE) 734
Fat calories (kc) 92	Calcium (mg) 158	Beta-carotene (RE) 1987
Cholesterol (mg) 81.7	Magnesium (mg) 71	Vitamin C (mg) 45
Saturated fat (g) 1.5	Zinc (mg) 1.4	Vitamin E (mg) 7.8
Polyunsaturated fat (g) 5.9	Selenium (mcg) 0	Thiamin B_1 (mg) 0.2
Monounsaturated fat (g) 2.5	Potassium (mg) 504	Riboflavin B_2 (mg) 0.4
Fiber (g) 4.0	Flavonoids (mg) 3.1	Niacin B_3 (mg) 5.9
Carbohydrates (g) 25.8	Lycopene (mg) 3.1	Vitamin B_6 (mg) 0.2
Sugar (g) 3.2	Fish (oz) 4.5	Folic acid (mcg) 33
Protein (g) 19.5	Nuts (oz) 0	Vitamin B_{12} (mcg) 3.4

Meaty Tofu and Stir-Fried Bok Choy over Udon Noodles

Preparation time: 12 minutes	*4 servings*
Cooking time: 8 minutes	*387 calories per serving, 24% from fat*

RealAge effect if eaten 12 times a year:	**RealAge-effect ingredients:**
Stocked with potassium and magnesium, this dish makes your RealAge 3.0 days younger.	Buckwheat noodles, tofu, sesame oil, garlic, bok choy, carrots (magnesium, calcium, potassium, beta-carotene, vitamin C, fiber, healthy protein, healthy fat, folic acid)

ingredients

8 ounces udon noodles (thick Japanese buckwheat noodles)

2 tablespoons seasoned black bean paste

2 tablespoons mirin (rice wine)

10 ounces firm-style tofu, such as White Wave brand

3 teaspoons dark sesame oil

4 garlic cloves, minced

1 small head or ½ large head bok choy, sliced ¼ inch thick, stems and leaves separated

2 cups julienned carrots (packaged or from the supermarket salad bar)

¼ cup julienned daikon or red radish (optional)

preparation

Cook noodles according to package directions. Meanwhile, combine black bean paste and mirin; mix well. Press the block of tofu between paper towels to absorb excess moisture. Cut tofu into ¾-inch slices; cut slices into 1-inch squares. Toss tofu with 2 tablespoons black bean mixture and set aside.

Heat a large, deep nonstick skillet over medium-high heat. Add 1 teaspoon of the oil, the garlic, and the bok choy stems; stir-fry 2 minutes. Add bok choy leaves, carrots, and tofu mixture; stir-fry 2 minutes or until the vegetables are crisp-tender. Salt to taste.

Drain noodles; toss with remaining black bean mixture and remaining 2 teaspoons sesame oil. Transfer to serving plates. Spoon tofu mixture over noodles; if desired, garnish with radish.

substitutions: Hoisin or teriyaki sauce may replace black bean sauce—both will make the dish much sweeter but still tasty. Whole wheat wide ribbon pasta—like a fettuccine—can replace buckwheat noodles. Black bean garlic sauce can replace the black bean sauce. Look for black bean garlic sauce, mirin, and udon noodles in the Asian section of your supermarket.

tips: Pickled ginger, also located in the ethnic section of your supermarket, adds a new sweet-sour dimension to this dish. Sprinkle a little pickled ginger on top, or just drizzle the juice from the jar, to make this dish really pop. The juice, which is usually just vinegar with a little salt and sugar, makes a big difference.

nutritional analysis

Total fat (g) 10.3	Sodium (mg) 1087	Vitamin A (RE) 1567
Fat calories (kc) 93.1	Calcium (mg) 213	Beta-carotene (RE) 9404
Cholesterol (mg) 0	Magnesium (mg) 106	Vitamin C (mg) 39
Saturated fat (g) 1.5	Zinc (mg) 1.7	Vitamin E (mg) 1.5
Polyunsaturated fat (g) 5.2	Selenium (mcg) 4	Thiamin B_1 (mg) 0.3
Monounsaturated fat (g) 2.8	Potassium (mg) 659	Riboflavin B_2 (mg) 0.2
Fiber (g) 5.5	Flavonoids (mg) 0.7	Niacin B_3 (mg) 1.5
Carbohydrates (g) 56.9	Lycopene (mg) 0	Vitamin B_6 (mg) 0.3
Sugar (g) 5.7	Fish (oz) 0	Folic acid (mcg) 84
Protein (g) 19.7	Nuts (oz) 0	Vitamin B_{12} (mcg) 0

Persian Kidney Beans

■　■　■　■

Preparation time: 10 minutes	*4 servings (approximately 5½ cups total)*
Cooking time: 18 minutes	*311 calories per serving, 8% from fat*

RealAge effect if eaten 12 times a year:	**RealAge-effect ingredients:**
6.7 days younger	Olive oil, onion, garlic, orange juice, tomato paste, beans (fiber, flavonoids, lycopene, potassium, vitamin C, folic acid)

ingredients

1½ teaspoons olive oil

1 cup finely chopped white or yellow onion

3 garlic cloves, minced

1 teaspoon each salt and ground cumin

¼ teaspoon cinnamon

1 cup fresh orange juice

2 tablespoons fresh lime juice

2 tablespoons tomato paste

1 teaspoon bottled or fresh seeded, minced, red jalapeño chile

3 cans (16 ounces each) red kidney beans, rinsed and drained

½ teaspoon each finely shredded lime peel and orange peel (zest)

¼ cup freshly grated Romano cheese (optional)

preparation

Heat a large saucepan or Dutch oven over medium heat. Add oil, then onion. Cook 5 minutes, stirring occasionally. Add garlic, salt, cumin, and cinnamon; continue to cook 3 minutes. Add orange and lime juices, tomato paste, and chile; simmer uncovered 5 minutes.

Add beans; bring to a boil. Reduce heat; simmer uncovered 5 minutes, stirring occasionally. Ladle into shallow bowls; top with lime and orange zests, and, if desired, cheese.

substitutions: Kidney beans accept all sorts of flavorings easily. Most beans do—black beans make an especially good substitute and could be combined with kidney beans, as could garbanzo beans.

tips: One lime provides enough juice and peel for this recipe. Grating the zest before squeezing the citrus saves the trouble of trying to get color and flavor from a slippery, misshapen fruit. Basmati and brown rice both make easy accompaniments; look for quick-cooking versions. For quick tacos, serve the beans with warm corn tortillas and top with grated cheese.

nutritional analysis

Total fat (g) 2.4	Sodium (mg) 1098	Vitamin A (RE) 34
Fat calories (kc) 21.6	Calcium (mg) 55	Beta-carotene (RE) 207
Cholesterol (mg) 0	Magnesium (mg) 21	Vitamin C (mg) 45
Saturated fat (g) 0.4	Zinc (mg) 1.1	Vitamin E (mg) 0.36
Polyunsaturated fat (g) 0.3	Selenium (mcg) 3	Thiamin B_1 (mg) 0.15
Monounsaturated fat (g) 1.5	Potassium (mg) 582	Riboflavin B_2 (mg) 0.09
Fiber (g) 7.1	Flavonoids (mg) 4.6	Niacin B_3 (mg) 1.3
Carbohydrates (g) 31.6	Lycopene (mg) 2.1	Vitamin B_6 (mg) 0.6
Sugar (g) 7.6	Fish (oz) 0	Folic acid (mcg) 60
Protein (g) 8.1	Nuts (oz) 0	Vitamin B_{12} (mcg) 0

Worcestershire Winter Vegetables with Currant-Studded Bulgur

■ ■ ■ ■

Preparation time: 10 minutes	*4 servings*
Cooking time: 20 minutes	*449 calories per serving, 18% from fat*

RealAge effect if eaten 12 times a year:	**RealAge-effect ingredients:**
You are 7.3 days younger because of the high fiber and low calories in this filling, nutrient-dense dish.	Whole grains, currants, cauliflower, broccoli rabe, beans, olive oil (fiber, healthy protein, healthy fat, potassium, magnesium, zinc, selenium, antioxidants, vitamin B$_3$, vitamin B$_6$, folic acid)

ingredients

2¼ cups low-salt chicken broth

1 cup coarse-grain bulgur, such as Bob's Red Mill brand

⅓ cup currants

3 cups (1-inch) cauliflower florets (10 ounces)

3 cups coarsely chopped broccoli rabe (rapini) (8 ounces)

2 tablespoons extra-virgin olive oil

½ teaspoon salt

½ teaspoon freshly ground black pepper

2 tablespoons Worcestershire sauce

1 can (16 or 19 ounces) cannellini beans, drained

preparation

Bring 2 cups of the broth to a boil in a medium saucepan. Stir in bulgur and currants; simmer 1 minute, stirring frequently. Remove from heat, cover, and let stand 15 to 18 minutes or until liquid is absorbed.

Meanwhile, heat broiler. Combine cauliflower and broccoli rabe in a shallow roasting pan. Drizzle 1 tablespoon of the oil over vegetables; toss well to coat. Broil 3 to 4 inches from heat source 7 minutes or until vegetables are browned and crisp-tender. Sprinkle vegetables with salt and pepper.

In a large bowl, combine remaining ¼ cup broth and Worcestershire sauce;

mix well. Add the broiled vegetable mixture; mix well. Add beans; mix well. Fluff bulgur with a fork and transfer to serving plates; top with vegetable mixture. Gently drizzle remaining 1 tablespoon oil over all.

substitutions: Broccoli florets or chopped broccolini may replace broccoli rabe: The dish will not be bitter at all, and the cooking time is about the same.

tips: Broccoli rabe needs to be cooked to be delicious. Here, we broiled it to intensify the flavor, but it also sautés beautifully. Try it with a splash of olive oil, a handful of garlic, and some halved grape tomatoes. Spread the topping over a pizza shell, sprinkle some real Parmigiano-Reggiano cheese, toss it in the oven or on the grill for 10 minutes, and you've got pizza to go!

nutritional analysis

Total fat (g) 9.1	Sodium (mg) 568	Vitamin A (RE) 89
Fat calories (kc) 82	Calcium (mg) 145	Beta-carotene (RE) 528
Cholesterol (mg) 0.6	Magnesium (mg) 152	Vitamin C (mg) 107
Saturated fat (g) 1.4	Zinc (mg) 2.6	Vitamin E (mg) 1.5
Polyunsaturated fat (g) 2.2	Selenium (mcg) 22	Thiamin B_1 (mg) 0.4
Monounsaturated fat (g) 5.2	Potassium (mg) 1348	Riboflavin B_2 (mg) 0.3
Fiber (g) 19.4	Flavonoids (mg) 2.8	Niacin B_3 (mg) 5.8
Carbohydrates (g) 75.3	Lycopene (mg) 0	Vitamin B_6 (mg) 1.1
Sugar (g) 12.7	Fish (oz) 0	Folic acid (mcg) 149
Protein (g) 22.5	Nuts (oz) 0	Vitamin B_{12} (mcg) 0.1

FOR DESSERT OR SNACK

Simon's Popcorn

■ ■ ■ ■

| Preparation time: 1 minute | 4 servings |
| Cooking time: 5 minutes | 61 calories per serving, 10% from fat |

RealAge effect if eaten 12 times a year:	RealAge-effect ingredients:
No RealAge effect, except to save you from the aging that other styles of popcorn can cause because of trans fat or saturated fats.	Corn (fiber)

ingredients

½ cup popcorn kernels

Butter-, olive oil-, or garlic-flavored cooking oil spray

Garlic salt, or cinnamon and sugar (optional)

preparation

Place popcorn in a 2½-quart microwave-safe container; cover and cook at high power 4 to 5 minutes or until popcorn is popped but not scorched. After 3 minutes, if the microwave oven does not have a turntable, use oven mitts to shake the covered container. Pour the popcorn onto a sheet pan (see tips) and coat with cooking oil spray. To flavor the popcorn, sprinkle on your favorite seasoning—garlic salt or cinnamon and sugar.

tips: Yes, a sheet pan has no sides or very shallow sides, so you're thinking the popcorn's going to spill all over the place and make a mess, plus get cold. Then you've got to put it in a bowl from a flat, mostly sideless sheet. However, this really works. Try it. This recipe makes a great low-calorie snack with flavor.

nutritional analysis

Total fat (g) 0.8	Sodium (mg) 0	Vitamin A (RE) 0
Fat calories (kc) 7.2	Calcium (mg) 1	Beta-carotene (RE) 0
Cholesterol (mg) 0	Magnesium (mg) 0	Vitamin C (mg) 0
Saturated fat (g) 0.1	Zinc (mg) 0.5	Vitamin E (mg) 0
Polyunsaturated fat (g) 0.5	Selenium (mcg) 1	Thiamin B_1 (mg) 0
Monounsaturated fat (g) 0.2	Potassium (mg) 0	Riboflavin B_2 (mg) 0.01
Fiber (g) 0.4	Flavonoids (mg) 0	Niacin B_3 (mg) 0.1
Carbohydrates (g) 10.0	Lycopene (mg) 0	Vitamin B_6 (mg) 0.01
Sugar (g) 0	Fish (oz) 0	Folic acid (mcg) 0
Protein (g) 1.0	Nuts (oz) 0	Vitamin B_{12} (mcg) 0

10

The **RealAge** Garden

As you become a RealAge gourmet cook and appreciate the enormous difference that really fresh produce and herbs can make in the taste of a dish, you may consider growing some of the ingredients yourself (3 Kitchen IQ points). Nothing beats the great taste and feeling of pride you'll experience when serving and eating them. Now, I'm much better at cooking and treating and motivating patients than I am at gardening. But I have enjoyed the little bit of gardening I've done. This chapter reviews some of the secrets great chefs use to produce fresh products locally—how they do it themselves. Not all of us will choose this RealAge kitchen option, but if you already grow your own, or if you want to start, here are some tricks that should make your RealAge younger.

Some of us find gardening too time-consuming or too complicated. Even though the exercise of gardening, learning a new skill, and possibly acquiring new friends almost always make your RealAge younger, you may be intimidated by the prospect of gardening. Perhaps you think you don't have enough space for a garden. Don't let these issues stop you if you really are interested in learning to garden. Just take that first small step and learn the basics.

Whether you have a backyard garden, keep a windowsill herb garden, or buy fresh garden produce at a farmers' market, you can get the most out of fresh produce by making the delicious dishes in this book.

Soil

The key to successful gardening is having nutrient-rich soil. You might want to start a compost pile right away. Onto this pile you toss your uncooked kitchen scraps—coffee grounds, egg shells, potato peels, apple cores—which eventually break down to become nutrients for your garden. These nutrients help produce food that is rich in taste. You might also visit an organic garden in your area—possibly gaining new friends—to see how it's done. Or, you might want to take a composting class to learn just how to make sure your garden soil has the right amounts of nitrogen, phosphate, and the other essential elements. Meeting a new challenge makes your RealAge even younger.

Tools

Your RealAge will be younger if you invest in quality tools for the garden. You don't need that many. The essentials are a garden spade, a digging fork, a garden rake, plant supports, a trowel, and a hoe. Before buying a tool, go through the motions of using it to make sure it "feels right" in your hands and doesn't strain your neck or back (making your RealAge older). Having all six essential garden tools is worth *1 Kitchen IQ point,* and testing them before buying is worth *2 Kitchen IQ points.*

Climate

Climate is everything! It determines your growing season and what will grow when. Apples don't grow in Southern California nearly as well as they grow in southern Wisconsin because they need enough days of chill to bear fruit. And in upstate New York, we've never seen (outside) an avocado tree (unlike Florida!). If you live in northern Montana, your garden in June will look different than if you live in southern Texas. A friend in Tucson replaced all the sandy soil in his garden with potting soil, so he could take advantage of the hot dry, Arizona air year-round.

The USDA has rated cold hardiness zones for gardening based on climate—mostly temperature. Often, a package of seeds or a seedling will tell you how hardy they are by naming the zone in which they grow best. But climate is not just cold hardiness. Climate is also influenced by topographical features such as hills and valleys, large bodies of water (with a lake effect), urban heat effect, wind, canopies—all of which can give rise to the nooks and crannies of microclimates.

To know what kinds of plants you can grow in your climate, ask at a local nursery—the sales people are usually very helpful. Go to a gardening club and ask other gardeners. Experiment with container gardening—it works, especially inside, no matter what the outside climate!

Getting Started

- **Start small.** Begin by planting just one type of vegetable in a small plot, just a few square feet, or in a planter, with potting soil. This keeps the work down to a manageable level.

- **Choose the vegetables your family loves best.** If you're starting small, never plant anything that a member of your family dislikes. You might as well grow something everyone will enjoy.

- **Start with the easiest crops.** Good choices for the beginner are radishes, green beans, cucumbers, or lettuce.

Choose the Right Location for Your Garden

- **Sun.** Find a place in your yard that gets plenty of sunshine. Four hours is enough for some vegetables, but many do better with more.

- **Access.** If you plant your crop in a place you pass every day, it will help you keep daily watch on its development.

- **Air.** You want a flow of fresh air but not a fierce wind. If you have problems with wind, consider erecting a wind barrier, or using a window box in a protected area.

- **Drainage.** Once you find an area that might be a good place for a garden, see what rain does to it. After a rain, check the soil in that area. If it stays muddy for a long time, drainage might not be adequate for a garden. Choosing another location might keep your RealAge younger by avoiding the stress of crop failure.

- **Water.** Make sure you can reach your plot with a garden hose. Mother Nature usually doesn't provide all the water you'll need. Water the ground below the vegetables, and try to avoid getting water on the leaves to prevent the spread of disease, and to keep blossoms intact.

Prepare Your Site

You can encourage good vegetable growth by removing any existing grass and weeds. Till the earth to aerate the soil and remove roots, rocks, and remaining parts of weeds. Spreading compost (about 1 inch thick) over the soil, so that it gets mixed in while you till, feeds your garden. Work from one end to the other, backing up so you never step on the tilled earth (which would cause it to lose the fluffy, air-filled texture your plants need to thrive). Rich soil smells good and clean, and is fun to run your hands through.

Start Planting

Once your plot has been prepared, it's time to start planting. Transplant baby plants you've bought at a nursery or have started yourself indoors, or plant seeds directly in the bed. The choice depends primarily on how long it will take the plants to grow, the expense involved, and the likelihood of success. Planting from seed takes longer, but seeds are less expensive than starter plants. With seeds you'll have the pleasure (and privilege) of seeing the plant grow from the beginning. Of course, animals may want to dig them up, especially vegetable seedlings; seedlings make good snacks for rabbits and squirrels. On the other hand, transplants are more likely than seeds to flourish in an amateur's hands.

In either case, you may want to put down landscaping cloth between rows to prevent weed growth. Such cloth is better than using an insecticide, and it reduces the need for time-consuming (and sometimes backbreaking) weeding.

If you decide to buy transplants from a nursery, ask a local gardening friend and expert to recommend the best local nursery. The second-best strategy is to find a nursery and its plants yourself, using the following questions:

1. Do the plants seem well cared for, with plenty of room and aeration?

2. Do the transplants have ample containers for their size? (Space to live is important to plants, just as it is to humans.) If there isn't enough space for a plant, the roots may become crowded. You can check for this by lifting the plant out of its container in the nursery. The soil should keep its shape, and you should see white tips on the roots, indicating they're healthy. Plants should not be root bound.

3. Are the plants healthy looking, free of yellowing or mottling? (Check the underside of the leaves.) Are they misshapen or infested?

If you decide to buy seeds instead of plants, check the date on the packet. Very old seeds may lose their ability to germinate. However, if you use only half a packet, you don't necessarily have to toss the rest. Seeds can last much longer than you'd expect, but if you want the best germination rates, use new seeds. Here's a general list of the approximate maximum viable life of some common vegetable seeds:

Beans, 3 years
Beets, 4 years
Broccoli, 3 years
Cabbage, 4 years
Carrots, 3 years
Cauliflower, 4 years
Corn, 2 years
Cucumbers, 5 years

Eggplant, 4 years
Lettuce, 6 years
Onions, 1 year
Peas, 3 years
Peppers, 2 years
Radishes, 5 years
Spinach, 3 years
Squash, 4 years

The success of growing from seed or transplants also depends on the vegetable itself. Beans and peas, for example, produce rather fragile seedlings that don't take well to transplanting. So, for those crops, planting seeds directly in the bed is the better method. Other vegetables, such as Brussels sprouts, aren't widely available as transplants, so this crop is another good seed choice. We're crazy about growing fresh herbs and spices, and cover that in the next chapter.

Managing Your Garden

Once your seeds or transplants are growing, you need to take care of your plot on a regular basis. The essentials of garden care are as follows:

• **Watering.** Many vegetables love soil that's moist—tomatoes and onions, especially. Try not to let the bed dry out completely. Watering varies with the plant—seek the advice of a local expert. Early morning seems like the time vegetables most like to receive water, and of course, it evaporates most slowly when the temperature is cool.

• **Mulching.** Mulch is a protective ground covering used to reduce evaporation, prevent erosion, control weeds, and enrich the soil. Shredded leaves or grass clippings make great mulch for your garden. If you use grass clippings, use only those from a lawn that has not been treated with chemical pesticides, fungicides, or herbicides. This will promote the success and vibrancy of your garden, and the health and youngest RealAge of those who consume its bounty.

• **Composting.** Compost is a mixture of decayed organic matter that is used for fertilizer. Continue to add organic uncooked kitchen waste to your compost pile. Also add soil and water, mixing them to encourage decay. By turning it over you aerate the pile to prevent mold and accelerate composting action. Keep the pile covered with a tarp so the rain doesn't wash the compost away, or consider purchasing a compost bin.

- **Weeding.** Weeds rob your vegetables of water, nutrients, and sunlight—three factors needed for successful crop growth. Although you don't have to eliminate every last weed from your garden, regular weeding keeps them under control and promotes good crop growth. Regular weeding means digging out as many weed roots as possible during the tilling process, and then pulling up weeds as they sprout among your vegetables.

- **Fertilizing.** If you have a good compost heap that you are using regularly to feed your garden, you may not need additional fertilization to have a great RealAge garden. However, if your garden is not filled with rich, organic soil, or if you're growing hungry plants—tomatoes, peppers, and onions are among the hungriest—you may want to supplement the soil's nutrients with a fertilizer. Several varieties exist, in both dry and liquid forms. Let a nursery help you choose the fertilizer that's best for your geographic area, crops, and other aspects of your garden. Fish emulsion, seaweed emulsion, and compost teas are especially effective and complement each other.

Obviously, this chapter does not provide an exhaustive discussion of gardening. But we'd love to help you find out more. If you're interested in learning more, see the Recommended Resources at the end of the book for gardening books that present much greater detail.

Sprouts

If you don't have a vegetable garden, or even enough room for a balcony or roof garden, but want to grow fresh food, a great place to start is with sprouts. Sprouts are full of protein and vitamin C, often lutein as well, and can be harvested all year long with minimal effort and expense. If you have children, enlisting their participation teaches them about the miracle of plant life and the fundamentals of good nutrition.

Alfalfa Sprouts

For alfalfa sprouts, all you need is a glass pint jar, cheesecloth, and a rubber band, or a glass pint jar that is fitted with a mesh wire top. If you are concerned about the risk of salmonella, you can rinse the seeds (and the jar they'll be growing in) in a solution of 1 tablespoon of bleach to a pint of water before starting the sprouting process. If this doesn't appeal to you, another way to safeguard against the risk of salmonella is to cook the sprouts. (Cooked bean sprouts are part of many wonderful Chinese dishes, such as stir-fries.)

To start, put a tablespoon of alfalfa seeds in the jar, fill it half full with room-temperature water, and let it sit overnight. The next day, drain the water. Rinse the seeds with lukewarm (not hot or cold) water and turn the jar upside down so that excess moisture can escape and the seeds can get oxygen.

Rinse the seeds with lukewarm water as described above two or three times a day. After a few days, the seeds will start to sprout. Be sure to shake the seeds gently to keep them separated as they grow. By about the fourth day, the sprouts will turn bright green, a signal that they are ready to eat. Past this point, the sprouts should be refrigerated.

Sprouts can become a staple in your lunchtime meal, to be added to salads and sandwiches for a delicious way to pack a nutritional punch.

Other Sprouts

Try sprouting different types of seeds and beans. Just be sure they have been grown organically (that is, they have not been treated with any chemical fungicides, herbicides, or pesticides, or chemical fertilizers that might inhibit growth or be toxic to you). Most seeds can be sprouted in the same way as alfalfa sprouts, although bigger seeds and beans (such as soybeans) will require a quart jar instead of a pint jar. It helps to store the seeds in a dark place with humidity that is not too cold. The cupboard under the kitchen sink is a good place. Be methodical about rinsing the seeds. If the water the beans are soaking in begins to bubble, that means the beans have been soaking for too long and fermentation has begun (toss these and start again).

What other seeds and beans can you try? Mustard seeds, soybeans, sunflower seeds, chia seeds, lima beans, fava beans, wheat kernels, rye kernels, and lentils are all good possibilities. Be creative.

11

Herbs
and Spices

The goal of the RealAge kitchen is to help you create great-tasting food that makes your arteries and immune system younger. In no way does a kitchen do this better than by having herbs and spices on hand. They accentuate food perfectly, turning merely "okay" dishes into truly delicious ones. Also, substituting the exciting taste of an herb for that of aging fat or a lot of salt is a smart way to make your RealAge younger while earning the title of great chef. This chapter shows some of the common and not-so-common combinations of herbs and spices that will make your dishes taste fabulous. Some of these herbs and spices are ones you can grow, which can enhance your pleasure, thus making your RealAge younger in two ways. But learning how to use herbs and spices to substitute for immune-system and artery-aging fats is the first step. Here's how.

A RealAge-smart kitchen isn't complete without herbs and spices. Herbs have been used for centuries for culinary and medicinal purposes. Chervil has a well-known association with French cuisine. Garlic is best known for its use in Mediterranean foods, and curry powder will suggest a Thai or an Indian flavor. While an herb is a leaf, a spice is usually a berry, seed, root, flower, stem, or pod. Sometimes we use both from the same plant. For example, I use the leaf (herb) from Chinese parsley (which is called cilantro) and the seed (spice) from the same plant (which is called coriander). They are wonderful together or apart, in the same dish or in separate dishes!

Fresh herbs are usually used at the end of cooking or as a garnish. Choose fresh herbs that have a bright color and firm leaves. Fresh herbs should be washed in cold water and blotted dry. To store herbs, cut ½ to 1 inch from the end of the stems and place them in a glass of water in the refrigerator. You can also store the leaves rolled in a moist paper towel in the vegetable compartment of your refrigerator. They should stay fresh for about five days. We hope you'll be using them frequently in your RealAge kitchen—any leftovers can be quickly chopped and frozen. We think herbs are key to making RealAge food taste fabulous.

Herbs can be dried for later use or for decoration. Just tie small bunches together and place them upside down in a paper bag that has been punctured with holes. The top of the bag should be tied tight and hung in a warm, airy place. (The bag prevents light from ruining the leaves and catches the leaves that drop.) Dried herbs are more potent than fresh herbs and generally (but not always) should be added at the beginning of cooking.

Store dried spices and herbs in airtight glass containers in a cool, dry place. They should last about six months. The general rule for substituting fresh herbs and dried herbs in a recipe is to use ½ teaspoon of ground dried herbs or 1 teaspoon of dried leaves for every 1 tablespoon of finely chopped fresh herb required. Buy just enough dried herbs for a six-month supply—usually found in a small jar or tin in the supermarket. (The bigger containers may look like a better value, but they're not if the herbs and spices are kept too long and go stale.)

Three Good Rules for Herbs and Spices

Here are three good, general rules regarding the use of herbs and spices in food. Using any of them adds to your *Kitchen IQ points*.

- **Herbs are best fresh; spices are best dried** (1 Kitchen IQ point). If you can find an herb fresh, use it. If you can find spices dried, use them.

- **Use the memory aids "Fresh-quick-fresh" and "Dried-slow-dried"** (1 Kitchen IQ point). If your food is fresh and cooked only briefly, use fresh herbs. If your food started out as dried (from beans and legumes, for example) or is to cook for more than a few minutes, use dried herbs and spices.

- **More of the same color is better.** If you have more than one herb or spice of the same color, and want to use them both, go ahead and try. Often herbs or spices of the same color complement each other and make the dish taste even better.

Growing Your Own Herbs

If you have considered a vegetable garden but don't have the space or don't feel up to the challenge, by all means try growing herbs. Herbs and spices are relatively easy to grow—many started out as weeds that were tasted by a few brave souls. After none of these testers became seriously ill, the herbs worked their way into cooking.

You can keep an herb garden and fresh herbs always at hand for cooking with just a small amount of space, such as an interior windowsill. Herbs do well in almost any soil, and take few nutrients from the soil. Although an inside kitchen windowsill may seem like the easiest place for a potted herb or two, keep an eye on it; some herbs wilt with the heat of the kitchen and would rather be outdoors.

As with any indoor plant, you must guard against overwatering. Soak the herbs once or twice a week and make sure the pots have good drainage. If you live in an arid climate, you might also want to mist the leaves. Putting the pots outside during the summer helps the plants become hardy and extends their lives. Many herbs are annuals, and must be planted anew each year. All of the following are excellent candidates for an indoor herb garden: basil, coriander, thyme, rosemary, and sage. Almost all fresh herbs freeze well. Just cut whole sprigs and wrap them tightly in a double layer of plastic wrap.

The RealAge Herb and Spice Chart

The following chart shows the herbs and spices we keep on our shelves and use in our recipes. We have suggested pairings for each herb and spice. Sometimes we've suggested alternatives: you may want a related but slightly different flavor, or, you may need a substitute. These are some favorites, but feel free to experiment with others. Expand your horizons and start making food more exciting and flavorful.

Herb or Spice	Characteristics	Soups, Stews	Fruits, Salads, Vegetables	Breads, Desserts Whole Grains	Sauces, Oils, Drinks, Misc.	Meat, Fish, or Other
Allspice	Allspice is a berry native to the West Indies and South America. Its flavor is a mixture of cinnamon, clove, juniper berry, and nutmeg. Although allspice is available as whole or ground berries, we recommend grinding whole berries as needed, for more potent flavor. *Alternative:* Equal parts clove, cinnamon, and nutmeg.	Consommé; bean, fish, tomato.	*Salads:* Tofu, mushroom, pasta. *Vegetables:* Beets, black beans, carrots, parsnips, peas, spinach, sweet potatoes, turnips.	*Breads:* Quick breads, stuffing. *Desserts:* Baked apples, chocolate, fruit, gingerbread, pumpkin, spice cakes. *Whole grains:* Bulgur, couscous, polenta, rice.	Barbecue, chocolate, meat, or tomato sauces.	Tofu, legumes, poached fish, turkey.
Basil	Basil tastes like a hint of orange zest; it also comes in scented varieties (lemon, cinnamon, and licorice). Basil often accompanies tomatoes, complements the flavor of garlic, and is a key ingredient in pesto. Basil is pungent, and the flavor tends to become stronger as cooked. It is available fresh or dried but use fresh, as dried basil lacks the aromatic quality of the fresh. *Alternative:* Mint with a little marjoram or lemon verbena.	Bean or tomato soups or stews.	*Fruit:* Peaches. *Vegetables:* Most summer vegetables, asparagus, beets, cabbage, celery, cucumbers, eggplant, mushrooms, onion, peas, potatoes, spinach, squash, rutabaga, tomatoes.	*Breads:* Cheese bread, corn bread, muffins, stuffing. *Whole grains:* Couscous, pasta, polenta.	Marinades, oils, pesto, vinegars.	Beans, fish (halibut, mackerel, salmon, tuna), tofu, legumes.

Herb or Spice	Characteristics	Soups, Stews	Fruits, Salads, Vegetables	Breads, Desserts Whole Grains	Sauces, Oils, Drinks, Misc.	Meat, Fish, or Other
Bay leaf	Bay leaves have a pungent and deep flavor. They are needed for stews and soups to create a strong base flavor. This is one herb that is usually found dried rather than fresh. Bay leaves should be added early in the cooking process and, if you like, left in while serving. Use one bay leaf per quart of liquid. *Alternative:* Thyme.	Most soups and stews.	*Vegetables:* Artichokes, beets, carrots, potatoes, tomatoes.	*Breads:* Stuffing. *Whole grains:* Store a leaf or two in a jar of rice to add flavor.	Marinades, vinegars.	Tofu, legumes, beans, poached fish.
Caraway seeds	Caraway seeds have a nutty, licorice-like flavor. They are widely used in German and Austrian foods and are a good accompaniment for winter vegetables.	Bean, cabbage, potato, or tomato soups or stews.	*Salads:* Coleslaw, cucumber, potato, tomato. *Vegetables:* Beets, cabbage, carrots, celery, cucumbers, onions, potatoes, sauerkraut, turnips, winter squash.	*Breads:* Rye, pumpernickel. *Desserts:* Apple pie and spice cake and cookies. *Whole grains:* Noodles.	Cheese sauces, salad dressings, tomato sauces.	Beans, legumes, sausage.
Cardamom	Cardamom has a spicy, lemon-ginger flavor that goes well with fall vegetables. It is available in whole pod or ground seed. Once ground, cardamom quickly loses its flavor, so grind it right before use. *Alternative:* Cinnamon or cloves.	Bean or pea soups or stews.	*Salads:* Melon, pasta, whole grain, bulgur, brown rice. *Vegetables:* Carrots, pumpkin, squash, sweet potatoes.	*Breads:* Cheese bread. *Desserts:* Baked apples, fruit, ices, and spice cake and cookies. *Whole grains:* Bulgur, couscous, noodles, polenta, rice.	Barbecue sauces, relishes.	Lentils, beans, sausage.

Herb or Spice	Characteristics	Soups, Stews	Fruits, Salads, Vegetables	Breads, Desserts Whole Grains	Sauces, Oils, Drinks, Misc.	Meat, Fish, or Other
Cayenne pepper	Cayenne pepper, also known as red pepper, is made from a variety of chiles. Add cayenne pepper to main and side dishes for an extra kick.	Chili; bean, tomato, potato, or vegetable soups or stews	*Vegetables:* Beans, cabbage, carrots, cucumbers, green beans, greens, lima beans, potatoes, spinach.	*Whole grains:* Pasta, polenta, rice.	Barbecue, cheese, meat, or chili sauces; curries; mustards; salsas.	Beans, tofu, most fish and shellfish, legumes, poultry.
Chervil	Chervil has a hint of anise and parsley. It is an indispensable herb in French cuisine and is suitable anywhere parsley is called for. It is available fresh or dried. Chervil is also part of *fines herbes* (a mixture of chives, parsley, tarragon, and chervil), which goes well with sautéed vegetables. *Alternative:* Parsley and chopped fennel greens.	Potato or vegetable soups or stews.	*Salads:* Egg, fruit, tuna. *Vegetables:* Asparagus, beets, carrots, eggplant, peas, spinach, tomatoes.	*Whole grains:* Bulgur, couscous, polenta, rice.	Butter sauces, vinegars.	Beans, tofu, egg, all fish and shellfish, legumes.
Chili powder	Chili powder is a commercial mixture of dried chiles, garlic, oregano, cumin, coriander, and cloves. Chili powder is used frequently in, of course, chili, but not authentic Mexican or Thai food. Avoid chili powder that is mostly salt. True chili powder is simply ground dried chiles.	Chili; bean, tomato, or vegetable soups or stews.	*Salads:* Bean, egg, mixed vegetable. *Vegetables:* Corn, eggplant, tomatoes.	*Breads:* Savory breads, stuffing. *Whole grains:* Pasta, polenta, rice.	Barbecue, cheese, meat, or chili sauces; marinades.	Beans, tofu, most fish and shellfish, legumes, sausage, turkey.
Chives	Chives have a mild onion flavor. Cut them close to serving time so they don't lose their crispness. Use	Broth-based or vegetable soups or stews.	*Salads:* Mixed green. *Vegetables:* Asparagus,	*Whole grains:* Couscous, basmati rice.	Blend chives with cream cheese or yogurt or	Many egg white dishes (omelets, scrambled

Herb or Spice	Characteristics	Soups, Stews	Fruits, Salads, Vegetables	Breads, Desserts Whole Grains	Sauces, Oils, Drinks, Misc.	Meat, Fish, or Other
	them in any dish you would use onion, and whenever you want a dash of color. *Alternative:* Scallion tops.		cauliflower, potatoes, tomatoes.		cheese, or sprinkle chives on baked potatoes.	eggs); fish and shellfish.
Cilantro	Cilantro is the leaf of Chinese parsley. It has been described as a mix of orange peel and sage. It pairs well with highly spiced foods. *Alternative:* For shape, flat-leaf parsley; and for flavor, spicy basil.	Most soups.	*Salads:* Fruit, rice, corn.	*Whole grains:* Couscous, noodles, rice.	Guacamole, salsas.	Beans, legumes, poultry.
Cinnamon	Although cinnamon is best known for its use in sweet foods, it also adds an exotic sweet-spicy flavor to meats and stews. Cinnamon is available in whole sticks or ground. *Alternative:* Canela (not true cinnamon, but tree bark all the same, and milder and softer than Indonesian cinnamon).	Bean or tofu soups or stews.	*Salads:* Fruit. *Vegetables:* Beets, carrots, lentils, onions, pumpkin, squash, sweet potatoes.	*Breads:* Quick breads. *Desserts:* Most desserts—cakes, compotes, cookies, fruit, and puddings. *Whole grains:* Bulgur, couscous, rice.	Chutneys; marinades; tea, cider, coffee, eggnog, hot chocolate, mulled wine.	Tofu, beans, legumes.
Cloves	Cloves have a deep, minty flavor and are used to season savory and sweet dishes. They are available whole or ground. Put a few cloves in an onion and simmer it in soups.	Bean, tofu, onion, or potato soups or stews.	*Salads:* Fruit. *Vegetables:* Beets, baked beans, carrots, squash, sweet potatoes.	*Breads:* Quick breads. *Desserts:* Chocolate, fruit, gingerbread, pumpkin, and spice cakes and cookies. *Whole grains:* Polenta.	Chutneys; jams; marinades; mulled wine, cider, hot chocolate.	Tofu, legumes.
Coriander	Coriander is known for its seeds (coriander) and leaves (cilantro); they do not resemble each other	Stocks; tofu or pea soups or stews.	*Vegetables:* Beets, cauliflower, onions,	*Whole grains:* Couscous, polenta, rice.	Cheese, chocolate, or fruit sauces; mulled wine.	Beans, tofu, legumes, sausage (even

Herb or Spice	Characteristics	Soups, Stews	Fruits, Salads, Vegetables	Breads, Desserts Whole Grains	Sauces, Oils, Drinks, Misc.	Meat, Fish, or Other
	in flavor. The seeds have a lemon-orange flavor, a little like curry, of which they are a component.		potatoes, spinach, tomatoes.			turkey sausage).
Cumin	Cumin, a member of the parsley family, is shaped like a fennel seed. There are at least three types of cumin: amber, white, and black. The first two are interchangeable, but black is more peppery in taste. Available in whole or ground seed.	Chili; bean, carrot, tofu, or vegetable soups or stews.	*Vegetables:* Cabbage, lentils, pumpkin, tomatoes.	*Desserts:* Fruit pies. *Whole grains:* Rice.	Barbecue, meat, fish, or tomato sauces or marinades.	Beans, tofu, fish (halibut, salmon, tuna) and shellfish, legumes.
Curry powder	Curry powder has a distinct flavor and aroma. It is a blend of 20 pungent spices, herbs, and seeds and is widely used in Indian cooking.	Consommé; bean, tofu, pea, tomato, or vegetable soups or stews.	*Salads:* Tofu, egg, fruit, pasta, seafood, vegetable. *Vegetables:* Beets, black beans, carrots, sweet potatoes, turnips, winter squash.	*Breads:* Savory breads. *Whole grains:* Couscous, noodles, rice.	Chutneys, salad dressings.	Beans, tofu, eggs, most fish and shellfish, legumes, turkey.
Dill	Dill is slightly grassy, with a hint of caraway, aniseseed, and fennel. The seed, flower, and leaf are all used; seeds and leaves can be used interchangeably. A yogurt-dill sauce is a good accompaniment for fresh or grilled vegetables. *Alternative:* Caraway.	Bean, split pea, or tomato soups or stews.	*Salads:* Cucumber, potato. *Vegetables:* Asparagus, beets, Brussels sprouts, cabbage, green beans, peas, potatoes.	*Breads:* Savory breads. *Whole grains:* Couscous, pasta, polenta, rice.	Marinades and vinegars. Also, blend dill with cottage cheese, silken tofu, or part-skim ricotta for a sandwich filling. Use the flower for pickling.	Beans, tofu, eggs, most fish and shellfish.
Epazote (worm-seed)	Epazote is a magical love-it-or-hate-it herb from Mexico. It grows without restraint, has tiny seeds	Bean or legume soups or stews, like hominy.	*Salads:* Jicama, cucumber, tomato.	Corn bread.	Cook epazote with beans of all kinds and then blend	Beans, legumes, eggs.

Herb or Spice	Characteristics	Soups, Stews	Fruits, Salads, Vegetables	Breads, Desserts Whole Grains	Sauces, Oils, Drinks, Misc.	Meat, Fish, or Other
	that are intensely flavorful (pungent), and is available both fresh and dried at specialty markets. It is best fresh, and a little goes a long way. You will get some of its flavor from dried leaves, although we don't recommend cooking with them, except in pots of black and Anasazi and pinto beans, where epazote shines, fresh or dried.				them with garlic and chile for a dip. Mince a little into fresh tomato or tomatillo salsas.	
Fennel	Fennel leaves have a fragrant anise seed flavor. There are two types of fennel: Florence (bulbing) and common. Common fennel, the type most used in the U.S., has oval seeds. The seeds have a more concentrated flavor than the leaf and flower. Fennel makes an interesting substitute for celery as a cooked and raw vegetable. *Alternative:* Dill or caraway.	Minestrone; cabbage, fish, meat, potato, or tomato soups or stews.	*Salads:* Bean salads, coleslaw. *Vegetables:* Cabbage, cucumber, onions, peas, sauerkraut, ratatouille, summer squash.	*Breads:* Savory breads, pizzas. *Desserts:* Fruit dishes with apples and pears, pumpkin, and spice cake and cookies. *Whole grains:* Pasta, polenta, rice.	Marinades, oils, vinegars.	Beans, tofu, legumes, chicken, sausage.
Garam masala	Like curry, garam masala is a pungent and aromatic mixture of spices. In India, the mixture varies from region to region. It can be spicy or mild, hot or sweet. Usually it does not contain salt.	All kinds of soups and stews, from summer squash to red wine and bean-based.	For almost all vegetables, garam masala is cooked with, instead of sprinkled on, the vegetable.	*Whole grains:* For rice, bulgur, and couscous, an exciting change from curry.		Beans, legumes, eggs, fish, shellfish.
Garlic	Garlic is very strong, so use it sparingly. For many	Garlic gives a strong flavor	Almost all vegetables.	*Whole grains:* Almost all	Oil, pesto, marinades,	Tofu, most fish and shellfish,

Herb or Spice	Characteristics	Soups, Stews	Fruits, Salads, Vegetables	Breads, Desserts Whole Grains	Sauces, Oils, Drinks, Misc.	Meat, Fish, or Other
	dishes, one fresh, uncooked clove is sufficient. Roast garlic for a sweeter taste, and use it as a spread.	to most stews and soups.		pastas and grains. As a spread on bread.	vinegars, wine sauces, salsas.	meats, legumes.
Ginger	Ginger has a fresh, distinct, bright, slightly sharp flavor.	Bean, tofu, fish, or tomato soups, stir-fries or stews.	*Salads:* Tofu, fruit, pasta, rice, shrimp. *Vegetables:* Cabbage, carrots, lentils, squash.	*Breads:* Gingerbread, quick breads. *Desserts:* Cookies, cakes. *Whole grains:* Polenta, rice.	Chutneys; cheese, chocolate, or fruit sauces; marinades; salsas; hot chocolate. Combine ginger, sesame oil, garlic, brown sugar, soy sauce, and red pepper flakes for a marinade.	Beans, tofu, legumes, most fish and shellfish.
Lemon balm	Lemon balm, or sweet balm, has a fresh, delicate, lemon fragrance and flavor. Mince and freeze in ice cubes, and add to drinks. Lemon balm is a good addition to mixed green salads.	Light broth-based soups and stews.	*Vegetables:* Asparagus.	*Desserts:* Custards, ice cream.	Marinades; vinegars; fruit drinks, herbal teas, wine cups.	Fish, shellfish, most poultry, legumes.
Lemon-grass	Lemongrass is widely used in Asian cooking. It adds a nice flavor to light soups and is available fresh or dried.	Light, broth-based soups and stews.	*Salads:* Mixed green salads.	*Desserts:* Sorbet, gelée.	Herbal teas.	Poultry.
Lemon verbena	Lemon verbena has a delicate, distinct lemon flavor and taste. Use several leaves: it's elegant and a nice surprise. Use it fresh, not dried. *Alternative:* Lemongrass or lemon zest.	Gazpacho.	*Salads:* Fruit, mixed green salads. *Vegetables:* Asparagus.	*Desserts:* Ice cream, sherbet, sorbet.	Fruit drinks, herbal teas, punch.	Shellfish.

Herb or Spice	Characteristics	Soups, Stews	Fruits, Salads, Vegetables	Breads, Desserts Whole Grains	Sauces, Oils, Drinks, Misc.	Meat, Fish, or Other
Lovage	Lovage has a celery flavor but is a bit spicier and licorice-like. It is often used as a celery substitute. The leaves are used for seasoning, and the stalk is eaten like celery. Add it to potatoes and corn for a different twist. Use it fresh. *Alternative:* Celery or celery leaves and flat-leaf parsley.	Meat broths, vegetable soups or stews.	*Salads:* Mixed green salads. *Vegetables:* Corn, potatoes, tomatoes.	Tabouleh.	Marinades.	Most fish and shellfish, and poultry.
Mace	Mace is the membrane that covers nutmeg, and therefore tastes and smells similar to nutmeg. Mace adds a wonderful taste to cakes. It is not as sharp, and is almost always available dried and ground. *Alternative:* Nutmeg.	Tomato-based soups.	*Vegetables:* Beans, broccoli, Brussels sprouts, cabbage, green beans, lentils, spinach.	*Breads:* Quick breads. *Desserts:* Fruit, chocolate, and spice cakes and cookies. *Whole grains:* Noodles, polenta, rice.	Chutneys, mulled wine, eggnog.	Beans, tofu, legumes, sausage, shellfish.
Marjoram	Marjoram is often confused with oregano because of the similar flavor. Marjoram is milder and less spicy. Of the many species, the most common in America is sweet marjoram, which is referred to simply as marjoram. It is a sweet summer herb with a distinctive savory flavor. The leaves are used fresh or dried—both work well. *Alternative:* Sweet basil or mint.	Bean or tofu soups or stews.	*Salads:* Egg, fruit, mixed green salads. *Vegetables:* Brussels sprouts, cabbage, carrots, celery, corn, eggplant, green beans, peas, potatoes, spinach, summer squash, tomatoes, potatoes.	*Breads:* Savory breads, Bruschetta, French toast. *Whole grains:* Bulgur, noodles, rice (especially for stuffed green and red peppers).	Oils, vinegars.	Tofu, most fish and shellfish.

Herb or Spice	Characteristics	Soups, Stews	Fruits, Salads, Vegetables	Breads, Desserts Whole Grains	Sauces, Oils, Drinks, Misc.	Meat, Fish, or Other
Mint	Of the many varieties of mint, peppermint and spearmint are the most common. Mint is a sweet, fresh, aromatic herb. The leaves are used fresh or dried. Mint is also often used as a garnish for drinks and desserts. (Although both dried and fresh are used, fresh is far preferable.)	Lentil or pea soups or stews.	*Salads:* Cucumber, fruit, mixed green salads. *Vegetables:* Cabbage, carrots, celery, corn, green beans, lentils, peas, potatoes, spinach, summer squash, tomatoes.	*Desserts:* Chocolate cakes, rich desserts.	Mint sauce, oils, salad dressings, salsas, vinegars.	Tofu, fish, legumes.
Mustard	Mustard seed has a pleasantly bitter, sharp taste and, when ground, is used to thicken and flavor sauces. A mustard-based sauce complements cauliflower and broccoli nicely.	Bean, potato, or sorrel soups or stews.	*Salads:* Egg, meat, mixed green, and potato salads. *Vegetables:* Beans, beets, broccoli, Brussels sprouts, cabbage, cauliflower, cucumbers, green beans, potatoes.	*Breads:* Cheese breads. *Whole grains:* Polenta.	Chutneys, relishes, marinades, salad dressings, sauces.	Beans, poultry, tofu, eggs, most fish and shellfish, legumes.
Nutmeg	Nutmeg is often used as a topping for eggnog. It has a delicate, warm spicy flavor. Try it in pancakes or French toast for a spicy flavor. Try to buy whole nutmegs: they last forever, grate easily, and have much better flavor than ground nutmeg.	Bean, black bean, tofu, pea, potato, squash, or tomato soups or stews.	*Vegetables:* Potatoes, spinach, squash.	*Desserts:* Chocolate, custard, fruit, gingerbread, pie, pumpkin, and spice cake and cookies. *Whole grains:* Bulgur, couscous, polenta, rice.	Cheese and chocolate sauces; chutneys; marinades; coffee, eggnog, mulled wine.	Beans, tofu, legumes, turkey.

Herb or Spice	Characteristics	Soups, Stews	Fruits, Salads, Vegetables	Breads, Desserts Whole Grains	Sauces, Oils, Drinks, Misc.	Meat, Fish, or Other
Oregano	Oregano, a member of the mint family, is commonly used in Greek foods with lemon. Oregano is similar to marjoram but is not as sweet, and has a sharper flavor and aroma. The leaves are used fresh or dried: Both work well, for different purposes. *Alternative:* Marjoram.	Chili; minestrone; bean, lentil, onion, or tomato soups or stews.	*Salads:* Bean, egg, potato. *Vegetables:* Broccoli, cabbage, green beans, potatoes, tomatoes.	*Breads:* Rolls, stuffing. *Whole grains:* Pasta, pizza (Italian foods), polenta, rice.	Salad dressings, oils, vinegars, salsas.	Beans, tofu, most fish and shellfish, turkey.
Paprika	Paprika is a dried red pepper. There are a few types, but Hungarian paprika has the best flavor, sweet or hot. Try both, in small quantities. *Alternative:* Ground red pepper (cayenne) in smaller amounts.	Bean, meat, or vegetable soups or stews.	*Salads:* Can be used as a garnish for almost any salad. *Vegetables:* Goes well with almost any vegetable.	Almost all pastas, grains, rice.	Almost any sauce, spread, salad dressing, or salsa.	Beans, tofu, eggs, fish, turkey.
Parsley	Parsley has a mild, peppery flavor and is used frequently as a garnish. Parsley is very versatile and goes with almost any dish. The most common parsley used in the U.S. is curly-leaf parsley. Whenever you can, buy flat-leaf (Italian) parsley fresh: the flavor is cleaner. The leaves are used fresh or dried, and parsley freezes well. After a meal, for fresh breath, chew the parsley garnish.	Almost all soups and stews.	*Salads:* Egg, mixed green, and potato salads; tabouleh. *Vegetables:* Cabbage, carrots, lentils, peas, potatoes, tomatoes.	*Breads:* Bruschetta, crostini, stuffing. *Whole grains:* Almost all pastas and grains.	Chimichurri. Also, with minced garlic and lemon zest as a garnish. Addition to pesto, with sweet basil.	Beans, tofu, fish, and shellfish.
Pepper	Pepper is a very versatile spice and goes with almost any dish. It is available in black or	Almost all soups and stews.	*Salads:* Almost all salads. *Vegetables:* Almost all	*Breads:* Stuffing. *Whole grains:* Most pastas	Marinades, salad dressings, tomato juice.	Most fish and shellfish, meats, poultry.

Herb or Spice	Characteristics	Soups, Stews	Fruits, Salads, Vegetables	Breads, Desserts Whole Grains	Sauces, Oils, Drinks, Misc.	Meat, Fish, or Other
	white. Black is more rich and pungent than white, which is slightly hot. Available whole or ground. Buy whole peppercorns and grind them in a pepper mill as needed. White pepper can be used in sauces when you don't want black flecks to appear, or when you want more heat.		vegetables.	and grains.		
Rosemary	Rosemary is a strong, aromatic herb. The flavor can be described as pine mixed with mint. The leaves are used fresh or dried. *Alternative:* Oregano or sweet basil leaves, because of their pungent flavor.	Tofu, fish, pea, potato, or spinach soups or stews.	*Salads:* Fruit. *Vegetables:* Green beans, white beans, peas, potatoes, salt potatoes.	*Breads:* Stuffing. *Whole grains:* Polenta, rice.	Marinades, oils, vinegars, spreads (try with roasted shallots and Gorgonzola).	Beans, most fish and shellfish, chicken, tofu, legumes.
Saffron	Saffron is an expensive spice because it must be harvested by hand from crocus flowers. You don't need much for great sunrise color and exotic flavor. Generally, the deeper the reddish-brown color, the finer the quality. Buy whole saffron, not ground or mixed with other herbs, and keep it in a tightly covered container in a cool, dark place. *Alternative:* Turmeric can provide some of the color and perfume of saffron.	Bouillabaisse; tofu, fish, paella, tomato soups or stews.	*Salads:* Tofu, egg, pasta, seafood, tomato. *Vegetables:* Carrots, corn, green beans, onions, potatoes, tomatoes, winter squash.	*Breads:* Savory and quick breads. *Desserts:* Cakes and cookies. *Whole grains:* Bulgur, couscous, noodles, polenta, rice, grain dishes.	Marinades, mayonnaise, relishes, vinegars.	Beans, tofu, legumes, most fish and shellfish (especially paella).

Herb or Spice	Characteristics	Soups, Stews	Fruits, Salads, Vegetables	Breads, Desserts Whole Grains	Sauces, Oils, Drinks, Misc.	Meat, Fish, or Other
Sage	Sage has a smoky, musky flavor and is used in stuffings. The leaves and flower are used fresh or dried. *Alternative:* Summer savory or thyme.	Chowders; minestrone; tofu, legume, or potato soups or stews.	*Vegetables:* Asparagus, Brussels sprouts, corn, green beans, tomatoes.	*Breads:* Stuffing.	Sauces for fish; vinegars.	Legumes, most fish and shellfish, sausage.
Savory	Savory has two varieties: summer and winter. Summer savory has a milder taste, but both have a strong flavor—a mix of thyme and mint. Savory is so frequently used with beans, its nickname is "the bean herb." The leaves are used fresh or dried. *Alternative:* Sweet marjoram.	Consommé; lentil, pea, potato, tomato, or vegetable soups or stews.	*Salads:* Bean, tofu, mixed green, potato, tuna. *Vegetables:* Artichokes, asparagus, Brussels sprouts, cabbage, green beans, lentils, peas, potatoes, tomatoes.	*Whole grains:* Almost all grains and pastas.	Most gravies and sauces, marinades, vinegars.	Beans, fish and shellfish, tofu, legumes, most poultry.
Sesame seeds	Sesame seeds have a nutty, slightly sweet flavor. They, too, come in white and black; the taste difference is subtle, but the color contrast is terrific. Toast them to bring out their flavor.	As a garnish for many soups with a dark color, especially vegetable-based.	*Salads:* Tofu, mixed green, potato, tomato. *Vegetables:* Beans, carrots, corn, eggplant, green beans, spinach.	*Breads:* Breads, rolls. *Desserts:* Cakes, cookies. *Whole grains:* Noodles.	Hummus as a dip; garnish for sautéed greens.	Beans, tofu, legumes.
Sorrel	Sorrel is an acidic, lemony herb that intensifies in flavor as it is cooked. It adds the perfect flavor to eggs and potatoes, or mixed as part of mesclun. Use it in split pea soup for a fresh flavor. Buy it fresh only.	Cream-based, pea, or vegetable soups or stews.	*Salads:* Mixed green salads. *Vegetables:* Lentils, parsnips, potatoes, spinach. Also, sorrel can be cooked as a vegetable, like spinach.	*Breads:* Savory breads.	Addition to pesto; infused vinegar.	Eggs, tofu, legumes.

Covering All the Bases

Many people avoid a vegetarian diet because they're afraid they won't get all the nutrients they need. It's true that if you're not eating meat, you will need to pay special attention to your intake of vitamins, amino acids, and minerals. However, this can be accomplished quite simply with delicious foods, and taking the right vitamins and minerals at the right times. If you eat lots of whole grains (such as wheat and oats and brown rice) and lots of soy (or fish and low-fat dairy products), you'll almost certainly be fine. But for optimum intake of vitamins—to slow aging, not just to avoid deficiency disease—you'll almost certainly need a multivitamin twice a day.

Getting enough protein is another common concern. Salmon, soy burgers, low-fat dairy products, and many legumes such as lima and kidney beans are all delicious and great sources of protein. If you also include fortified breakfast cereals, spinach, raisins, and other nutrient-rich foods, you'll be making yourself younger while meeting your dietary needs.

Because meat contains zinc, iron, vitamin B_6, and vitamin B_{12}, if you're not eating meat, make sure you're getting these nutrients in other foods or in your vitamins. Wheat germ, wheat bran, crab, tofu, sunflower seeds, almonds, and tuna all contain zinc. Whole grains, nuts, and legumes contain vitamin B_6. In addition, vitamin B_6 can be found in peanut butter, green beans, bananas, artichokes, and whole wheat spaghetti. Salmon, shrimp, nonfat yogurt, and eggs all contain vitamin B_{12}.

If you're getting your protein mainly through nonmeat foods, eat a wide variety so you make the most of the nutrients these foods do offer. Strict vegetarians or vegans who eat no meat whatsoever should consult a physician and a dietitian to ensure they're getting all the nutrients they need. Taking daily multivitamins can also help make your RealAge younger and provide the energy you desire. Since antioxidant vitamins usually become pro-oxidant, taking too much, or taking the vitamins like C all at one time, may not make your RealAge as young as taking one-half your vitamins twice a day.

Multivitamins to Hit the RealAge Optimum

When you shop for a multivitamin, the first thing to do is read the label. The multivitamin should have the usual DVs of the vitamins and minerals we've talked about. Then you need to supplement that amount so that you reach the RAOs for each vitamin and mineral listed below. The vitamins are sequential from A through F. Then you have to remember four minerals (sorry, there's no shortcut). Just photocopy this list and take it with you when you go to buy your multi.

A	More than 5,000 IU is too much (even as beta-carotene, keep your total from non-food sources low)
B_6	4 mg a day
B_{12}	800 mcg a day
C	400 mg × 3 (remember it's water soluble, so you need several doses over the day), or 1,200 mg a day
D	600 IU a day
E	400 or 800 IU a day (some would say that mixed tocopherols are better than the usual "E" provided— the synthetic alpha tocopherol)
F (folate)	800 mcg a day (folic acid or folate, or folicin is sometimes listed as vitamin B_9)
Calcium	1,200 mg a day in divided doses (1,600 mg for women). You cannot absorb more than 600 mg at a time.
Magnesium	400 mg a day
Selenium	200 mcg a day
Potassium	Four fruits plus a normal diet should do it
Lycopene	10 tablespoons of tomato sauce a week should do it.
Lutein	A leafy green vegetable a day should do it
Iron	At a different time, if at all. Recommend none if you are not a vegetarian or a female in the menstruating years; for all menstruating females, 15mg a day (30 mg if you are trying to get pregnant or are pregnant); if female or vegetarian, you can obtain a yearly test for

your hematocrit and hemoglobin levels to see if you need iron supplementation. Take iron at a time separated by at least 2 hours from the time you take calcium and vitamin C.

If you take a statin drug such as prevastatin, lovastatin, atorvastatin (Lipitor), or others, the data is beginning to indicate you might want to take only 50 mg of vitamin C, 50 IU of vitamin E, and add 100 mg coenzyme Q-10, all twice a day.

Before you go to purchase your vitamins, check your cupboard and evaluate what you already have. Check expiration dates. Throw away the vitamins that contain more than you need in one day. If you're worried about arterial aging, make sure you get the antioxidant vitamins E and C and the homocysteine-lowering folate, as well as lutein and lycopene. If you're concerned about osteoporosis, arthritis, or immune aging, pay careful attention to your intake of calcium, magnesium, selenium, lycopene, and vitamins B_6, B_{12}, and D, and avoid excesses of vitamin A.

Organic versus Nonorganic Foods

Organic foods are understood to be grown without artificial chemical fertilizers, herbicides, fungicides, or pesticides, but today no standard inspection system exists to assure the consumer that these criteria are being met. With the recent (late 2002) final ruling from the U.S. government mandating a single, national standard for certification of "organic" foods, the coming years will be a better time than ever to buy organic foods. Of course, whether or not to spend the extra money for organic foods is each person's decision. The argument in favor of doing so is compelling, and consists of five major assertions:

1. Organic food is more nutritious. What has been long suspected is finally being proven: organic produce is more nutritious than its nonorganic counterparts. As reported in the *Journal of Alternative and Complementary Medicine* (2001), a review of forty-one studies comparing the vitamin and mineral content of organic versus nonorganic foods showed that, in the vast majority of cases, organic foods contained higher levels of vitamins and minerals, particularly magnesium (29% more), vitamin C (27% more), and iron (21% more).

2. Production of organic foods involves more humane treatment of animals.
Organically raised livestock must be allowed access to pasture. By contrast, many
nonorganically raised chickens are caged, sometimes in tiny spaces, and their feet never
once touch the ground during their lifetime. In addition, organically raised livestock
are not given growth hormones. Although the effects of these hormonal growth pro-
moters on the consuming public have not yet been proven, it's easy to imagine why it's
best to avoid added hormones.

3. Organic foods taste better. Many people believe that, across the board, organic
vegetables and fruits are more flavorful, fragrant, and delicious than nonorganic foods.
If you really want your dishes to pack a big flavor punch, using organic ingredients (for
example, organic berries in a smoothie) may be your best bet.

4. Organic foods are grown with less use of pesticides. Instead of blasting crops
with chemical pesticides, fungicides, and herbicides, organic farmers use methods such
as crop rotation, companion planting, enriching cover crops, and the introduction of
beneficial insects to keep crops healthy. Organic farmers are barred from using processed sewage as fertilizer and, instead, use compost.

Fruits and vegetables vary in the amount of pesticide they retain. So, it's a good
investment to buy organic versions of the conventional produce with the most pesticide residue. According to the Environmental Working Group, using FDA and EPA
data, the following fruits and vegetables commonly contain the highest levels of pesticide residue: strawberries, bell peppers, spinach, cherries, peaches, Mexican cantaloupe, celery, apples, apricots, green beans, imported grapes, and cucumbers.

Strawberries and bell peppers top the list as retaining the very highest levels of pesticide and should therefore *always* be bought in their organic form. Remember to wash
all produce very well (a minimum of three times in warm water). If you can't get organic
versions of the above foods, substitute foods that commonly don't retain a lot of pesticide residue. These include avocados, corn, onions, sweet potatoes, cauliflower, Brussels
sprouts, grapes (U.S. grown), bananas, plums, green onions, watermelon, and broccoli.

5. Organic foods are better for the environment. Less use of pesticides is not only
better for us, it's better for the environment. In addition, organic farmers guard against
soil depletion, soil erosion, and many other environmental hazards that result from
nonorganic farming practices that do damage to our planet.

One reason people sometimes choose not to buy organic foods is, of course, a financial one. Organic foods are usually more expensive than nonorganic foods. However, like so many aspects of the RealAge lifestyle, buying pesticide-free, nutrient-rich organic food is an investment. Your own health and the well-being of the planet are at stake. Put another way, you can pay now or you can pay later. Since late October 2002, under the USDA's National Organic Program, all food purporting to be "organic" must be labeled in one of the following three ways:

1. "100% Organic": Certifies that the food contains only organic ingredients, with the exception of water and salt.

2. "Organic": Certifies that the food contains "at least" 95 percent organic ingredients, with the exception of water and salt.

3. "Made with Organic Ingredients": Foods that contain at least 70 percent organic ingredients. The remaining nonorganic ingredients cannot have been produced by means of certain prohibited methods, such as fertilization with sewage sludge or the inclusion of genetically engineered materials.

Buy Local, Eat Global, Think Fabulous Food

One way to increase taste, and perhaps ensure your food is organic, is to buy local. When you support your local farmers, you are helping your community while making yourself younger. Because of the freshness, you gain the same nutrients with even better taste. It's easy, too! A trip to a farmers' market is a delightful experience for your senses and can inspire you to try new vegetarian recipes. The aroma of fresh herbs and flowers fills the air, and bold, beautiful colors please the eye. A trip to the market can help you learn how always to make the place you eat a sensuous, special place. The market bustles with excited visitors looking for the ripest produce and the freshest herbs. There are so many sights to take in, you may not know where to start. To begin, walk around and survey the whole landscape. However, if the market is huge, like the one at Madison, Wisconsin, which stretches for more than half a mile, just plunge right in.

The Farmers' Market

Here's why you should shop at a farmers' market.

FOR FRESHNESS

For fruits and vegetables, time is of the essence. Some produce starts to lose sweetness the moment it leaves the plant. Some nutrients dissipate over time. A good source of vitamin C at the time of harvest may contain little vitamin C at the supermarket. So, the faster the food gets to you, the greater its potential for peak freshness and the more plentiful the vitamins and nutrients that keep your RealAge young.

Many national supermarket chains use local or even regional suppliers only infrequently. (The P & C and Wegmans supermarket chains are an exception: all their stores, I understand, have a section with local produce. The P & C where we teach a course for medical students about nutrition and cooking is truly fabulous.) Typically, produce often travels very far to reach you. Too often, produce (for example, bananas and most tomatoes) is picked green and then gassed to give the appearance of ripeness. To increase its moisture retention and shelf life at the supermarket, some produce is waxed. Apples and pears are sometimes held in storage for months before they reach you. Fruits you buy out of season—in February and March—definitely reflect storage: they don't have much flavor but may have a whole lot of great texture. While they still have great nutrients, that bland taste makes it harder for you to use them to make your RealAge younger. However, there are two solutions: freezing them when in season and eating them fresh in season.

Produce at a farmers' market is as fresh, or fresher, than produce in most supermarkets. Farmers and their families sell directly to you. Vegetables are crisp when they're supposed to be, and soft and tender when that's right, too. They're not gassed and they're not waxed. In flavor, they're head and shoulders above the produce in many supermarkets.

FOR ORGANIC METHODS

The farmers' market is a good place to shop for organic produce. If you choose carefully and ask the farmer, you can avoid synthetic chemical fungicides, pesticides, and herbicides. Some small farmers grow organically but cannot afford the USDA's labeling process.

For Savings

Produce at a farmers' market is often less expensive than equivalent produce in a supermarket because there's no middleman and no cost of storage, transportation, and marketing or merchandising.

For Information

Farmers are a great source of information. They can tell you how their fruit was grown, how the weather and pests have affected their crops, and what kinds of chemicals, if any, were used. They can also tell you if their soybeans, corn, and potatoes were genetically modified. Farmers can give tips on how to tell what's ripe and what's not. Often they'll even share their family recipes.

For Samples

Farmers very often let you sample foods before buying, a practice that's not usually welcome at the supermarket. Ask for samples of freshly baked bread, homemade blackberry jam, Mutsu apple, and Bartlett pear, or whatever is in season and you'd like to try.

To Support the Local Economy

When you buy locally, you're supporting your local farmers and the local economy.

Go to the farmers' market whenever possible, but if you can, get there early—within 30 minutes of opening. You'll avoid crowds (less stress keeps you young) and get the pick of the crops. Sometimes farmers bring only a small quantity of certain fruits, vegetables, and herbs, and this quantity doesn't last long. At a farmers' market, the early bird gets the best choices. Also, if the weather is hot, a morning visit is better, since it's cooler and the produce hasn't been sitting all day in the heat. If you can't make it in the morning and you're shopping for quantity, you can try to shop within 30 minutes of closing, when the farmers are packing up. Faced with hauling their goods home, they're more likely to give you a break on price.

We recommend you take your own cloth bags or a big, lightweight basket that has sturdy handles. Expandable net bags are also useful. Having your own bag means you won't have to juggle a lot of small bags. After you're done shopping, head right home *(4 Kitchen IQ points)*. Nothing ruins the quality of produce like the trunk of a car on a sweltering day. If you can't go home right away, pack your purchases in a cooler to keep them fresh. (A cooler is a great addition to any trip to a farmers' market.)

The produce is so inviting, you might be tempted to buy too much. The solution is have a list, but keep it flexible. Buy what you need, but don't pass up great items that aren't on your list—a new cress you've never tried, an unusual apricot you can smell from 10 feet away, or a huge bundle of purslane (a delicious cooking green that's high in omega-3 fatty acids) that's going for 50 cents a bunch. By all means, take advantage of these opportunities.

How do you find out if there's a farmers' market in your area? It's easy. Just go to the Web sites listed under "Internet Resources" at the back of this book.

Community-Supported Agriculture

Community-supported agriculture (CSA) is an exciting concept that might be of interest to you. It's a mutually beneficial relationship between local farmers and local consumers. Farmers provide fresh and nutritious food and, at the same time, protect the land. Consumers purchase shares in the farm, in return for in-season fruits and vegetables. So, the farmer grows the food while community members support the farm and share the harvest. Simple, huh?

Almost every state buys 85 to 90 percent of its food from either another state or another country. For example, most strawberries consumed in the United States are grown in California. How fresh can strawberries be if they have to be shipped to Michigan or Maine (both of which, by the way, have wonderful strawberries when they're in season)? New York State is another area where great juicy fruit and vegetables are grown, but because of mass-market techniques, these are rarely available to home-state consumers. Community-supported agriculture was developed, in part, to address these issues. Why purchase produce from afar when it can be grown locally and delivered at peak freshness and, at the same time, help the local economy?

The idea of community-supported agriculture arose almost thirty years ago in Japan. A group of people were tired of paying too much for imported produce. They had a little land—why shouldn't they farm for themselves? They started growing their own crops, calling the concept *teikei*—"putting the farmer's face on food." CSA farms then caught on in Europe, and the concept moved to the United States in the late 1970s. Today, there are almost a thousand CSA farms in North America.

How Do CSA Farms Come into Being?

CSA farms can start out as existing farms. They can also be established by land trusts, religious orders, food banks, and other institutions. In addition, CSA farms have been improvised by groups of consumers who have an interest in farming.

Here's one story about the start of a CSA farm. In the late 1960s, John Peterson took over his family's farm. However, overwhelmed by debt, he had to sell off much of the land. After dabbling in other careers for many years, he returned to the farm. He converted most of the land to CSA, began an internship program for prospective farmers, and started growing organic vegetables. Eventually he was able to form a group that purchased adjoining commercial land and converted it to farm use. By 2002 he had approximately eight hundred partner-customers in the Chicago area, with plans for future growth.

How Does a CSA Farm Work?

A farmer develops a budget showing what it would cost to run the farm for a year. The budget is divided by the number of people for whom the farm will supply food—each will receive a share. Consumers then purchase shares of the harvest, often a weekly supply from June through October, depending on locale. Some CSA farms offer winter supplies and some start as early as spring. Although some CSA farms ask their members to harvest the crops, or to pick up the crops after harvest, the usual arrangement is to deliver the harvest to the member.

Shareholders pay a single sum to belong to the CSA farm and receive crops in return. This yearly sum covers the cost of seed, labor, and other expenses in producing the crop. Some risk exists for both the shareholder and the farmer. If crops are destroyed or the weather isn't right, shareholders and farmers may not get the crops they had hoped for. If hornworms are plentiful, tomatoes may suffer. If it doesn't rain for two weeks, all the broccoli may wilt and suffer stunted growth. Nevertheless, a CSA farm can make the RealAge of your community younger.

Community-Supported Agriculture Has Many Benefits

CSA Brings Farming Back to the Community. CSA reaffirms the basic connection between farmers and their community. The community relies on the farmer for food, and the farmer relies on the community for support, both financial and physical. Unfortunately, family farms are currently slipping away while corporate farms are taking over. Then, because produce has to be shipped so far, the tie is not to the local community, but to distant places.

CSA Addresses Health and Environmental Concerns. With careful planning and thoughtfulness, and using the time-honored methods of crop rotation, application of beneficial insects, and promotion of soil health and conservation, a small farm can produce a wonderful crop using few, if any, additives.

In contrast, corporate farming often relies on a considerable amount of synthetic chemical pesticides, herbicides, fungicides, and other additives, and on genetic engineering of crops. Why is this? Consumers demand produce that is good-looking and uniform in shape and color, yet low in price. More important, all kinds of produce must be available at any time of the year. As a result, produce has to be grown in distant locales and must be easy to pack and ship. Corporate farming therefore resorts to the quickest and easiest ways to produce crops—often those entailing the use of additives. These additives might not only harm our health but also might harm our soil and water supply.

The CSA Concept Has Educational Value. Most Americans don't know how or where their food is grown. Too many children think that snap peas and carrots come from a box in the freezer section of the supermarket. The CSA concept is a terrific way to correct those misconceptions, to understand how what you put into the earth turns into what you harvest to eat, and to help members realize connections with one another, and with the practice of sustainable agriculture.

CHECK FOR CSA FARMS IN YOUR AREA

If you want to become involved, visit a CSA farm. If you decide the idea is right for you, you can join a farm, complete an internship on a farm, or even start your own. Check http://www.nal.usda.gov/afsic/csa/ or http://www.csacenter.org/csaorgs.htm for information.

I've put a great deal of information into this chapter—information about the benefits of vegetarianism, of organic food, of local produce, and of consumer-supported agriculture. Remember, RealAge is a currency that let's you know the value of your choices—no one will do all of them, no one will have a kitchen with a perfect IQ. But you ought to know the values of your choices. Like walking, you can start small and build if you think you'd like to try something.

Keep in mind that you don't have to be *perfect* at anything to gain benefits—not perfect at fats, not perfect at meat, not a perfect vegetarian. An occasional slip doesn't mean you should give up and go back to eating porterhouse steaks three times a week. Being a part-time vegetarian who eats a diet rich in fruits, vegetables, whole grains, fish, and chicken is a great start and makes you substantially younger.

And congratulations! You've just completed *Cooking the RealAge Way.* Whether you started as a pro or as a rookie, as Mike did, I hope this book helps you increase your Kitchen IQ substantially and that you've chosen some RealAge recipes that taste fabulous. If so, you are on your way to controlling your genes and looking and feeling younger. ENJOY THE ENERGY.

Recommended References

Books

Aloni, Nicole. *Secrets from a Caterer's Kitchen.* New York: HP Books, 2000.

Berk, Sally Ann. *The Farmer's Market Guide and Cookbook.* New York: Black Dog and Leventhal, 1996.

Bittman, Mark. *How to Cook Everything.* New York: Macmillan, 1998.

Bown, Deni. *New Encyclopedia of Herbs and Their Uses.* The Herb Society of America. New York: Dorling Kindersley, 2001.

Boxer, Aravelli, and Philippa Back. *The Herb Book.* New York: Smithmark, 1980.

Bremness, Lesley. *Herbs.* New York: Dorling Kindersley, 1990.

Brennan, Georgeanne. *Williams-Sonoma Cooking from the Farmer's Market.* San Francisco: Weldon Owen, 1999.

Bridge, Fred, and Jean Tibbetts. *The Well-Tooled Kitchen.* New York: William Morrow, 1991.

Brody, Lora. *Lora Brody Plugged In.* New York: William Morrow, 1998.

Clingerman, Polly. *The Kitchen Companion.* Gaithersburg, Md.: The American Cooking Guild, 1994.

Conran, Terence, and A. M. Clevely. *The Chef's Garden.* San Francisco: SOMA Books, 1999.

Cunningham, Marion. *The Fannie Farmer Cookbook,* 13th ed. New York: Alfred A. Knopf, 2000.

Ettlinger, Steve. *The Kitchenware Book.* New York: Macmillan, 1992.

Fletcher, Janet. *Fresh from the Farmer's Market.* San Francisco: Chronicle Books, 1997.

Garland, Sarah. *The Herb Garden.* New York: Penguin Books, 1984.

Ginsberg, Beth, and Michael Milken. *The Taste for Living Cookbook.* New York: Allen and Osborne, 1998.

Groh, T., and S. McFadden. *Farms of Tomorrow Revisited: Community Supported Farms-Farm Supported Communities.* San Francisco: Biodynamic Farming and Gardening Association, 1992.

Henderson, E. *Sharing the Harvest: A Guide to Community Supported Agriculture.* White River Junction, Vt.: Chelsea Green, 1999.

Herbst, Sharon. *The New Food Lover's Companion.* Hauppauge, N.Y.: Barron's, 1995.

Hooker, Monique. *Cooking with the Seasons.* New York: Henry Holt, 1997.

Jones, Jeanne. *Canyon Ranch Cooking.* New York: HarperCollins, 1998.

Kafka, Barbara. *Roasting.* New York: HarperCollins, 1995.

Katzen, Mollie. *Mollie Katzen's Vegetable Heaven.* New York: Hyperion, 1997.

———. *The Moosewood Cookbook.* New York: Ten Speed Press, 1992.

Kinderlehrer, Jane. *Confessions of a Sneaky Organic Cook.* Emmaus, Pa.: Rodale Press, 1971.

Larson Duyff, R. *The American Dietetic Association Complete Food and Nutrition Guide,* 2nd ed. New York: John Wiley, 2002.

Looker, Dan. *Farmers for the Future.* Ames: Iowa State University Press, 1996.

Madison, Deborah. *Local Flavors.* New York: Random House, 2002.

———. *Vegetarian Cooking for Everyone.* New York: Broadway Books, 1997.

Merchant, G. *The Harvest Collection: A Vegetarian Cookbook for All Seasons.* Garden City Park, N.J.: Avery Publishing, 1994.

Meyers, Perla. *Fresh from the Garden.* New York: Clarkson Potter, 1996.

Olney, Judith. *The Farm Market Cookbook.* New York: Doubleday, 1991.

Ornish, Dean. *Eat More, Weigh Less.* New York: HarperCollins, 1993.

———. *Everyday Cooking with Dr. Dean Ornish.* New York: HarperCollins, 1996.

Rombauer, Irma S., Marion Rombauer Becker, and Ethan Becker. *The All New Joy of Cooking.* New York: Scribners, 1997.

Thomas, Pamela. *Greenmarket: The Complete Guide to New York City's Farmer's Markets.* New York: Stewart, Tabori & Chang, 1999.

Thompson, Sylvia. *The Kitchen Garden Cookbook.* New York: Bantam Books, 1995.

Tolley, Emelie, and Chris Mead. *Cooking with Herbs.* New York: Clarkson Potter, 1989.

———. *The Herbal Pantry.* New York: Clarkson Potter, 1992.

Vegetables: Rodale Organic Gardening Basics. Emmaus, Pa.: Rodale Press, 2000.

Von Starkloff Rombauer, Irma, Irma S. Rombauer, and Marion Becker. *The Joy of Cooking.* Indianapolis: Bobbs-Merrill Co., 1975.

Waters, Alice. *Chez Panisse Vegetables.* New York: HarperCollins, 1996.

Williams, Chuck. *The Williams-Sonoma Cookbook and Guide to Kitchenware.* New York: Random House, 1986.

Internet Resources

www.ag.uiuc.edu/~robsond/solutions/horticulture/fruits.html

This site has general information on fruits.

www.ams.usda.gov/farmersmarkets/map.htm

This is a good place to find a farmers' market in your area. It provides all of the listings for the state at one time.

www.ams.usda.gov/howtobuy/fveg.htm

This site has useful information on how to buy fresh produce.

www.angelic-organics.com

This is the Web site for the CSA farm story shared in the article.

www.biodynamics.com

This Web site for the Biodynamic Farming and Gardening Association lists many organic farms and CSAs nationwide.

www.botanical.com

This site features reliable research and news on herbs and other plants.

www.ces.ncsu.edu/hil/veg-index.html

This site gives information on planting and harvesting vegetables.

www.csacenter.org/csaorgs.htm

The best single site for locating CSAs, ordering, and organizations and Web sites related to Community-Supported Agriculture

www.epicurious.com

This site lists tools of the trade—equipment you can't live without—and advice on how to outfit a basic kitchen. There's also "Kitchen Counsel," a discussion board for cooking-related questions.

www.food.epicurious.com/run/fooddictionary/home

Use this dictionary to find out more about foods (peak season, storage, use) and cooking terms.

www.farmersmarketonline.com/communit.htm

This is a good general overview of community-supported agriculture, how it got started, and how it works. This site also contains information on a CSA networking list and research grants.

www.farmersmarketonline.com/openair.htm

This site has good general information on farmers' markets, with links to specific markets and harvest charts for some areas.

www.food.homearts.com

This is a fun site that helps you match wines with food.

www.goodcooking.com//jjvherb.htm

This excellent page serves the chef who wants to garden, and the gardener who wants to cook.

www.nal.usda.gov/afsic/csa

This is the main page for the Alternative Farming Systems Information Center of the National Agriculture Library (a part of the U.S. Department of Agriculture), and the main page for resources for community-supported agriculture.

www.nal.usda.gov/afsic/csa/csaorgs.htm

The Alternative Farming Systems Information Center of the National Agriculture Library (a part of the U.S. Department of Agriculture) describes organizations and Web sites related to community-supported agriculture.

www.nal.usda.gov/afsic/csa/csastate.htm

The Alternative Farming Systems Information Center of the National Agriculture Library (a part of the U.S. Department of Agriculture) locates farms in your state.

www.nutrition.cornell.edu/foodguide/quiz.html

Quiz: "Are You a Regional or Seasonal Eater?"

www.nutrition.cornell.edu/foodguide/seasoning.html

This site has tips on how to eat seasonally.

www.realage.com

This site is our "home" site, featuring the latest information on choices that make your RealAge younger. Click on the RealAge cafe button to see more about Cooking the RealAge way, or "my fitness plan" to see exercises on strength, for example. It is a rich site for those who want to live younger.

www.seasonalchef.com

This site is interesting for its interviews with chefs and farmers on seasonal produce.

www.talksoy.com

Created by the United Soybean Board, this site gives a good description of the different types of soy foods and how they can be used.

www.umass.edu/umext/csa/about.html

The University of Massachusetts Extension provides a good overview of CSA.

www.unl.edu/pubs/horticulture/g271.htm

This site has information on when to harvest fruits and vegetables.

Index

acidification, 115–16
aflatoxin, 83
aging, 1, 4, 6
    of arteries, 7–8, 9–10, 13,
        334
    and blood sugar, 125
    controlling rate of, 2
    food choices and, 12, 19
    of immune system, 8–9
    and iron, 73–74
    premature, 4–5
    and sense of smell, 116
alcohol, 16, 135
alfalfa sprouts, 317
allspice, 321
almonds, 13
aluminum foil, 105
amino acids, 335
Anasazi beans, 78
ancho chiles, 79
antioxidants, 86, 107, 141,
    335
appetizers, 139
apple(s), 239–40, 340
    double, cinnamon
      smoothie, 250–51
    sweet baked, with cherries
      and citrus, 277–78

sweet potato pancakes with
    cinnamon and, 254–55
    triple, sauté, 278–79
applesauce, 77
appliances, 63
apricot, 177
    breakfast polenta, 251–52
arborio rice, 81
arrowroot, 77–78
arteries, 7–8, 9–10, 13, 90, 334
arthritis, 9, 129
artichoke hearts, 78
artichokes, 145–46
    baking, 97–98
arugula, 146
    grilled portobello
      mushroom barley pilaf
      with pine nuts and,
      270–71
asparagus, 147
    and coriander-crusted sea
      bass over sweet potato
      purée, 268–70
    Keith's, 174
    roasted, roasted chicken
      with pesto gemelli and,
      166–67
    and shiitake mushroom

frittata with smoked
    salmon, 154–55
autumn produce, 239–49
avocado, 13, 147–48
    in Donna's basic
      guacamole, 215–16
    -mango salsa, double
      sesame salmon with,
      263–65
    smoky posole with
      chipotle chiles and,
      214–15
    two-bean chili with salsa
      and, 260–61

baby food, 126–27
bacteria, 106
baked goods, 13–14, 97
baking, 96–98
    RealAge tips for, 97–98
baking pans, 64
baking powder, 78
baking soda, 78
balsamic vinegar, 87–88,
    115–16, 139–40
banana(s):
    in caramelized ripe tropical
      fruit, 234–35